Neurology: A Case-Based Approach

Neurology: A Case-Based Approach

Editor: Steven Graham

AMERICAN
MEDICAL PUBLISHERS
www.americanmedicalpublishers.com

AMERICAN
MEDICAL PUBLISHERS
www.americanmedicalpublishers.com

Cataloging-in-Publication Data

Neurology : a case-based approach / edited by Steven Graham.
p. cm.
Includes bibliographical references and index.
ISBN 978-1-63927-318-8
1. Neurology. 2. Nervous system--Diseases. 3. Nervous system--Diseases--Case studies. I. Graham, Steven.
RC346 .N48 2022
616.8--dc23

American Medical Publishers,
41 Flatbush Avenue,
1st Floor, New York,
NY 11217, USA

ISBN 978-1-63927-318-8 (Hardback)

Contents

Preface

The main aim of this book is to educate learners and enhance their research focus by presenting diverse topics covering this vast field. This is an advanced book which compiles significant studies by distinguished experts in the area of analysis. This book addresses successive solutions to the challenges arising in the area of application, along with it; the book provides scope for future developments.

The branch of medicine that deals with the disorders of the nervous system is referred to as neurology. It focuses on the diseases of central and peripheral nervous systems as well as their coverings and blood vessels. The most common symptoms of these disorders occur due to structural, electrical and biochemical abnormalities in the brain. Such disorders can result in paralysis, muscle weakness, seizures, confusion and loss of sensation. The examination of nervous system disorders is based on the physical examination. It analyzes the mental health and functioning of the cranial nerves, sensation, reflexes and strength. This book contains some path-breaking studies in the field of neurology. Some of the diverse topics covered in this book address the varied disorders that fall under this category. It will serve as a valuable source of reference for graduate and post graduate students.

It was a great honour to edit this book, though there were challenges, as it involved a lot of communication and networking between me and the editorial team. However, the end result was this all-inclusive book covering diverse themes in the field.

Finally, it is important to acknowledge the efforts of the contributors for their excellent chapters, through which a wide variety of issues have been addressed. I would also like to thank my colleagues for their valuable feedback during the making of this book.

Editor

1

A limb-girdle myopathy phenotype of *RUNX2* mutation in a patient with cleidocranial dysplasia

Sung-Ju Hsueh[1], Ni-Chung Lee[2], Shu-Hua Yang[3], Han-I Lin[1] and Chin-Hsien Lin[1*]

Abstract

Background: Cleidocranial dysplasia (CCD) is a rare hereditary disorder that arises from heterozygous loss of function mutations in the runt-related transcription factor 2 (*RUNX2*) gene. As *RUNX2* is mainly expressed in osteoblasts, CCD typically affects the skeletal and dental systems. Few studies have investigated *RUNX2* mutation effects on non-skeletal systems. Here, we describe limb-girdle myopathy, an uncommon phenotype of CCD, in a patient with a heterozygous missense mutation (p.R225Q) in the *RUNX2* gene.

Case presentation: A 58 year-old man presented with progressive back pain and six months of weakness in the proximal parts of all four limbs. Physical examinations showed that he was short in stature (height, 164.4 cm; weight, 79.1 kg) with a dysmorphic face, including hypertelorism, midface hypoplasia, and chin protrusion. At a young age, he had received orthodontic surgery, due to dental abnormalities. Neurological examinations revealed sloping shoulders, weakness, and atrophy in the proximal areas of the arms, shoulder girdle muscles, and legs. The deep tendon reflex and sensory system were normal. Radiological examinations revealed mild scoliosis, shortened clavicles, and a depressed skull bone, which were consistent with a clinical diagnosis of CCD. Electromyography (EMG) studies showed myogenic polyphasic waves in the deltoid, biceps brachii, and rectus femoris muscles. Instead, the EMG findings were normal in the first dorsal interosseous, tibialis anterior and facial muscles. The EMG findings were compatible with a limb-girdle pattern with facial sparing. The patient's family history showed his father and eldest daughter with similar dysmorphic faces, skeletal disorders and proximal upper extremity weakness. We sequenced the *RUNX2* gene and discovered a heterozygous missense mutation (c.G674A, p.R225Q), which altered the C-terminal end of the RUNX2 protein. This mutation was predicted to inactivate the protein and might affect its interactions with other proteins. This mutation co-segregated with the disease phenotypes in the family.

Conclusions: We described limb-girdle myopathy in a patient with CCD that carried a heterozygous *RUNX2* missense mutation. This uncommon phenotype expanded the phenotypic spectrum of the *RUNX2* p.R225Q mutation. The role of *RUNX2* in myogenic development merits future studies. Our findings remind clinicians that myopathic patients with myopathies combined with facial dysmorphism and shortened clavicles should consider the diagnosis of CCD.

Keywords: Cleidocranial dysplasia, RUNX2, Myopathy, Neurological system, Case report

* Correspondence: chlin@ntu.edu.tw
[1]Department of Neurology, National Taiwan University Hospital, No. 7, Chung-Shan South Road, Taipei 100, Taiwan
Full list of author information is available at the end of the article

Background

Cleidocranial dysplasia (CCD, OMIM 119600) is a rare skeletal disorder of autosomal dominant inheritance with an estimated incidence of 1/1,000,000 [1]. The main clinical features of CCD include persistent, open cranial sutures with bulging calvaria; hypoplasia or aplasia of the clavicles; dental anomalies; a short middle phalanx in the fifth finger; and associated vertebral anomalies [2]. This condition is primarily caused by mutations in the gene that encodes runt-related transcription factor 2 (RUNX2, MIM #600211), located on chromosome 6p21 [3]. The *RUNX2* gene encodes a 521 amino-acid protein with a highly conserved region of 128 amino acids (runt domain), an N-terminal stretch of glutamine/alanine repeats (Q/A domain), and a C-terminal proline/serine/threonine-rich (PST) domain [2]. The RUNX2 protein functions mainly in osteoblast differentiation and regulation [4], which contributes to the skeletal and dental abnormalities observed in CCD. In addition to its expression in osteoblasts, the RUNX2 protein is also present in non-osteoblast cells, including skeletal and smooth muscle cells [5], T cells [6], sperm cells, and neurons [7]. However, few patients with CCD manifest extra-skeletal manifestations. Here, we describe limb-girdle myopathy, an uncommon phenotype in CCD, in a patient with a heterozygous missense mutation in the *RUNX2* gene.

Case presentation

We examined a 58-year-old man with no underlying medical conditions. He presented with progressive back pain and 6 months of weakness in the proximal parts of all four limbs. There was no diplopia, chocking, swallowing difficulty, drop neck, respiratory distress or other symptoms of heart failure while tracing back his history. Physical examinations showed he was short in stature, with a height of 164.4 cm and a weight of 79.1 kg. He had a dysmorphic face with hypertelorism, midface hypoplasia, and chin protrusion (Fig. 1a). He had received orthodontic surgery due to dental abnormalities while he was young. Neurological examinations revealed sloping shoulders, atrophy of the shoulder girdle muscles,

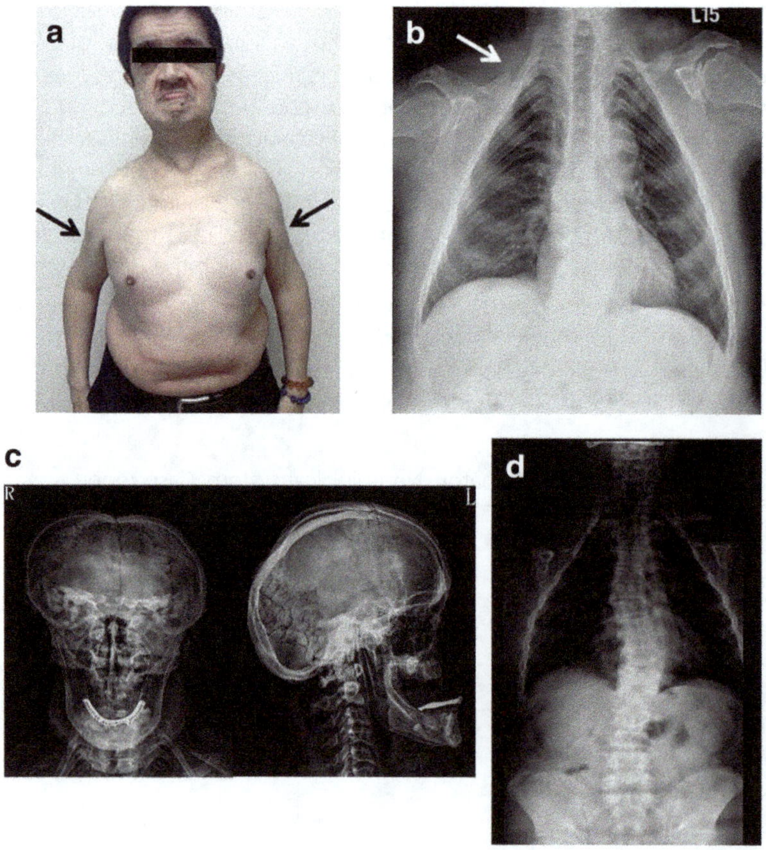

Fig. 1 Clinical pictures and radiologic findings for the index patient with CCD. **a** The photographs show a flat face, sunken nasal bridge, hypertelorism, chin protrusion, and sloping shoulders. Arrows indicate atrophy of bilateral shoulder girdle muscles. **b** Chest X-ray shows the absent right clavicle (arrow) and a hypoplastic left clavicle. **c** Skull X-ray shows wormian bones in the skull (left panel) and a hypoplastic maxilla (right panel). **d** Spine X-ray reveals mild scoliosis of the thoraco-lumbar spine

and symmetrical weakness in the proximal parts of the arms and legs. There was no facial weakness or limitation of extra-ocular movement. The deep tendon reflex and sensory systems were normal. Radiological examinations revealed wormian bones in the skull, the absence of the right clavicle, hypoplasia of the left clavicle, and mild scoliosis. These signs were consistent with the clinical diagnosis of CCD (Fig. 1b–d). Electromyography (EMG) revealed myogenic polyphasic waves of small amplitude and short-duration polyphasic waves at 400–500 μV in the bilateral biceps brachii, deltoid, infraspinatus, trapezius, and rectus femoris muscles. However, the EMG findings were normal in bilateral first dorsal interosseous, tibialis anterior and facial muscles. Magnetic resonance imaging (MRI) of the upper extremity showed atrophy associated with fatty infiltration of right deltoid and biceps brachii muscles without acute edematous changes, suggesting a chronic muscle insult (Fig. 2a, b). These findings indicated a limb-girdle distribution of chronic myopathy. Laboratory data, including the serum creatine kinase level, were normal. The thyroid function, tumor markers, and autoimmune profiles for survey of common metabolic and inflammatory myopathy were within normal limits. Muscle biopsy of right biceps brachii muscle was suggested but this suggestion was declined by the patient. The patient did not have symptoms of respiratory distress or heart failure sign. Cardiac echo showed normal cardiac contractility and the heart ejection fraction is within normal limits. The patient's family history showed that his father and eldest daughter had similar skeletal, dental disorders and proximal weakness of upper extremity (Fig. 3a). EMG findings of bilateral deltoid, biceps brachii and rectus femoris muscles of the proband's elder daughter also showed myopathic polyphasic waves. These observations suggest that the myopathy is not a sporadic condition associate with the patient but segregate with the skeletal problems within his family.

The patient initially presented with facial dysmorphism, sloping shoulders, atrophy, and weakness, predominantly over the shoulder girdle. Therefore, we analyzed the double homeobox *DUX4* gene for facioscapulohumeral muscular dystrophy. In addition, the radiologic findings and the patient's autosomal-dominant family history were consistent with CCD. Therefore, we also analyzed the *RUNX2* gene after the patient provided informed consent. Genomic DNA was extracted from peripheral whole blood for PCR analysis. We amplified exons 1 through 8 and the flanking intronic sequences of the *RUNX2* gene with eight pairs of PCR primers, designed as previously described [8]. Genetic analysis for the *DUX4* gene was performed as previously described [9]. The purified PCR products were sequenced in both directions at our on-site biochemistry sequencing facility with Big Dye Version 3.1 and a 3730 XL sequencer (Applied Biosystems, Foster City, CA). We found that the patient carried a heterozygous missense mutation (c.G674A, p.R225Q), located at the C-terminal end of the RUNX2 protein. This mutation was predicted to inactivate the protein, and it might also affect protein structural stability and interactions with other proteins. The reference sequence and base-pair numbers refer to GenBank accession numbers AF001443-AF001450 and NM_001024630. This mutation co-segregated with the disease phenotype in the patient's family (Fig. 3B). Research protocol was reviewed by the institutional ethics board committee of the National Taiwan University Hospital and all subjects gave informed consent.

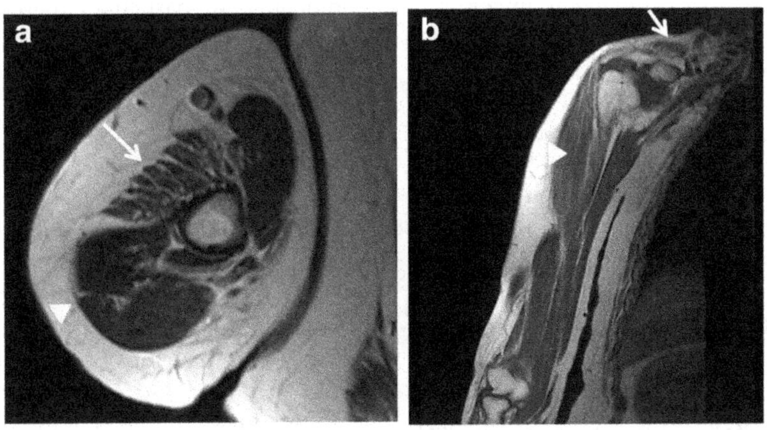

Fig. 2 MRI of right upper extremity of the index patient. **a** Coronal T1 weighted MRI shows atrophy and fatty infiltration of the deltoid (arrow), and biceps brachii (arrowhead) muscles. **b** Sagittal T1 weighted MRI displays concomitant atrophy and fatty infiltration of the trapezius (arrows) and biceps brachii (arrowhead) muscles

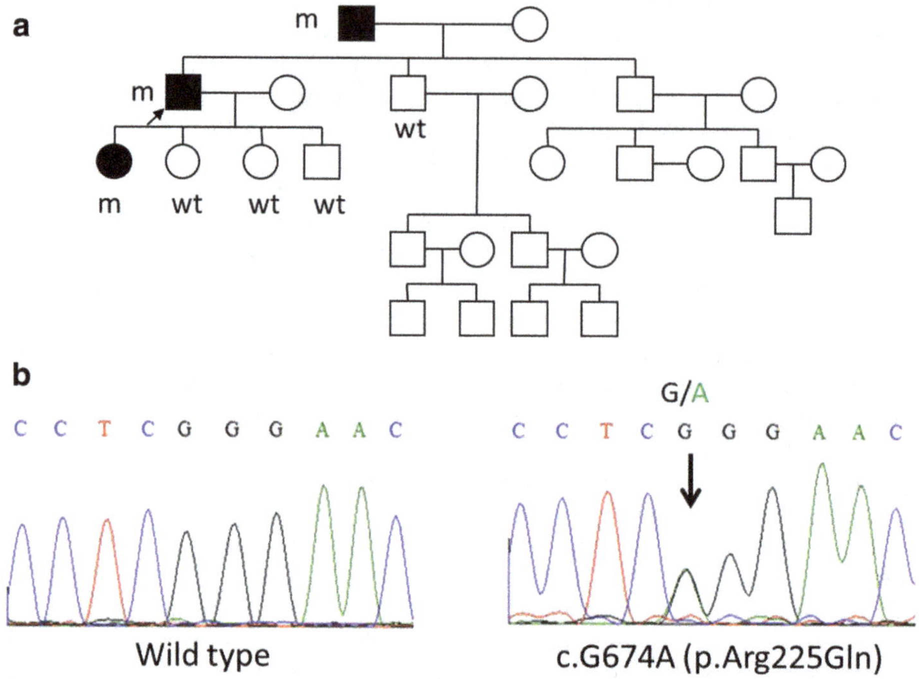

Fig. 3 Family pedigree and genetic analysis of the *RUNX2* gene of the index patient with CCD. **a** Family pedigree of the index family. Black symbols denote family members affected with CCD. The proband we described in the current study is marked with an arrow. m, mutated alleles; wt, normal alleles. **b** Chromatograms of direct sequencing of the *RUNX2* genomic sequence. Genetic analysis reveals a single nucleotide change (c.674G > A, p.Arg225Gln, right panel) compared to the wild type sequence (left panel). The mutations identified in this study were located in the indicated position

Conclusions

To date, variable *RUNX2* mutations have been described in subjects with CCD, including insertions, deletions, nonsense, and missense mutations. CCD has been reported in people of Mongoloid ethnicity, including Japanese, Korean, Chinese, and Taiwanese [10–13]. In most cases, patients present with classical skeletal and dental abnormalities that appear in childhood. Here, we described a patient with CCD that exhibited an uncommon initial manifestation of late-onset, limb-girdle myopathy, due to a missense mutation (c.G674A, p.R225Q) in the *RUNX2* gene.

The missense mutation, p.R225Q, located at the C-terminal end of the runt domain, is a known mutational hotspot in the *RUNX2* gene [14, 15]. The runt domain is a highly conserved DNA-binding domain, which binds to a consensus DNA sequence. The runt domain also mediates binding to CBFβ, an unrelated partner protein that does not interact directly with DNA, but enhances the DNA-binding affinity of the RUNX protein [16]. In our patient, the substitution of Arg225 with glutamine abolished the positive charge of the protein at this position, which was predicted to impair the DNA binding ability of RUNX2 [15]. Therefore, the p.R225Q mutation can cause severe phenotypes in CCD.

The p.R225Q mutation was previously reported in a Taiwanese patient with sporadic CCD. The age of onset was 8 years old, and the patient presented with classical bone phenotypes that had appeared in childhood [10]. This mutation was later reported in a teenage Korean patient with sporadic CCD, who also presented with dental and skeletal problems [11]. Those carriers of the *RUNX2* p.R225Q mutation reported no neurological complaints; in particular, there were no symptoms or signs of myopathy. In addition, a nearby nucleotide missense mutation, which changed the same amino acid, c.C673T (p.R225W), was previously described in one Italian family, but no atypical features were reported [17]. Those observations reinforced the notion that Arg225 played a vital role in the function of the RUNX2 protein, and the mutation carriers most commonly exhibited childhood or juvenile onset of dental or skeletal abnormalities, without neurological system involvement.

Notably, the patient in the present study initially presented with an upper extremity, predominant limb-girdle myopathy. As extra-skeletal presentation, especially myopathy, is not common in patients with CCD, we performed computerized English language literature searches to identify case reports of myopathy or other related neurological presentations in patients with CCD,

Table 1 Clinical and genetic findings in three CCD patents presented with myopathy

Subjects/reference	Classical CCD	Involvement of weakness	Other neurological signs	EMG findings	MRI findings	Muscle biopsy	*RUNX2* mutation
Case 7, Tessa et al., 2003 [17]	+	Limb-girdle myopathy	Conductive deafness	N.A.	N.A.	N.A.	Exon 2-intron junction (IVS2 + 2 T > A)
Case 4, Tessa et al., 2003 [17]	+	Limb-girdle myopathy	-	N.A.	N.A.	N.A.	c.389G > A (W130X)
Index patient of the current study	+	Limb-girdle myopathy	-	Short-duration, small-amplitude polyphasic waves	Atrophy with fatty infiltration patterns	N.A.	c.674G > A (R255Q)

CCD cleidocranial dysplasia, *EMG* electromyography, *MRI* magnetic resonance imaging, *N.A.* not available

making use of the following databases: PubMed (from 1975), and Ovid MEDLINE (from 1975). We used the following main key words for searches: cleidocranial dysplasia, myopathy, weakness, atrophy and neurological symptoms. For each selected article, the clinical descriptions of study subjects were carefully reviewed. After carefully reviewing more than 500 case studies, 13 studies reported their CCD patients present with muscle weakness. Among these 15 reported cases, 2 were found to carry *FIG 4* gene mutation without *RUNX2* gene mutations, 1 patient was diagnosed as Ritscher-Schinzel syndrome, 2 subjects' weakness were secondary to cervical myelopathy, 8 cases were lacking of detailed descriptions of the weakness and the remaining 2 cases presented with limb-girdle myopathy (Table 1). In those cases, CCD was related to the c.G389A nonsense mutation (p.W130X) and a mutation in the exon 2-intron junction splice site (IVS2 + 2 T > A) [17]. The p.W130X mutation produced a protein predicted to lack 390 amino acids, including part of the runt and PST domains. The subject with the IVS2 + 2 T > A mutation exhibited mild conductive deafness, in addition to myopathy. Histological and histochemical analyses of a muscle biopsy specimen from the patient that carried the p.W130X mutation revealed minor, non-specific, myopathic changes [17]. These observations, combined with our findings, suggested that muscular weakness was not associated with mutations in any particular protein domain; thus, muscle weakness might be related to the loss of function of the gene product. Recent studies have shown that the expression of the *RUNX2* transcription factor may not be limited to osteoblasts and mesenchymal stem cells; expression was also found in non-osteoblast cells [5–7]. Several lines of evidence have indicated that RUNX2 also plays an important role in adipogenesis and skeletal muscle differentiation [18, 19]. RUNX2 stimulated the trans-differentiation of primary skeletal myoblasts into a mineralizing osteoblastic phenotype. RUNX2 also prevented myogenesis and myotube formation via the suppression of MyoD and myogenin transcripts [19]. Thus, RUNX2 broadly modulates cellular fates, including the fate of skeletal muscle cells. Therefore, we hypothesized that mutations in the *RUNX2* gene may lead to damaging effects in muscle cell maturation, which result in myopathy.

In summary, this case study described an uncommon phenotype of late-onset limb-girdle distribution myopathy in a patient with CCD, associated with a *RUNX2* p.Arg225Gln mutation. Considering the role of the *RUNX2* transcription factor in myogenesis, it is not surprising that a carrier of the *RUNX2* mutation presented with extra-skeletal features. Our findings extended the phenotypic spectrum of the *RUNX2* p.R225Q mutation, from typical dental/skeletal abnormalities to a limb-girdle pattern of myopathy. Our results also remind clinicians that patients with myopathies that present with facial dysmorphism and dental or skeletal deformities should be differentially diagnosed for CCD.

Abbreviations

CCD: Cleidocranial dysplasia; RUNX2: Runt-related transcription factor 2

Acknowledgements

We thank the patient in this case study and his family for participating in the study. We are also grateful to the staff of the Second Core Lab, Department of Medical Research, National Taiwan University Hospital, for technical support during the study.

Funding

This work was supported by the Ministry of Science and Technology (grant number: MOST 104-2314-B-002-175-MY2).

Authors' contributions

Study concept and design: CH Lin. Acquisition of data: SJ Hsueh, NC Lee, SY Yang, and HI Lin. Analysis and interpretation of data: SJ Hsueh, HI Lin, and CH Lin. Drafting of the manuscript: SJ Hsueh and CH Lin. Critical revision of the manuscript for important intellectual content: SJ Hsueh and CH Lin. Study supervision: CH Lin. All authors read and approved the final manuscript.

Competing interests

The authors declare that they have no competing interests.

Author details
[1]Department of Neurology, National Taiwan University Hospital, No. 7, Chung-Shan South Road, Taipei 100, Taiwan. [2]Department of Medical Genetics, National Taiwan University Hospital, Taipei 100, Taiwan. [3]Department of Orthopedics, National Taiwan University Hospital, No. 7, Chung-Shan South Road, Taipei 100, Taiwan.

References

1. Brueton LA, Reeve A, Ellis R, Husband P, Thompson EM, Kingston HM. Apparent cleidocranial dysplasia associated with abnormalities of 8q22 in three individuals. Am J Med Genet. 1992;43:612–8.
2. Mundlos S. Cleidocranial dysplasia: clinical and molecular genetics. J Med Genet. 1999;36:177–82.
3. Lee B, Thirunavukkarasu K, Zhou L, Pastore L, Baldini A, Hecht J, et al. Missense mutations abolishing DNA binding of the osteoblast-specific transcription factor OSF2/CBFA1 in cleidocranial dysplasia. Nat Genet. 1997;16:307–10.
4. Komori T. Regulation of osteoblast differentiation by transcription factors. J Cell Biochem. 2006;99:1233–9.
5. Tanaka T, Sato H, Doi H, Yoshida CA, Shimizu T, Matsui H, et al. Runx2 represses myocardin-mediated differentiation and facilitates osteogenic conversion of vascular smooth muscle cells. Mol Cell Biol. 2008;28:1147–60.
6. Satake M, Nomura S, Yamaguchi-Iwai Y, Takahama Y, Hashimoto Y, Niki M, et al. Expression of the Runt domain-encoding PEBP2 alpha genes in T cells during thymic development. Mol Cell Biol. 1995;15:1662–70.
7. Jeong JH, Jin JS, Kim HN, Kang SM, Liu JC, Lengner CJ, et al. Expression of Runx2 transcription factor in non-skeletal tissues, sperm and brain. J Cell Physiol. 2008;217:511–7.
8. Mundlos S, Otto F, Mundlos C, Mulliken JB, Aylsworth AS, Albright S, et al. Mutations involving the transcription factor CBFA1 cause cleidocranial dysplasia. Cell. 1997;89:773–9.
9. Lemmers R, Miller DG, van der Maarel SM. Facioscapulohumeral Muscular Dystrophy, in GeneReviews(R), R.A. Pagon, et al., Editors. University of Washington: Seattle; 1993.
10. Lin WD, Lin SP, Wang CH, Tsai Y, Chen CP, Tsai FJ. RUNX2 mutations in Taiwanese patients with cleidocranial dysplasia. Genet Mol Biol. 2011;34:201–4.
11. Lee KE, Seymen F, Ko J, Yildirim M, Tuna EB, Gencay K, et al. RUNX2 mutations in cleidocranial dysplasia. Genet Mol Res. 2013;12:4567–74.
12. Wu LZ, Su WQ, Liu YF, Ge X, Zhang Y, Wang XJ. Role of the RUNX2 p.R225Q mutation in cleidocranial dysplasia: a rare presentation and an analysis of the RUNX2 protein structure. Genet Mol Res. 2014;13:1187–94.
13. Shibata A, Machida J, Yamaguchi S, Kimura M, Tatematsu T, Miyachi H, et al. Characterisation of novel RUNX2 mutation with alanine tract expansion from Japanese cleidocranial dysplasia patient. Mutagenesis. 2016;31:61–7.
14. Otto F, Kanegane H, Mundlos S. Mutations in the RUNX2 gene in patients with cleidocranial dysplasia. Hum Mutat. 2002;19:209–16.
15. Yoshida T, Kanegane H, Osato M, Yanagida M, Miyawaki T, Ito Y, et al. Functional analysis of RUNX2 mutations in Japanese patients with cleidocranial dysplasia demonstrates novel genotype-phenotype correlations. Am J Hum Genet. 2002;71:724–38.
16. Bartfeld D, Shimon L, Couture GC, Rabinovich D, Frolow F, Levanon D, et al. DNA recognition by the RUNX1 transcription factor is mediated by an allosteric transition in the RUNT domain and by DNA bending. Structure. 2002;10:1395–407.
17. Tessa A, Salvi S, Casali C, Garavelli L, Digilio MC, Dotti MT, et al. Six novel mutations of the RUNX2 gene in Italian patients with cleidocranial dysplasia. Hum Mutat. 2003;22:104.
18. Enomoto H, Furuichi T, Zanma A, Yamana K, Yoshida C, Sumitani S, et al. Runx2 deficiency in chondrocytes causes adipogenic changes in vitro. J Cell Sci. 2004;117:417–25.
19. Gersbach CA, Byers BA, Pavlath GK, García AJ. Runx2/Cbfa1 stimulates transdifferentiation of primary skeletal myoblasts into a mineralizing osteoblastic phenotype. Exp Cell Res. 2004;300:406–17.

2

Rapidly progressive psychotic symptoms triggered by infection in a patient with methylenetetrahydrofolate reductase deficiency

Shin Iida[1], Masataka Nakamura[1*], Shinya Asayama[1], Takenobu Kunieda[1], Satoshi Kaneko[1], Hitoshi Osaka[2] and Hirofumi Kusaka[1]

Abstract

Background: Methylenetetrahydrofolate reductase (MTHFR) deficiency is a rare inborn error of metabolism inherited in autosomal recessive pattern and is associated with a wide spectrum of neurological abnormalities.

Case presentation: We herein describe a 15-year-old boy with MTHFR deficiency who presented with a slowly progressive decline of school performance and a spastic gait. Rapidly deteriorating psychosis and repetitive seizures triggered by a febrile infection prompted neurological investigation. He had significantly elevated total plasma homocysteine and urinary homocystine levels, as well as a decreased plasma methionine level. Brain magnetic resonance imaging (MRI) revealed leukoencephalopathy. DNA gene sequencing showed c.446_447 del GC ins TT and c.137G > A, and c.665C > T heterozygous mutations in the MTHFR gene of the patient. Oral administration of betaine drastically improved his clinical symptoms within a few months. After 8 months of treatment, his total plasma homocysteine level moderately decreased; and the plasma methionine concentration became normalized. Furthermore, the white matter lesions on MRI had disappeared.

Conclusion: This patient demonstrates the possibility that MTHFR deficiency should be considered in mentally retarded adolescents who display an abnormally elevated plasma level of homocysteine in association with progressive neurological dysfunction and leukoencephalopathy. Febrile infections may be an aggravating factor in patients with MTHFR deficiency.

Keywords: MTHFR, Betaine, Spastic paraplegia, Psychosis, Leukoencephalopathy

Background

5,10-Methylenetetrahydrofolate reductase (MTHFR) deficiency is a rare autosomal recessive disease. The enzyme MTHFR catalyzes the conversion of 5,10-methylenetetrahydrofolate to 5-methyltetrahydrofolate, which serves as a methyl donor in the remethylation of homocysteine to methionine (Fig. 1). Therefore, patients with this deficiency show hyperhomocysteinemia, hypomethioninaemia and usually low folate levels. A broad spectrum of clinical symptoms can appear neonatally, in early or late childhood, or even in the adult. The infantile presentation is the most clinically severe and includes hypotonia, seizures, apneas and/or coma. Adolescents or adults may present with mental retardation, motor and gait disturbance, seizures, psychiatric manifestations, and thrombosis [1]. We herein report the case of a 15-year-old patient with MTHFR deficiency presenting with a slowly progressive mental decline and spastic paraplegia, followed by rapidly progressive psychosis and repetitive seizures triggered by infection that successfully responded to betaine treatment.

* Correspondence: nakamuma@hirakata.kmu.ac.jp
[1]Department of Neurology, Kansai Medical University, 2-5-1, Shinmachi, Hirakata, Osaka 5731010, Japan

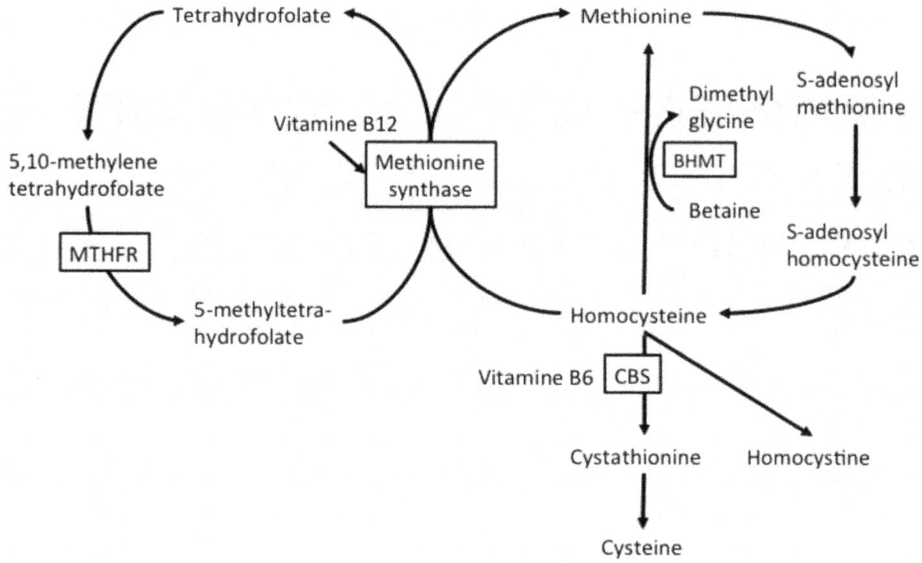

Fig. 1 An overview of methionine and homocysteine metabolism. MTHFR, Methylenetetrahydrofolate reductase; CBS, cystathionine beta-synthase; BHMT, betaine-homocysteine S-methyltransferase

Case presentation

A 15-year-old Japanese boy was referred to our hospital for rapidly progressive psychiatric and neurological symptoms. His growth and development had been normal until the age of 11, when he began to experience academic difficulties.

At the age of 13 years, he visited a local hospital because of a 6-month history of slowly progressive difficulty in walking. Neurological examination revealed a spastic gait and marked lower limb hyper-reflexia. However, brain and spinal magnetic resonance imaging (MRI) showed no abnormalities. His total plasma homocysteine level was 216 nmol/ml (normal, 3.7-12.5 nmol/ml); and serum folic acid and cobalamine levels were 1.7 ng/ml (normal, 3.6–12.9 ng/ml) and 397 pg/ml (normal, 233–914 pg/ml), respectively. The plasma concentrations of very-long-chain fatty acids were all within normal limits. Based on a tentative diagnosis of subacute combined degeneration of the spinal cord secondary to folic acid deficiency, folic acid (15 mg/day) therapy was started. However, his gait disturbance gradually worsened.

At the age of 15 years, he began to show deficits in motivation and effort. One week later, he was immediately admitted to a hospital because of a high fever and acute diarrhea with vomiting caused by viral gastroenteritis that had started the previous evening. After admission, he rapidly developed psychotic symptoms, particularly delusions and auditory hallucinations. His general condition was improved by rehydration, and he was discharged 3 days later with a diagnosis of hospital-induced delirium. However, his psychotic symptoms, such as depression, delusions, hallucinations, and anorexia, worsened over the next 2 weeks. Furthermore, he experienced several episodes of generalized convulsions, for which levetiracetam was prescribed (1000 mg/day). He was repeatedly in and out of another local hospital because of dehydration due to a refusal to eat caused by his psychotic state or convulsions. He was treated with risperidone for a month, but still suffered from delusions, hallucination, and failure to eat. A brain MRI showed generalized atrophy and hyperintensity in the white matter around the posterior horns of the lateral ventricles on T2-weighted and fluid-attenuated inversion recovery (FLAIR) images (Fig. 2a-c). An electroencephalogram showed a diffusely low-amplitude background activity without epileptic discharge. The results of a nerve conduction study and biochemical examination including lysosomal enzymatic activities were both normal. He became severely apathetic and bedridden within two months after infectious gastroenteritis. Therefore, he was transferred to our hospital for further investigation.

On admission, no abnormal facial appearance or skeletal anomalies were noted. Neurological examination revealed a fluctuating level of consciousness with confusion, delusion, and abnormal behavior. Cranial nerves were normal. Marked spasticity of the lower limbs was noticed, with hyper-reflexia in both arms and legs. There was also sustained clonus at the ankles following sudden passive dorsiflexion of the foot. However, pathological reflexes (Babinski and Chaddock signs) were negative. Serum folic acid and cobalamine levels were elevated (more than 20 ng/ml and 1120 pg/ml, respectively). Plasma amino acid analysis showed an elevated level of total homocysteine (229.9 nmol/ml) and a decreased methionine

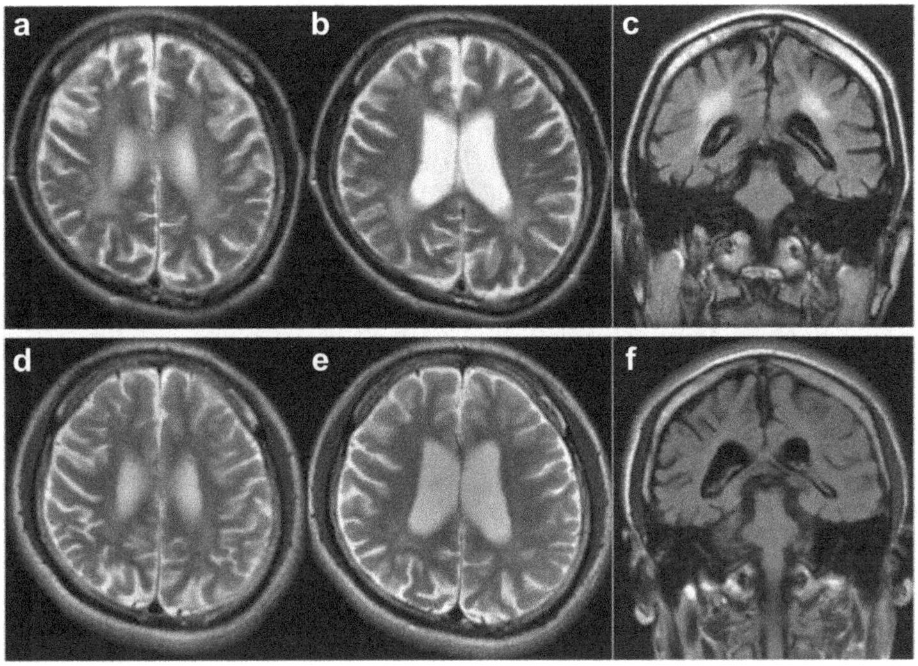

Fig. 2 **a-c** Axial and coronal T2 weighted magnetic resonance imaging (MRI) images and axial fluid-attenuated inversion recovery (FLAIR) MRI image obtained at age 15 reveal a high-intensity area in the white matter around the posterior horns of the lateral ventricles. **d-f** Axial and coronal T2 weighted MRI images and FLAIR MRI image obtained at age 16 (8 months after betaine treatment) show resolution of the hyper-intensity in the white matter

level (10.9 nmol/ml; normal, 19.2-32.7 nmol/ml). Cerebrospinal fluid analysis indicated normal values. Gas chromatographic-mass spectrometric urinary metabolome analysis revealed a markedly elevated urinary homocystine level of 19.7 mmol/mol total creatinine (normal, not detected) and undetectable urinary methionine levels (−3.0 standard deviation; SD). His urinary methylmalonic acid level was normal (−0.3 SD). These results of the amino acid analyses were highly suggestive of MTHFR deficiency. Therefore, MTHFR gene sequencing was undertaken; and the results showed compound heterozygous mutations c.446_447 del GC ins TT (p.Gly149Val) and c.137G > A (p.Arg46Gln). In addition, heterozygous c. 665C > T (p.Ala222Val) polymorphism was noted. Multivitamins including vitamins B1, B6, and B12 (750 μg/day) as well as folic acid were administered. Subsequently, oral substitution treatment with betaine was initiated at a dosage of 3 g/day, which was slowly increased to 9 g/day. Over a few months, consciousness, delusion, and abnormal behavior dramatically improved, and he became able to sit in a wheelchair. After 8 months of therapy, the earlier white matter hyperintensities on T2-weighted and FLAIR images had resolved (Fig. 2d-f). Moreover, his total plasma homocysteine level had decreased to around half of its initial value (91.2 nmol/ml); and the plasma methionine level had normalized (20.4 nmol/ml). Thereafter, low specific activity of MTHFR was observed in skin fibroblasts cultured from the patient (2.8 nmol/h/mg protein; normal control values in 75 normal subjects, 25.3 ± 8.9 nmol/h/mg protein). MTHFR gene sequencing of his mother revealed mutation c.137G > A and polymorphism c. 665C > T, both in the heterozygous state. Following 2 years of clinical follow-up, the patient had no psychiatric symptoms (apathy, delusion or hallucination) or relapse, and he became able to stand up and walk with the aid of a walker.

Discussion

Our patient had two compound missense mutations, c.446_447 del GC ins TT and c.137G > A, in the heterozygous state in addition to a c. 665C > T functional polymorphism. The tandem missense mutation c.446_447 del GC ins TT had already been described in Japanese patients with MTHFR deficiency [2–4]. These patients had a homozygous or heterozygous mutation and displayed decreased MTHFR activity. The MTHFR gene polymorphism c. 665C > T is also known to be associated with reduced enzyme activity [5]. Genetic analysis of the present patient's mother revealed the presence of c.137G > A and c. 665C > T, indicating that pathogenicity of our patient could have been due to the combined effect of tandem missense mutation c.446_447 del GC ins TT and common polymorphism c. 665C > T.

Newborn screening for homocystinuria is based on the identification of an increased level of plasma methionine. MTHFR deficiency causes a low methionine level and is therefore not detected by current screening. Unless clinicians maintain a high index of suspicion and are aware of varied clinical presentations, this diagnosis is often missed. The clinical presentation and age at onset of MTHFR deficiency varies greatly depending on the degree of enzyme deficiency [6]. Patients with severe MTHFR deficiency (0-20% residual enzyme activity) in infancy or adolescence present with developmental delay, severe mental retardation, motor and gait dysfunction, seizures, psychiatric disturbances, and other neurological abnormalities. Our patient displayed decreased MTHFR activity (11% of control activity) and had a clinical pattern and age at presentation consistent with a severe deficiency.

Previously, rapidly deteriorating psychosis was reported in the case of adolesecent- or adult-onset MTHFR deficiency [7–10]. The reason for rapid deterioration in these patients is not known; but the lack of dietary supplements, the use of nitrous oxide during general anesthesia, and long-term use of the antiepileptic drug phenytoin have been reported as risk factors for acute neurological deterioration [3, 11]. So, we speculate that the change in nutritional status through reductions in dietary intake and intestinal absorption due to gastroenteritis might have been responsible for the rapid deterioration seen in our patient. Moreover, prolonged undernutrition due to refusal to eat could have aggravated his psychiatric symptoms. Another possible cause is that the common MTHFR gene polymorphism (c. 665C > T) increases the thermolability of the enzyme [5]. Thus, a high fever may potentially worsen psychiatric symptoms by causing inactivation of the enzyme activity. Therefore, febrile infections may be an aggravating factor in patients with MTHFR deficiency.

The biochemical therapeutic goals in MTHFR deficiency are aimed at reducing plasma homocysteine and normalizing methionine levels. Betaine is an endogenous catabolite of choline, and high doses of betaine are the mainstay of therapy for patients with MTHFR deficiency. The beneficial effect of betaine is mediated through betaine-homocysteine methyltransferase with the use of an alternate methyl donor for remethylation of homocysteine to methionine (Fig. 1) [12]. Indeed, betaine supplementation has been shown to decrease homocysteine levels and normalize methionine levels in patients with MTHFR deficiency [12]. Folic acid and supplementation with vitamins B6 and B12 also play key roles in converting homocysteine into methionine. As expected in our case, the supplementation with betaine and multi-vitamins resulted in a moderate decrease in the level of total plasma homocysteine and normalization of plasma methionine, that were associated with the disappearance of psychosis and leukoencephalopathy and the recovery of motor functions.

Conclusions

We reported the case of a school-aged boy with severe MTHFR deficiency who presented with a slowly progressive mental decline and spastic paraplegia and who later developed rapidly progressive psychosis and repetitive seizures following infectious gastroenteritis. Patients with MTHFR deficiency are sensitive to febrile infections, which may trigger new-onset neurological or psychic symptoms, or worsen existing symptoms. Since MTHFR deficiency is one of the treatable metabolic disorders not identified by current newborn mass screening, we should consider the possibility of MTHFR deficiency in adolescents with mental retardation who display abnormally elevated homocysteine in association with progressive neurological or psychiatric dysfunction and leukoencephalopathy.

Abbreviations

FLAIR: Fluid-attenuated inversion recovery; MRI: Magnetic resonance imaging; MTHFR: Methylenetetrahydrofolate reductase; SD: Standard deviation

Acknowledgements

We thank Dr. med. Matthias Baumgartne (Division for Metabolic Disease, University Children's Hospital Zurich) and Dr. Tomiko Kuhara (Japan Clinical Metabolomics Institute) for measurement of the MTHFR enzyme activity and metabolomics analysis, respectively.

Funding

We received no funding support.

Authors' contributions

SI wrote the draft manuscript. MN acquired the data, drafted the manuscript, created the figure, and revised the manuscript. SA and TK were involved in drafting of the manuscript. SK, HO, and HK revised the manuscript for important intellectual content. All authors read and approved the final manuscript.

Competing interests

The authors declare that they have no competing interests.

Author details

[1]Department of Neurology, Kansai Medical University, 2-5-1, Shinmachi, Hirakata, Osaka 5731010, Japan. [2]Department of Pediatrics, Jichi Medical School, 3311-1, Yakushiji, Shimotsuke-shi, Tochigi 3290498, Japan.

References

1. Ogierde Baulny H, Gérard M, Saudubray JM, Zittoun J. Remethylation defects: guidelines for clinical diagnosis and treatment. Eur J Pediatr. 1998;157 Suppl 2:S77–83.

2. Tsuji M, Takagi A, Sameshima K, Iai M, Yamashita S, Shinbo H, et al. 5,10-Methylenetetrahydrofolate reductase deficiency with progressive polyneuropathy in an infant. Brain Dev. 2011;33:521–4.
3. Arai M, Osaka H. Acute leukoencephalopathy possibly induced by phenytoin intoxication in an adult patient with methylenetetrahydrofolate reductase deficiency. Epilepsia. 2011;52:e58–61.
4. Yano H, Nakaso K, Yasui K, Wakutani Y, Nakayasu H, Kowa H, et al. Mutations of the MTHFR gene (428C > T and [458G > T + 459C > T]) markedly decrease MTHFR enzyme activity. Neurogenetics. 2004;5:135–40.
5. Frosst P, Blom HJ, Milos R, Goyette P, Sheppard CA, Matthews RG, et al. A candidate genetic risk factor for vascular disease: a common mutation in methylenetetrahydrofolate reductase. Nat Genet. 1995;10:111–3.
6. Goyette P, Frosst P, Rosenblatt DS, Rozen R. Seven novel mutations in the methylenetetrahydrofolate reductase gene and genotype/phenotype correlations in severe methylenetetrahydrofolate reductase deficiency. Am J Hum Genet. 1995;56:1052–9.
7. Freeman JM, Finkelstein JD, Mudd SH. Folate-responsive homocystinuria and "schizophrenia". A defect in methylation due to deficient 5,10-methylenetetrahydrofolate reductase activity. N Engl J Med. 1975;292:491–6.
8. Birnbaum T, Blom HJ, Prokisch H, Hartig M, Klopstock T. Methylenetetrahydrofolate reductase deficiency (homocystinuria type II) as a rare cause of rapidly progressive tetraspasticity and psychosis in a previously healthy adult. J Neurol. 2008;255:1845–6.
9. Michot JM, Sedel F, Giraudier S, Smiejan JM, Papo T. Psychosis, paraplegia and coma revealing methylenetetrahydrofolate reductase deficiency in a 56-year-old woman. J Neurol Neurosurg Psychiatry. 2008;79:963–4.
10. Pasquier F, Lebert F, Petit H, Zittoun J, Marquet J. Methylenetetrahydrofolate reductase deficiency revealed by a neuropathy in a psychotic adult. J Neurol Neurosurg Psychiatry. 1994;57:765–6.
11. Selzer RR, Rosenblatt DS, Laxova R, Hogan K. Adverse effect of nitrous oxide in a child with 5,10-methylenetetrahydrofolate reductase deficiency. N Engl J Med. 2003;349:45–50.
12. Strauss KA, Morton DH, Puffenberger EG, Hendrickson C, Robinson DL, Wagner C, et al. Prevention of brain disease from severe 5,10-methylenetetrahydrofolate reductase deficiency. Mol Genet Metab. 2007;91:165–75.

Short-term motor learning through non-immersive virtual reality task in individuals with down syndrome

Carlos Bandeira de Mello Monteiro[1,2], Talita Dias da Silva[1,3*], Luiz Carlos de Abreu[2], Felipe Fregni[4,5], Luciano Vieira de Araujo[1], Fernando Henrique Inocêncio Borba Ferreira[1] and Claudio Leone[2]

Abstract

Background: Down syndrome (DS) has unique physical, motor and cognitive characteristics. Despite cognitive and motor difficulties, there is a possibility of intervention based on the knowledge of motor learning. However, it is important to study the motor learning process in individuals with DS during a virtual reality task to justify the use of virtual reality to organize intervention programs. The aim of this study was to analyze the motor learning process in individuals with DS during a virtual reality task.

Methods: A total of 40 individuals participated in this study, 20 of whom had DS (24 males and 8 females, mean age of 19 years, ranging between 14 and 30 yrs.) and 20 typically developing individuals (TD) who were matched by age and gender to the individuals with DS. To examine this issue, we used software that uses 3D images and reproduced a coincidence-timing task.

Results: The results showed that all individuals improved performance in the virtual task, but the individuals with DS that started the task with worse performance showed higher difference from the beginning. Besides that, they were able to retain and transfer the performance with increase of speed of the task.

Conclusion: Individuals with DS are able to learn movements from virtual tasks, even though the movement time was higher compared to the TD individuals. The results showed that individuals with DS who started with low performance improved coincidence- timing task with virtual objects, but were less accurate than typically developing individuals.

Keywords: Down syndrome, Virtual reality, Rehabilitation, User-computer interface, Physical therapy modalities

Background

Down syndrome (DS) is typically characterized by an additional chromosome, or trisomy 21 (Hsa21), with incidence of 1 in 750 live births and is considered one of the most frequent cause of learning difficulties [1].

The alterations made by individuals with DS may pose difficulties in functionality and independence to perform activities of daily living even during adulthood. Mancini et al. [2] reported that individuals with DS have less functional performance than individuals without motor and cognitive dysfunction with alterations in cognitive, motor areas and social function.

Due to the importance of learning motor skills for individuals with DS, it is important that practitioners use the knowledge derived from motor learning, which will enable an intervention program based on scientific evidence from this area of expertise. Examining how motor skill learning can be enhanced in individuals with DS is not only of theoretical interest, but may also have important practical implications for the lives of those affected by DS [3].

Some studies about motor learning in DS [3–6] were found, as well as a study about how individuals perform in a timing coincident task in a real environment using

* Correspondence: ft.talitadias@gmail.com
[1]School of Arts, Sciences and Humanities, University of São Paulo, Av. Arlindo Béttio, 1000, Ermelino Matarazzo, São Paulo 03828-000, Brazil
[3]Harvard School of Public Health, Harvard University, Boston, MA, USA
Full list of author information is available at the end of the article

Bassin Anticipatory timing and the results showed that it is a good tool to evaluate improvement on motor performance in people with DS [7] but little was found on motor learning in a virtual reality task in individuals with DS [8]. Recently, with the growing accessibility of computer-assisted technology, rehabilitation programs increasingly use virtual reality environments to enhance dedicated practice, thus, to study the use of virtual reality becomes essential [9–12]. Also, the use of the real task (Bassin Anticipatory timing) present some difficulties to be used worldwide considering its size, weight and price, in addition if someone needs to import the equipment, they must anticipate going through bureaucratic red tape, a long waiting time and difficulty for technical support. Thus, it is important to verify the performance of DS individuals in a virtual task using a computer that can offer visual and auditory feedback and facilitate the use of a coincident timing assessment for rehabilitation professionals to predict the anticipatory timing. Virtual task with 3D images has been used in different devices and represent the future in technology promoting independence and functionality in the daily life tasks for individuals with DS.

Given this background, the aim of the current study was to assess the motor learning capacity of individuals with DS in a non-immersive virtual reality task. Based upon the above deliberations, we hypothesized that individuals with DS will improve their coincident time of movement during acquisition in a 3D task, in addition to maintaining performance for the retention phase and transfer the performance with an increase of speed, however with lower performance and more variability when compared to the control group.

Methods

Participants

A total of 40 individuals participated in this study, 20 of whom had DS (11 males and 9 females, mean age = 19 years, ranging between 14 and 30 yrs.) and 20 typically developing individuals (TD) who were matched by age and gender to the individuals with DS. Criteria for inclusion were a medical diagnosis of DS and the ability to understand the task. The ability to understand the task was: after two demonstrations from the experimenter (one showing right reach and other showing wrong reach) the participant had two attempts to show if he/she understood the task. All participants were from school program and alphabetized. Exclusion criteria were disorders in cognitive function that would prevent comprehension of the experimental instruction.

Material and apparatus

This study used software that uses 3D images to reproduce a coincidence-timing task developed and tested by the Department of Electronic System Engineering of the Polytechnic School, University of São Paulo (EP/USP) (see also Silva et al. [13] and de Mello Monteiro et al. [14]) and upgraded by the Laboratory of Information Systems from the University of São Paulo.

This software enabled the coincidence-timing task to be done by pressing the space key on a keyboard. The coincident timing task was based on the Bassin Anticipation Timer [7, 15–21] and consisted of a task used worldwide by many authors (see Chiviacowsky et al. [3]; de Mello Monteiro et al. [14]; Corrêa et al. [18]) aiming to assess and verify motor learning considering the performance obtained by decreasing the errors, or the variability of errors.

To this end, 10 3D–cubes were displayed simultaneously in a vertical column on a monitor. The cubes created turned on (i.e., changed from blue to green) and off sequentially (from top to bottom) until the target cube (i.e., the tenth cube) was reached. The task for the participant was to press the space bar on the keyboard in the exact time to hitting the target object (Fig. 1).

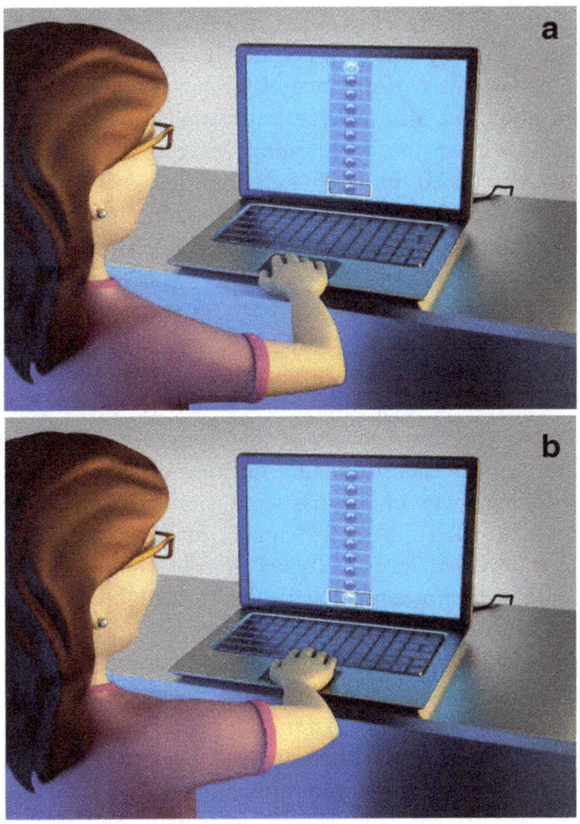

Fig. 1 Coincident timing task using 3D image: initial position (**a**) and final position **b**

Procedure and design

Participants performed the task individually in a quiet room with only the researcher who gave the instructions to the individual present. The computer was placed on a table. The participants were seated in chair, which was adjusted in height according to the needs of the individual. Also a footrest was available, if required. After being seated, the experimenter explained the task verbally equally for all participants and as mentioned before gave two demonstrations of how to perform the coincidence-timing tasks and two trials as tests for the participant, as a way to access the comprehension of the task. These attempts did not count for the experiment. The participants were instructed to place the preferred hand on a mark in front of the target (the location was individually adjusted but ranged from 2 to 4 cm from the target keyboard). Once the first top cube turned on, the individual had to move his or her hand to either touch the target key on the keyboard, exactly at the moment coinciding with the bottom target cube turning on. During the tasks, the experimenter did not provide any encouragement or reward. Different sounds were provided as feedback for a hit or miss during acquisition, retention and transfer, the range of error being −200 to 200 ms. We chose auditory feedback because it is viable and better differentiated by the computer, and is described as a widely used form with evidence of effectiveness as sensorial feedback [22].

The primary purpose of practice is considered not only to facilitate the performance of temporary effects during acquisition but also provide improved durable performance (assigned to the learning) of the retention and transfer tests. To this end, "Retention test" was used as a way to measure the capacity to maintain the same performance acquired with the practice after a period with no contact with the task and "Transfer test" was used to assess the capacity to maintain the same performance acquired with practice when changing something in the task; it evaluates the ability to transfer the performance in a similar task or environment.

During the three phases of the study, we used blocks of 5 attempts each to ensure fairness in the evaluation of performances of the participant, as used in several studies [3, 14, 18]. All participants made 20 trial acquisitions (divided into 4 blocks), 5 trial retentions after 10 min with no contact with the task (1 block) and 5 trial transfers immediately after retention trials (1 block). Thus, each participant had 32 trials (2 test trials – that did not count for the study; 20 acquisition trials; 5 retention trials; 5 transfer trials). During acquisition and retention trials, the cubes simulated a dropped light movement with the turning on and off of the lights in an interval of 400 ms between positions change, while during transfer light movement was increased with 300 ms between positions.

Data analysis

The dependent variable used was the timing error, i.e., constant error (CE), absolute error (AE) and variable error (VE).

Constant error (CE)

The calculation of CE was done by the simple arithmetic average of the error values, considering the algebraic sign (negative or positive) in a series of attempts (block of trials). It represents the direction of error if it is late or early.

$$CE = [\Sigma(Xi{-}T)/N]$$

In which: Σ = sum, i = number of attempts, Xi – score of the trial i, T = distance from the target, N = number of trials.

Absolute error (AE)

The individual values of AE were used with no algebraic sign (all values are positive) before proceeding to the calculation of average. The absolute error represents the individual as well as combinations effects of tasks characteristics [23]. AE represents the accuracy measurement.

$$\mathrm{AE} = [\Sigma\ (|\ \mathrm{Xi}{-}\mathrm{T})/\mathrm{N}]$$

In which: Σ = sum, | = "absolute value of", i = number of attempts, Xi – score of the trial i, T = distance from the target, N = number of trials.

Variable error (VE)

To calculate the variable error, we squared the difference between each score and the individual CE mean, then sum all and divided by the number of trials. Then we compute the square root of this number. It represents the variability of error.

$$VE = \sqrt{\left[\sum (Xi{-}CE)^2/N\right]}$$

In which: Σ = sum, i = number of attempts, Xi– score of the trial i, CE = constant error, N = number of trials.

The timing error was defined as the time difference between the moment the target cube switched on (arrival time) and the moment at which the keyboard was touched. The dependent variable for the CE was submitted to a 2 (group: DS and TD) by 2 (blocks) ANOVA, repeated measures were utilized for the last factor.

The cognitive and motor function in people with DS is very different within them, so we divided the groups in order to find out if the performance on the first block would be related to the comprehension of the task, affecting the performance. For AE and VE the groups were divided by two subgroups according to the performance in the first acquisition block (10 individuals with best movement time: Performance Group A and 10 individuals with worse movement time: Performance Group B) the dependent variables were submitted to a 2 (group: DS and TD), by 2 (performance groups: A and B) by 2 (blocks) ANOVA, repeated measures were utilized for the last factor. For the factor block separate comparisons were made for acquisition (first acquisition block A1 versus final acquisition block A4), retention (A4 versus retention block R) and transfer (A4 versus transfer block T). Post hoc comparisons were carried out using Tukey-HSD test ($p < .05$).

Results

The t-test found no statistical difference for age between groups of best movement time and worst movement time for both DS-group (18.4 ± 5; 20.5 ± 3, $p = 0.154$, respectively) and TD-group (19.3 ± 4; 18.8 ± 4, $p = 0.400$, respectively).

Acquisition

Constant error

Figure 2 present the CE's during acquisition tasks among the DS- and TD-groups. The ANOVA did not reveal any effect or interaction for Block. However, a significant main effect for Group was found, $F(1, 38) = 6.62$, $p = .014$, $\eta^2 = .15$. It suggests that a difference in movement time between groups occurred, in other words DS-group had a much larger constant error (M = 193 ms) than TD-group (M = 6 ms) and in both groups the directional trend was late in movement.

Absolute error

The pattern of absolute errors is illustrated in Fig. 3. Significant effects were found for Group $F(1, 36) = 75.2$, $p < .001$, $\eta^2 = .68$, Performance Group $F(1, 36) = 11.7$, $p = .002$, $\eta^2 = .25$ and Block, $F(1, 36) = 12.4$, $p = .001$, $\eta^2 = .26$, and interactions for Group by Performance Group $F(1, 36) = 5.18$, $p = .029$, $\eta^2 = .13$, Blocks by Performance Group $F(1, 36) = 13.1$, $p = .001$, $\eta^2 = .27$, Blocks by Group $F(1, 36) = 4.66$, $p = .038$, $\eta^2 = .12$ and Blocks by Performance Group by Group $F(1, 36) = 6.65$, $p = .014$, $\eta^2 = .16$. It indicates that DS- group had a much larger absolute error (M = 434 ms) than TD- group (M = 123 ms) and the Performance Group B has a much larger absolute error (M = 340 ms) than the Performance Group A (M = 217 ms). The post hoc test showed that this difference can be attributed to the DS-group that had a larger movement time in the Performance Group B (M = 536 ms) than in the Performance Group A (M = 332 ms), while for the TD-group this difference did not occurr (M = 143 ms versus 103 ms, respectively).

For Blocks, in the final block the movement time was smaller (M = 226 ms) when compared to the first block of acquisition (M = 331 ms) in both groups. The post hoc test showed that this difference can be attributed to the DS-group that showed worse performance in the first block of acquisition- Performance Group B (M = 714 ms) when compared to the final block of acquisition (M = 359 ms), for the other three groups this difference did not occurred.

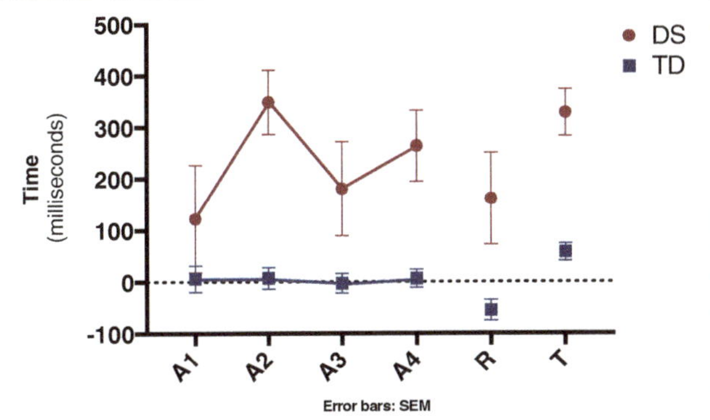

Fig. 2 Constant error between groups on acquisition, retention and transfer blocks. A1-A4- refers to four acquisition blocks; R- refers to retention block; T- refers to tranfer block; DS- Down syndrome; TD- typical development; SEM- standard error of mean

Variable error

Similar to the absolute error, significant effects were found for Group $F(1, 36) = 35.5$, $p < .001$, $\eta^2 = .50$, Performance Group $F(1, 36) = 35.4$, $p < .001$, $\eta^2 = .50$ and Block, $F(1, 36) = 33.0$, $p < .001$, $\eta^2 = .48$, and interactions for Group by Performance Group $F(1, 36) = 14.5$, $p = .001$, $\eta^2 = .29$, Blocks by Group $F(1, 36) = 20.6$, $p < .001$, $\eta^2 = .36$, Blocks by Performance Group $F(1, 36) = 14.1$, $p = .001$, $\eta^2 = .28$, and Blocks by Performance Group by Group $F(1, 36) = 8.64$, $p = .006$, $\eta^2 = .19$. It indicates that DS- group had a much larger variable error (M = 107 ms) than TD- group (M = 39 ms) and the Performance Group B has a much larger variable error (M = 107 ms) than the Performance Group A (M = 39 ms). The post hoc test showed that this difference can be attributed to the DS-group that had a larger movement time -Performance Group B (M = 163 ms) than in the Performance Group A (M = 51 ms), while for the TD-group this difference did not occur (M = 51 versus 27 ms, respectively).

For Blocks, in the final block of acquisition the movement time was smaller (M = 37 ms) when compared to the first block of acquisition (M = 109 ms) in both groups. The post hoc test showed that this difference can be attributed to the DS-group that showed worse performance in the first block of acquisition -Performance Group B (M = 268 ms) when compared to the final block of acquisition (M = 57 ms), for the other three groups this difference did not occurred (Fig. 4).

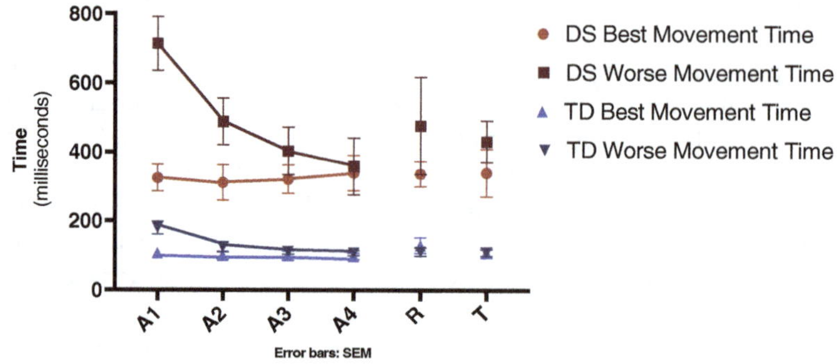

Fig. 3 Absolute error between groups on acquisition, retention and transfer blocks. A1-A4- refers to four acquisition blocks; R- refers to retention block; T- refers to tranfer block; DS- Down syndrome; TD- typical development; SEM- standard error of mean

Retention

There was significant effect of Block only for constant error, $F(1, 38) = 5.05$, $p = .030$, $\eta^2 = .12$. The result indicates that in the final acquisition block the constant error was much larger (M = 135 ms) than the retention block (M = 53 ms), in addition, the directional trend was late in movement. For the absolute and variable error the ANOVA did not find any main effects and interactions, suggesting that the patterns of movement were no different during retention as compared to final acquisition block for absolute (DS- 407 to 349 ms and TD- 119 to 102 ms, respectively) and variable errors (DS- 55 to 43 ms and TD- 33 to 31 ms, respectively).

Transfer

Similarly to retention test, there was significant effect of Block only for constant error, $F(1, 38) = 6.44$, $p = .015$, $\eta^2 = .15$. This result indicates that in the transfer block the constant error was much larger (M = 135 ms) than the final acquisition block (M = 193 ms), in addition the directional trend was late in movement. For the absolute and variable error there were no significant effects of Block, suggesting that the patterns of movement were no different during transfer as compared to final acquisition block for absolute (DS- 385 to 349 ms and TD- 108 to 102 ms, respectively) and variable errors (DS- 58 to 43 ms and TD- 32 to 31 ms, respectively).

Discussion

The main objective of this study was to determine whether individuals with DS can learn a non-immersive virtual task, and if there is the ability to adapt new environmental demands through improved performance in the acquisition and transfer with increasing speed. Therefore, the chosen task was coincident timing with (3D) virtual object held on a computer screen.

According to the results, the initial hypothesis of improved performance in a virtual task was partly confirmed, it was found that only Down Syndrome in Performance Group B showed significant improvement in performance in the execution of the task between the first block (M = 714 ms) and the final block of the acquisition (M = 359 ms). Latash [24] says that performance of individuals with DS shows dramatic improvement with practice even in tasks that are very simple, and seem to offer little room for improvement, but our results show that for the task used, this improvement in performance occurred only with individuals with low performance in the beginning.

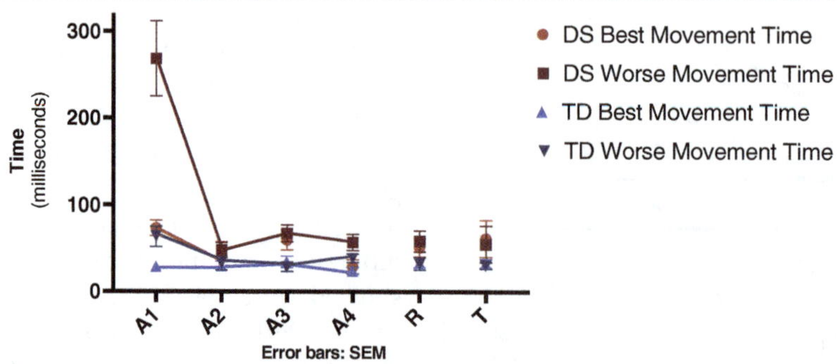

Fig. 4 Variable error between groups on acquisition, retention and transfer blocks. A1-A4- refers to four acquisition blocks; R- refers to retention block; T- refers to tranfer block; DS- Down syndrome; TD- typical development; SEM- standard error of mean

Based on the present findings, we can only speculate why the individuals with DS with high performance did not improve. Considering that the motor and cognitive function in people with DS are very different among them [25] even between DS from school programs (all alphabetized), probably the task was easier for the group with high performance and they already show the best score from the beginning of the protocol. This speculation can be supported by Malak et al. [26], who evaluated the association of the motor and cognitive development in children with DS and concluded that the motor development is associated with cognitive development, i.e. mental age.

However, the primary purpose of practice is not only to facilitate the performance of temporary effects during acquisition but also provide improved durable performance (assigned to the learning) of the retention and transfer tests. From the results obtained, there was no significant difference between the last block of acquisition with retention and transfer blocks in absolute error in both the TD (102 ms to 119 ms, respectively) group, as in DS (349 ms to 407 ms, respectively) group. That is, both groups maintained the ability to perform the task after a certain time without running.

It is important to note that the small number of repetitions was sufficient to improve performance, but only in the group with DS who had more difficulty in the beginning of the task. For this group, even considering an acquisition with few repetitions, participants underwent an initial phase - characterized by a greater number of errors, inconsistencies and high demand attention - until a later stage, which is characterized by greater consistency, fewer errors and likely reduced demand attention. Those DS individuals organized their reaching and aiming movements to achieve the precision dictated by the task demands, while optimizing movement speed and energy efficiency. When faced with unexpected changes to the task demands, they are usually very adept at adjusting their movement trajectories to accommodate the new environmental constraints [27].

Considering the results of the last acquisition block (TD = 102 ms and DS = 349 ms) with transfer block (TD = 108 ms and DS = 385 ms), there were no statistically significant differences between blocks in both groups. Therefore, a situation with increased speed of the task did not cause significant performance drop. Again, primarily participants with DS who started with low performance after practice showed good adaptability to a new situation in coincident timing task. Considering the variable error, except for the first block of the group with DS with worse performance, the variability of error is similar between DS and people with typical development.

Those findings are partly in line with the notion that DS individuals can improve their ability in a virtual computer task (see Berg et al. [28]), The recent development in the area of motor control allows researchers and practitioners to tap into these reserves and use quantitative indices of changes in motor synergies with practice to optimize training programs for DS individuals [24].

Comparing the DS and TD groups, it was found that the DS-group had worse performance in acquisition than the group with typical development. This difference was also observed in the phases of retention and transfer. In DS, inability to effectively control movement through online processing of information may account for the slowness that is characteristic of their performance. They likely have difficulties due to less time in deceleration of reaching, less anticipatory capacity, longer movement times [29] and stability challenges of ligamentous laxity and hypotonia (see Galli et al. [30] and Cisterna et al. [31]).

Another factor that may contribute to greater difficulty in performance in participants with DS is the movement pattern and strategy used to accomplish the task. Individuals with DS have difficulty performing precision goal-directed movement with any degree of speed or efficiency and the movement performed took twice as long to complete than TD person [27] and individuals with DS have preference for patterns of muscle activation characterized by higher levels of co-contraction, that is, simultaneous activation of muscle pairs acting at a joint in opposite directions ("agonist-antagonist muscle pairs") [32].

Considering the constant error and variable error, result indicates that in CE all individuals (DS and TD) had a trend to delay the movement. Masumoto et al. [33] evaluated adolescents with DS in a bimanual and unilateral tapping task and found also that they presented delay to reach the timing task. However in VE the DS-group had a much larger variable error (M = 107 ms) than TD- group (M = 39 ms), our findings confirm data from Torriani-Pasin et al. [7], even in a 3D task the individuals with Down syndrome tend to perform tasks in unstable and irregular coincidence of visual-motor systems, when compared to control subjects. Individuals with DS looked at experimental objects less frequently than their typically and children with typical development spent more time than DS in the highest visual stimulation complexity zone [34].

Another difficultly for DS individuals is in the deficit of the perceptual-motor abilities, which are responsible for the abilities that support the acquisition of several motor skills. Individuals with DS rely more on feedback control, whereas they have problems with movement planning and feed-forward control as showed by Kearney and Gentile [29] and Spanò et al. [35], the different strategy operated by individuals with DS leads to a different task performance. Probably DS has a deficit in voluntary motor commands and preprogramming of actions, which results in altered strategies of movement that enhance security and stability instead of efficiency of the performance [36].

Conclusions

Based on the present findings, individuals with DS are able to learn movements from virtual tasks, even though the movement time was higher compared to the TD individuals. The results showed that individuals with DS who started with low performance improved coincidence- timing task with virtual objects, but were less accurate than typically developing individuals.

Although individuals with DS having different exploratory actions, perceptual-motor abilities, pattern and movement strategies, results showed the ability to improve performance in non-immersive virtual tasks especially for individuals who have more difficulties, which can encourage the use of virtual environments in programs of motor habilitation in individuals with DS.

Limitations and future studies

As limitations of the study, we could not assess the cognitive function and mental age of the participants with DS or their access to computers or video games. This information could give more explanations about the difference between the groups with worse and better performance.

When compared to previous studies in this field, the present study included a rather heterogeneous population with a wide age range including adolescents and adults with different gender. Even though we cannot rule out the effects of these factors, it is believed that this did not affect the results to a great extent. Both groups were carefully matched for age and all participants in the DS group showed to be able to perform the task.

Moreover, the computer program we used limited the outcome parameters to non-immersive virtual task and we could not compare with a real task, probably transfer to a real task could have given even better insight into our findings. Therefore, for future studies it would be recommended to not only look at virtual task but also transfer for real environment since this could provide valuable information. Additionally, we suggest that this non-immersive task of virtual reality may be an option to be reproduced in others diseases with motor and cognitive disabilities.

Abbreviations

AE: Absolute Error; CE: Constant Error; DS: Down Syndrome; TD: Typical Development; VE: Variable Error

Acknowledgements

We acknowledge the participants in the study.

Funding

This study received financial support from the FAPESP (Fundação de Amparo à Pesquisa do Estado de São Paulo, process number 2012/16970-6 and 2013/00619-0).

Author's contributions

CBMM: drafted, designed and wrote the manuscript; TDS: study implementation, data collection, performed data analysis and interpretation; LCA: help with manuscript preparation; FF: help with data analysis and manuscript preparation; LVA: Software development and data interpretation; FHIBF: Software development and data interpretation; CL: help with data analysis and manuscript preparation. All authors read and approved the final manuscript.

Competing interests

The authors declare that they have no competing interests.

Author details

[1]School of Arts, Sciences and Humanities, University of São Paulo, Av. Arlindo Béttio, 1000, Ermelino Matarazzo, São Paulo 03828-000, Brazil. [2]School of Public Health, University of São Paulo, São Paulo, Brazil. [3]Harvard School of Public Health, Harvard University, Boston, MA, USA. [4]Center for Neurosciences (NEC), University of São Paulo, São Paulo, Brazil. [5]Spaulding Rehabilitation Hospital and Massachusetts General Hospital, Harvard Medical School, Boston, MA, USA.

References

1. Lana-Elola E, Watson-Scales SD, Fisher EM, Tybulewicz VL. Down syndrome: searching for the genetic culprits. Dis Model Mech. 2011;4:586–95.
2. Mancini MC, Silva PC, Gonçalves SC, Matins SM. Comparação do desempenho funcional de crianças portadoras de síndrome de Down e crianças com desenvolvimento normal aos 2 e 5 anos de idade. Arq Neuropsiquiatr. 2003;61:15–409.
3. Chiviacowsky S, Wulf G, Machado C, Rydberg N. Self-controlled feedback enhances learning in adults with down syndrome. Rev Bras Fisioter. 2012;16:191–6.
4. Latash ML, Kang N, Patterson D. Finger coordination in persons with down syndrome: atypical patterns of coordination and the effects of practice. Exp Brain Res. 2002;146:345–55.
5. Bussy G, Charrin E, Brun A, Curie A, des Portes V. Implicit procedural learning in fragile X and down syndrome. J Intellect Disabil Res. 2011;55:521–8.
6. Ringenbach SD, Mulvey GM, Chen CC, Jung ML. Unimanual and bimanual continuous movements benefit from visual instructions in persons with down syndrome. J Mot Behav. 2012;44:233–9.
7. Torriani-Pasin C, Bonuzzi GM, Soares MA, Antunes GL, Palma GC, Monteiro CBM, et al. Performance of down syndrome subjects during a coincident timing task. Int Arch Med. 2013;6:15.
8. Courbois Y, Farran EK, Lemahieu A, Blades M, Mengue-Topio H, Sockeel P. Wayfinding behaviour in down syndrome: a study with virtual environments. Res Dev Disabil. 2013;34:1825–31.
9. Barton GJ, Hawken MB, Foster RJ, Holmes G, Butler PB. The effects of virtual reality game training on trunk to pelvis coupling in a child with cerebral palsy. J Neuroeng Rehabil. 2013;10:15.
10. Burdea GC, Cioi D, Kale A, Janes WE, Ross SA, Engsberg JR. Robotics and gaming to improve ankle strength, motor control, and function in children with cerebral palsy–a case study series. IEEE Trans Neural Syst Rehabil Eng. 2013;21:165–73.
11. Mitchell L, Ziviani J, Oftedal S, Boyd R. The effect of virtual reality interventions on physical activity in children and adolescents with early brain injuries including cerebral palsy. Dev Med Child Neurol. 2012;54:667–71.
12. Riener R, Dislaki E, Keller U, Koenig A, Van Hedel H, Nagle A. Virtual reality aided training of combined arm and leg movements of children with CP. Stud Health Technol Inform. 2013;184:349–55.
13. Silva TD, Monteiro CBM, Hasue RH, Moura MCDS, Correa AGD, Ficheman IK, et al. Aprendizagem motora em tarefa virtual na Paralisia Cerebral. Temas Desenvolv. 2013;104:47–53.

14. de Mello Monteiro CB, Massetti T, Silva TD, van der Kamp J, de Abreu LC, Leone C, et al. Transfer of motor learning from virtual to natural environments in individuals with cerebral palsy. Res Dev Disabil. 2014;35:2430–7.
15. Shea CH, Ashby AA. Modifications to the Bassin anticipation timer. Res Q Exerc Sport. 1981;52:278–80.
16. Overdorf V, Page SJ, Schweighardt R, McGrath RE. Mental and physical practice schedules in acquisition and retention of novel timing skills. Percept Mot Skills. 2004;99:51–62.
17. Harrold D, Kozar B. Velocity, occlusion, and sex of subjects in coincidence of anticipation. Percept Mot Skills. 2002;94:914–20.
18. Corrêa UC, Oliveira PH, Oliveira JA, Freudenheim AM, Meira-Junior CM, Marinovic W, et al. "Timing" coincidente em tarefas complexas: estudo exploratório do desempenho de adultos de diferentes idades em diferentes velocidades de estímulo visual. Rev Bras Educ Fís Esporte. 2005;19:307–15.
19. Santos S, Corrêa UC, Freudenheim AM. Variabilidade de performance numa tarefa de "timing" antecipatório em indivíduos de diferentes faixas etárias. Rev Paul Educ Fís. 2003;17:154–62.
20. Williams K. Age difference on a coincident anticipation task: influence of stereotypic or "preferred" movement speed. J Mot Behav. 1985;17:389–410.
21. Williams LR, Jasiewicz JM, Simmons RW. Coincidence timing of finger, arm, and whole body movements. Percept Mot Skills. 2001;92:535–47.
22. Rosati G, Rodà A, Avanzini F, Masiero S. On the role of auditory feedback in robot-assisted movement training after stroke: review of the literature. Comput Intell Neurosci. 2013;2013:586138. doi:10.1155/2013/586138. Published online 2013 December 8
23. Duncan MJ, Stanley M, Smith M, Price MJ, Wright SL. Coincidence anticipation timing performance during an acute bout of brisk walking in older adults: effect of stimulus speed. Neural Plast. 2015;2015:210213. doi:10.1155/2015/210213.
24. Latash ML. Learning motor synergies by persons with down syndrome. J Intellect Disabil Res. 2007;51:962–71.
25. Rihtman T, Tekuzener E, Parush S, Tenenbaum A, Bachrach SJ, Ornoy A. Are the cognitive functions of children with down syndrome related to their participation? Dev Med Child Neurol. 2010 Jan;52(1):72–8.
26. Malak R, Kotwicka M, Krawczyk-Wasielewska A, Mojs E, Samborski W. Motor skills, cognitive development and balance functions of children with down syndrome. Ann Agric Environ Med. 2013;20(4):803–6.
27. Elliott D, Hansen S, Grierson LE, Lyons J, Bennett SJ, Hayes SJ. Goal-directed aiming: two components but multiple processes. Psychol Bull. 2010;136:1023–44.
28. Berg P, Becker T, Martian A, Primrose KD, Wingen J. Motor control outcomes following Nintendo Wii use by a child with down syndrome. Pediatr Phys Ther. 2012;24:78–84.
29. Kearney K, Gentile AM. Prehension in young children with down syndrome. Acta Psychol. 2003;112:3–16.
30. Galli M, Cimolin V, Rigoldi C, Pau M, Costici P, Albertini G. The effects of low arched feet on foot rotation during gait in children with down syndrome. J Intellect Disabil Res. 2014;58(8):758–64. doi:10.1111/jir.12087. Epub 2013 Aug 19
31. Cisterna B, Costanzo M, Scherini E, Zancanaro C, Malatesta M. Ultrastructural features of skeletal muscle in adult and aging Ts65Dn mice, a murine model of down syndrome. Muscles Ligaments Tendons J. 2014;3(4):287–94. eCollection 2013
32. Latash ML, Anson JG. Synergies in health and disease: relations to adaptive changes in motor coordination. Phys Ther. 2006;86:1151–60.
33. Masumoto J, Abe T, Inui N. Adolescents with down syndrome exhibit greater force and delay in onset of tapping movements. Percept Mot Skills. 2012;114(3):826–36.
34. Kawa R, Pisula E. Locomotor activity, object exploration and space preference in children with autism and down syndrome. Acta Neurobiol Exp. 2010;70:131–40.
35. Spanò M, Mercuri E, Randò T, Pantò T, Gagliano A, Henderson S, et al. Motor and perceptual-motor competence in children with down syndrome: variation in performance with age. Eur J Paediatr Neurol. 1999;3:7–13.
36. Vimercati SL, Galli M, Rigoldi C, Ancillao A, Albertini G. Motor strategies and motor programs during an arm tapping task in adults with down syndrome. Exp Brain Res. 2013;225:333–8.

4

Cortical laminar necrosis in dengue encephalitis

Ravindra Kumar Garg[1*], Imran Rizvi[1], Rajan Ingole[1], Amita Jain[2], Hardeep Singh Malhotra[1], Neeraj Kumar[1] and Dhruv Batra[1]

Abstract

Background: Dengue encephalitis is a rare neurological manifestation of dengue fever. Its clinical presentation is similar to other viral encephalitides and encephalopathy. No single specific finding on magnetic resonance imaging of dengue encephalitis has yet been documented. They are highly variable and atypical.

Case presentation: A 15-year boy presented with fever, the headache and altered sensorium of 12-day duration. On neurological examination, his Glasgow Coma Scale score was 10 (E3M4V3). There was no focal neurological deficit. Laboratory evaluation revealed leukopenia and marked thrombocytopenia. Dengue virus IgM antibody was positive both in serum and cerebrospinal fluid. Magnetic resonance imaging of the brain revealed signal changes in bilateral parietooccipital and left frontal regions (left hemisphere more involved than the right hemisphere). There was gyriform enhancement bilateral parietooccipital regions consistent with cortical laminar necrosis. Bilaterally diffuse subcortical white matter was also involved and subtle T2 hyperintensity involving both basal ganglia was noted. Gradient echo sequence revealed presence of hemorrhage in the subcortical white matter. Patient was treated conservatively and received platelet transfusion. Patient became fully conscious after 7 days.

Conclusion: In a patient with highly suggestive dengue e\ephalitis, we describe an unusual magnetic resonance imaging finding. This report is possibly the first instance of cortical laminar necrosis in such a setting.

Keywords: Cortical laminar necrosis, Encephalitis, Encephalopathy, Magnetic resonance imaging, Dengue virus, Case report

Background

Currently, dengue infection is endemic in more than 100 countries. The incidence of dengue has increased dramatically in recent decades. World Health Organization, currently, estimates that 390 million dengue infections occur per year, of which 96 million manifest clinically; about 2.5% of those affected dies. Dengue virus is a single-stranded RNA virus belonging to the *Flaviviridae* family. There are four serotypes of dengue virus (DENV-1 to DENV-4), of which serotypes DENV-2 and DENV-3 have been implicated most frequently in dengue fever. The involvement of the central nervous system has been described with all 3 classical types of dengue, dengue fever, dengue hemorrhagic fever, and dengue shock syndrome [1].

Encephalitis has been reported worldwide as a severe complication in patients infected by dengue virus. Dengue virus encephalitis often presents as acute encephalitis syndrome during dengue epidemics and can be seen in all 3 classical types of dengue. Indirect mechanisms such as impaired kidney and liver dysfunctions, hypoxic-ischemic insults, and other metabolic disorders can affect brain function and clinically present as encephalopathy. In addition to direct viral involvement of brain, there are several other pathologies like ischemic and hemorrhagic strokes, subdural hematoma, cerebral venous thrombosis, and acute disseminated encephalomyelitis that can affect the brain [2–6] (Table 1).

In most cases with dengue virus encephalitis, neuroimaging is normal [7]. Whenever, neuroimaging is abnormal, changes are usually non-specific in terms of etiology but may provide a hint towards the possible pathophysiological process. We report a case highly

* Correspondence: garg50@yahoo.com
[1]Department of Neurology, King George's Medical University, UP, Lucknow 226003, India
Full list of author information is available at the end of the article

Table 1 Neuroimaging spectrum of dengue-associated encephalitis/encephalopathy

Clinical syndrome	Neuroimaging features	Pathogenesis
Diffuse brain involvement		
Encephalopathy	Often normal	Impaired liver and renal dysfunction Ischemic-hypoxemic injury
Acute encephalitis	Usually normal; diffuse cortical and periventricular, hyperintensities	Direct viral invasion of brain
Acute hemorrhagic encephalitis	GRE sequence shows areas of blooming indicating hemorrhage	Direct viral invasion of brain
Acute disseminated encephalomyelitis	Periventricular white matter lesions	Post-infectious demyelination
Vascular complications		
Cerebral venous thrombosis	Thrombosis of venous system of brain	Severe dehydration and hypotension
Intracerebral hemorrhage	Cerebral parenchymal, subdural or subarachnoidal hematoma	Thrombocytopenia, disseminated intravascular coagulation and associated coagulopathies
Ischemic stroke	Multiple infarctions	Vasculitis, infective thromboembolism
Focal encephalitis		
Cerebellitis Rhombencephalitis	Hyperintensities in brainstem and cerebellum	Direct viral invasion

suggestive of dengue encephalitis with an unusual magnetic resonance imaging finding in brain.

Case presentation

A 15-year-old boy presented to our University Hospital, a tertiary care neurology facility, with fever, headache, and altered sensorium of 12-day duration. At admission, he was febrile (101 °F), with a pulse rate of 110/min and a blood pressure recording of 114/74 mmHg; his Glasgow Coma Scale score was 10 (E3M4V3). There were no petechiae or signs of bleeding over the skin or any mucosal surface. There was no focal neurological deficit and neurological examination was normal, including (absence of) signs of meningeal irritation. Laboratory evaluation revealed the following estimations: hemoglobin of 11 g/dl, total leukocyte count of 3300 cells/mm^3, and platelet count of 22,000 cells/mm^3 which dropped to 8000 cells/mm^3 on next day. His aspartate aminotransferase level was 155 U/L, alanine aminotransferase was 140 U/L and alkaline phosphatase was 56 U/L. Additional biochemical parameters, renal function tests, blood sugar, electrolytes, and arterial blood gas analysis, were normal. Malarial parasite was not detected in the peripheral blood smear. The cerebrospinal fluid examination, cytological and biochemical, was normal. IgM antibody against dengue virus was positive both in serum and cerebrospinal fluid; meanwhile, dengue NS1 antigen was negative. Electroencephalography revealed generalized slowing. On magnetic resonance imaging of the brain, signal changes were seen in bilateral parietooccipital and left frontal region (left hemisphere was more involved than the right hemisphere). There were diffuse subcortical white matter changes along with suggestion of hemorrhage on gradient echo sequence. Subtle hyperintensity on T2 W images was also noted in bilateral basal ganglia. Gadolinium-contrast study revealed a gyriform enhancement suggestive of cortical laminar necrosis (Fig. 1). He was managed conservatively and given platelet transfusion. The patient responded well to management and became fully conscious in 7 days.

Discussion

Cortical laminar necrosis is an imaging term classically used to describe high-intensity cortical lesions in a gyriform distribution on T1-weighted magnetic resonance imaging. Cortical laminar necrosis is, pathologically, characterized as necrosis of particular cortical laminae involving neurons, glial cells, and cerebral blood vessels. Cortical laminar necrosis is predominantly caused by hypoxia and metabolic disorders, like hypoglycemia, intoxication, hypoxic-ischemic encephalopathy, renal and hepatic dysfunction, but may also be seen in patients with encephalitis [8–10]. We describe the occurrence of cortical laminar necrosis in a setting highly suggestive of dengue infection, possibly the first instance, in a 15-year-old boy.

Dengue virus was, at large, considered a non-neurotropic virus. With an increase in awareness and improvement in laboratory techniques, dengue virus or dengue viral components are being isolated from brain tissue or from cerebrospinal fluid specimens [11–13]. The mechanism of dengue virus invasion of the central nervous system, and its consequences, is not completely understood. It is supposed that the neurological complications of dengue virus are caused by many mechanisms, singularly or in a combination, like systemic metabolic

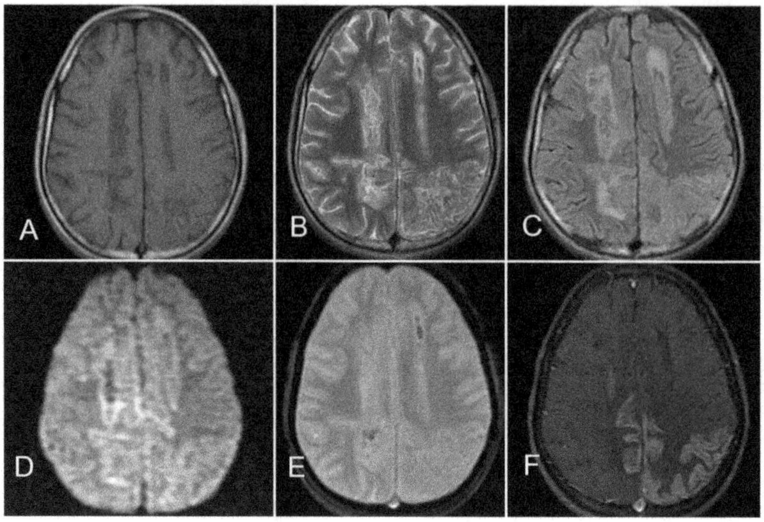

Fig. 1 Axial sections of MRI of the brain depict curvilinear hyperintense cortical lesions in bilateral parietal and occipital areas on T1 W (**a**), T2 W (**b**) and T2 fluid attenuated inversion recovery (**c**) sequences. Mild gyral diffusion restriction is noted on diffusion weighted sequence (**d**) while blooming is seen on gradient echo sequence (**e**). Post-contrast T1 W sequence (**f**) depicts gyral enhancement

abnormalities, liver and kidney dysfunctions, direct infection, post-infectious immune disorders, abnormal vascular permeability and flow abnormalities, and coagulopathies. Possibly, the virus enters the central nervous system via infected macrophages. In an experimental study, Bordignon and co-workers noted that a mutant dengue virus-1 escaped immune defense mechanism of the body and caused a severe meningo-encephalitis in mice [14]. In another study that included 84 patients with fatal dengue meningoencephalitis, dengue virus serology in cerebrospinal fluid specimens was positive in 50% of the patients. These findings indicate that dengue virus has neurotropic properties and actively invades central nervous system [11]. Dengue virus-associated cerebrospinal fluid pleocytosis, cerebral parenchymal inflammatory cell infiltrates, and intrathecal synthesis of dengue-specific antibodies also indicate active viral invasion of brain [15].

A wide variety of neuroimaging changes have been described in dengue encephalitis. Not all patients have neuroimaging abnormalities. Bhoi and co-workers, in a series of 20 patients, noted neuroimaging abnormalities in 50% of patients with dengue virus infection [16]. Multifocal hyperintensities in bilateral periventricular zones, including basal ganglia, may be seen on T2 W and fluid attenuated inversion recovery sequences [3]. Brainstem, cerebellum, corpus callosum and thalamus may also be involved [17]. In many patients with acute hemorrhagic encephalitis, gradient echo sequences reveal patchy areas of blooming suggestive of hemorrhage [18]. In many patients with dengue infection, encephalopathy is being attributed to acute disseminated encephalomyelitis. In such cases, T2-weighted magnetic resonance imaging reveals signal abnormalities in the subcortical and periventricular white matter, with or without gray matter involvement. Dengue-associated acute disseminated encephalomyelitis, being an immune mediated disorder of the central nervous system, has been shown to respond well to intravenous methylprednisolone [2].

In our case, we kept the possibility of direct dengue virus infection as the foremost cause of cortical laminar necrosis. Metabolic abnormalities, as depicted by *mildly* deranged liver functions, was kept as the next possibility. As the patient was hemodynamically stable, hypoxic-ischemic insult seems unlikely and the spatial distribution of lesions did not favor the occurrence of posterior leukoencephalopathy. Although evidence of blooming is known in patients with encephalitis, thrombocytopenia in the present scenario might have had a contributory role in the characteristic radiological presentation.

Diagnosis of dengue encephalitis is often not difficult in the setting of a dengue epidemic and a patient presenting with febrile encephalopathy and demonstration of anti-dengue IgM antibodies or dengue genomic material in serum and/or cerebrospinal fluid could be diagnosed as dengue encephalitis [19]. However, in low incidence areas and non-endemic zones, a high index of suspicion should be kept and an effort should be made to rule out other causes of viral encephalitis prevalent in that area [20]. Dengue NS-1 antigen might not be demonstrable in all cases especially those who present after 1 week of onset of symptoms. A low platelet count and altered liver and renal function may help in making diagnosis of dengue encephalitis/encephalopathy.

Conclusion

There is no characteristic neuroimaging finding in dengue encephalitis. Frequently, changes in white matter and deep gray matter have been described. We describe an unusual magnetic resonance imaging finding in a patient dengue encephalitis. Cortical laminar necrosis has never been described in dengue encephalitis.

Abbreviations

DENV: Dengue virus; RNA: Ribonucleic acid

Acknowledgement

None.

Funding

Not applicable.

Authors' contributions

RKG: Case evaluation, contributing in work up of the patient and writing the manuscript. IR: Case evaluation, contributing in work up of the patient and writing the manuscript. RI: Case evaluation, contributing in work up of the patient and writing the manuscript. AJ: Virological evaluation and manuscript review. HSM: Review of literature and writing the manuscript. NK: Review of literature and writing the manuscript. DB: Case evaluation, contributing in work up of the patient and writing the manuscript. All authors read and approved the final manuscript.

Competing interest

On behalf of all authors, the corresponding author states that there is no competing of interest.

Author details

[1]Department of Neurology, King George's Medical University, UP, Lucknow 226003, India. [2]Department of Microbiology, King George's Medical University, UP, Lucknow 226003, India.

References

1. World Health Organization. Dengue and severe dengue: Fact sheet, Updated July 2016. http://www.who.int/mediacentre/factsheets/fs117/en/; Assessed 28 Dec 2016.
2. Viswanathan S, Botross N, Rusli BN, Riad A. Acute disseminated encephalomyelitis complicating dengue infection with neuroimaging mimicking multiple sclerosis: a report of two cases. Mult Scler Relat Disord. 2016;10:112–5.
3. Porwal J, Chauhan A. Dengue encephalitis. J Assoc Physicians India. 2016;64: 99–100.
4. Vasanthi N, Vairamon PM, Gowtham T, Das AK. Unusual presentation of dengue fever-cerebral venous thrombosis. J Clin Diagn Res. 2015;9:OD09–10.
5. Sam JE, Gee TS, Nasser AW. Deadly intracranial bleed in patients with dengue fever: a series of nine patients and review of literature. J Neurosci Rural Pract. 2016;7:423–34.
6. Jayasinghe NS, Thalagala E, Wattegama M, Thirumavalavan K. Dengue fever with diffuse cerebral hemorrhages, subdural hematoma and cranial diabetes insipidus. BMC Res Notes. 2016;9:265.
7. Baldaçara L, Ferreira JR, Filho LC, Venturini RR, Coutinho OM, Camarço WC, Fernandes CC, Júnior EV. Behavior disorder after encephalitis caused by dengue. J Neuropsychiatry Clin Neurosci. 2013;25:E44.
8. Niwa T, Aida N, Shishikura A, Fujita K, Inoue T. Susceptibility-weighted imaging findings of cortical laminar necrosis in pediatric patients. AJNR Am J Neuroradiol. 2008;29(9):1795–8.
9. Liu X, Zhao X, Yang J, Han X, Ruan X, Du Y. Cortical laminar necrosis following the rapid correction of drug-induced hyponatremia. Neurol Sci. 2015;36:1725–7.
10. Rajasekharan C, Jithesh B, Renjith SW. Cortical laminar necrosis due to hypoglycaemic encephalopathy:-images in medicine. BMJ Case Rep. 2013.
11. Araújo FM, Araújo MS, Nogueira RM, Brilhante RS, Oliveira DN, Rocha MF, Cordeiro RA, Araújo RM, Sidrim JJ. Central nervous system involvement in dengue: a study in fatal cases from a dengue endemic area. Neurology. 2012;78:736–42.
12. Araújo FM, Brilhante RS, Cavalcanti LP, Rocha MF, Cordeiro RA, Perdigão AC, Miralles IS, Araújo LC, Araújo RM, Lima EG, Sidrim JJ. Detection of the dengue non-structural 1 antigen in cerebral spinal fluid samples using a commercially available enzyme-linked immunosorbent assay. J Virol Methods. 2011;177:128–31.
13. Miagostovich MP, Ramos RG, Nicol AF, Nogueira RM, Cuzzi-Maya T, Oliveira AV, Marchevsky RS, Mesquita RP, Schatzmayr HG. Retrospective study on dengue fatal cases. Clin Neuropathol. 1997;16:204–8.
14. Bordignon J, Strottmann DM, Mosimann AL, Probst CM, Stella V, Noronha L, Zanata SM, Dos Santos CN. Dengue neurovirulence in mice: identification of molecular signatures in the E and NS3 helicase domains. J Med Virol. 2007; 79:1506–17.
15. Puccioni-Sohler M, Soares CN, Papaiz-Alvarenga R, Castro MJ, Faria LC, Peralta JM. Neurologic dengue manifestations associated with intrathecal specific immune response. Neurology. 2009;73:1413–7.
16. Bhoi SK, Naik S, Kumar S, Phadke RV, Kalita J, Misra UK. Cranial imaging findings in dengue virus infection. J Neurol Sci. 2014;342:36–41.
17. Verma R, Bharti K, Mehta M, Bansod A. Rhombencephalitis associated with dengue fever. J Clin Virol. 2016;78:99–101.
18. Nadarajah J, Madhusudhan KS, Yadav AK, Gupta AK, Vikram NK. Acute hemorrhagic encephalitis: an unusual presentation of dengue viral infection. Indian J Radiol Imaging. 2015;25:52–5.
19. Soares CN, Faria LC, Peralta JM, de Freitas MR, Puccioni-Sohler M. Dengue infection: neurological manifestations and cerebrospinal fluid (CSF) analysis. J Neurol Sci. 2006;249:19–24.
20. Garg RK, Malhotra HS, Gupta A, Kumar N, Jain A. Concurrent dengue virus and Japanese encephalitis virus infection of the brain: is it co-infection or co-detection? Infection. 2012;40:589–93.

5

Clinical predictors for the prognosis of myasthenia gravis

Lili Wang*, Yun Zhang and Maolin He

Abstract

Background: Clinical predictors for myasthenia gravis relapse and ocular myasthenia gravis secondary generalization during the first two years after disease onset remain incompletely identified. This study attempts to investigate the clinical predictors for the prognosis of Myasthenia Gravis.

Methods: Eighty three patients with myasthenia gravis were concluded in this study. Baseline characteristics were analyzed as predictors.

Results: Relapse of myasthenia gravis developed in 26 patients (34%). Generalization developed in 34 ocular myasthenia gravis patients (85%). Other autoimmune diseases were observed more commonly in relapsed myasthenia gravis ($P = 0.012$). Second generalization group contained more late onset patients ($P = 0.021$). Ocular myasthenia gravis patients with thymus hyperplasia progressed more rapidly than those with other thymus pathology ($P = 0.027$). Single onset symptom of ocular myasthenia gravis such as ptosis or diplopia predicted early progression than concurrence of ptosis and diplopia ($P = 0.027$). Treatment effect including glucocorticoid, pyridostigmine, thymectomy, IVIG, immunosuppressive drugs did not show significant difference between the relapsed and non-relapsed groups. The treatment outcome also showed no difference between the single OMG and second generalized groups.

Conclusions: Occurrence of associated autoimmune disease can serve as a potential predictor for myasthenia gravis relapse. Either ptosis or diplopia, as well as thymic hyperplasia can predict generalization in the first six months.

Keywords: Myasthenia gravis, Prognosis, Ocular, Relapse

Background

Myasthenia Gravis (MG) is an autoimmune disorder targeting at neuromuscular junction by anti-acetylcholine receptor antibodies (AChR-Ab). Ocular symptoms were present in 40–50% of MG patients and ocular myasthenia gravis (OMG) developed to secondary generalized myasthenia gravis (SGMG) in 50%–80% of cases within the first 1 or 2 years [1, 2]. Studies suggested that late age of onset, high titers of anti-acetylcholine receptor (AChR) antibody and thymoma could increase the risk of secondary generalization. Early treatment with immunosuppressive drug such as corticosteroids and/or azathioprine, was suggested the possibility to reduce the risk of secondary generalization [3–6].

The clinical course of MG included remission, relapse, exacerbation and death. About 38% MG patients experienced remission [7]. One study demonstrated that early thymectomy and administration of prednisolone were more frequently seen in the complete remission cases than in the relapsed OMG patients. [7]. Anti-Kv1.4 antibody is a useful independent factor for predicting MG relapse [8]. Time of diagnosis after onset and age at onset (<40 years) were found to be predictive factors of remission. Gender seems to be an un-relevant factor for predicting MG [9]. Thymus hyperplasia was more common than other thymus pathologies in relapsed MG [9]. However, the prognostic value of thymoma on MG relapse remains inconclusive. In addition, less attention was paid on the effect of other autoimmune diseases and initial OMG symptoms of disease onset such as ptosis on one or both eyes, ptosis and diplopia concurrence or alone on both MG relapse and OMG second generalization. Our study aimed to explore the roles of these baseline clinical characters in the prediction of MG relapse and OMG secondary generalization.

* Correspondence: bitljq2012@163.com
Department of Neurology, Beijing Shijitan Hospital, Capital Medical University, Beijing 100038, People's Republic of China

Methods

Patients

This is a retrospective study. All patients recruited in this study were examined in the Neurology Department of Beijing Shijitan Hospital, Capital Medical University between January 2002 and October 2014. The diagnosis of MG was based on the combination of clinical and laboratory criteria [10]. Inclusion criteria consisted of fluctuating muscle weakness and one or more of the following results: (1) positive response to pyridostigmine; (2) more than 10% decreased amplitude of the compound muscle action potential in the repetitive nerve stimulation; (3) increased jitter on single-fiber electromyography (SFEMG); (4) positive AChR antibody assay. Patients with pregnancy, function failure of heart, lung, liver or kidney were excluded. The study was approved by the ethics committee of Beijing Shijitan Hospital,Capital Medical University and written informed consent was obtained from all of the patients in this study.

There were no unified criteria for the diagnosis of MG relapse [11, 12]. In this study, MG relapse was diagnosed with the reappearance of any symptoms and signs of extra-ocular, pharyngeal, neck, respiratory, axial or limb muscles weakness. The reappeared symptoms and signs should last more than 24 h. And the duration between the MG relapse and last remission should be more than 30 days. Based on these conditions, MG patients were categorized into two groups: relapsed group and non-relapsed group.

The clinical classification criteria of Myasthenia Gravis Foundation of America (MGFA) were used to rank disease severity [13]. Included MG patients were divided into MGFA Class I (OMG) and MGFA Class II-V (GMG) according to the symptoms at disease onset. OMG patients were further divided into two subgroups based on the generalization after two years of disease onset. The first subgroup remained ocular (OMG-R) and the second subgroup developed to secondary generalized MG (SGMG). SGMG patients were also divided into two subgroups based on the disease duration between the time of secondary generalization and the time of first symptom onset of OMG: ≤6 months group and 7–24 months group. Moreover, SGMG patients were also classified into three subgroups including limb group, bulbar group, both limb and bulbar group according to appearance of the first generalized symptoms.

Anti-AChR antibodies were measured by radioimmunoassay in the neuroimmunology laboratory of Peking Union Medical College Hospital. The result with the value greater than 2.966 nmol/L was considered abnormal. The diagnosis of thymic hyperplasia or thymoma was based on CT scan result. 73.5% patients undergoing thymectomy (n = 61) had available thymus histology result. Autoimmune thyroid diseases such as Graves'disease and antibody positive thyroid disease, were diagnosed on the basis of clinical features and laboratory examinations including serum thyroxin, serum thyroid stimulating hormone, thyroid peroxidase antibody, and thyroglobulin antibody levels. The diagnosis of Rheumatoid Arthritis was based on the guideline of The American College of Rheumatology (ACR).

Clinical predictors

Age, gender, thymus abnormality, autoimmune diseases and symptoms of disease onset were chosen as potential clinical predictors for MG prognosis. These potential clinical predictors were compared between relapsed and non-relapsed MG groups. In addition, they were also compared between pure OMG and secondary generalized MG groups. Furthermore, we compared the drug effect including glucocorticoid, pyridostigmine, thymectomy, IVIG, immunosuppressive drugs such as azathioprine, mycophenolate mofetil, cyclosporine A, tacrolimus, methotrexate, cyclophosphamide between the relapsed and non-relapsed MG groups. The treatment effect was also compared between single OMG and secondary generalized MG groups.

Statistical analysis

Statistical analysis was performed with SPSS 22 software (IBM, New York). Categorical variables were analyzed using the chi-square and Fisher exact test. Continuous variables were analyzed with correlation matrix. Multivariable logistic regression analysis was used to perform corrections. $P < 0.05$ was considered statistically significant.

Results

Predictors of MG relapse.

Eighty three patients fulfilled the inclusion criteria. There were 45 female and 38 male patients, with a median age of 39.8 ± 20.3 years old (from4 to 74 years). Fifty nine patients presented with only ocular signs and symptoms (OMG) at disease onset and twenty-four patients presented with generalized symptoms (GMG) at disease onset. These patients were divided into two groups: relapsed MG group (RMG, n = 26) and non-relapsed MG group (NRMG, n = 51) based on the prognosis after two years of disease onset. Unfortunately, information of six patients whether relapse or not was not available. The baseline clinical factors associated with MG relapse were examined by fisher exact test or Chi-square analysis. Results showed that there was no difference in gender, thymus abnormality, age, and first symptoms of disease onset between the two groups, but other autoimmune diseases such as Graves' disease and Rheumatoid Arthritis were observed more frequently in RMG group than in NRMG group (p = 0.012). Treatment outcome including glucocorticoid, pyridostigmine, thymectomy, IVIG, immunosuppressive drugs did not show significant difference between the relapsed and non-relapsed groups. The common clinical features of the RMG and NRMG patients were listed in Table 1.

In addition, 26 relapsed MG patients were further divided into three groups (≤6 months group, 7–12 months group, >12 months group) based on the duration between the time of relapse and the time of first symptom onset of MG. Eleven patients relapsed within the first 6 months after disease onset. Six patients relapsed in 7–12 months after disease onset, and 9 patients were classified into >12 month group. Fisher exact test or Chi-square analysis was used to evaluate associations of baseline characteristics including gender, age of disease onset, first symptom of disease onset, thymus abnormality, and other autoimmune diseases with the relapse time of MG. We found that no

Table 1 Relapse of myasthenia gravis

	RMG	NRMG	NA	*P*-value	Time of recurrence(month)			*P*-value
					≤6	7–12	>12	
Sample size	26	51	6		11	6	9	
Age of onset(year)[b]	26	51		0.176	11	6	9	0.464
Age of onset(year)[c]								
≤ 40	10	25		0.262	4	4	2	0.219
> 40	16	26			7	2	7	
Sex								
Male	11	27		0.261	4	3	4	0.851
Female	15	24			7	3	5	
Thymus								
Normal	2	8		0.739	1	1	0	0.339
Thymic hyperplasia	12	24			6	1	5	
Thymoma	9	15			3	2	4	
NA	3	4			1	2	0	
Other autoimmune disease								
No	15	43			6	4	5	
Yes	11	8		0.012	5	2	4	0.878
Symptom of onset								
OMG	21	34	4	0.152	11	4	6	0.103
GMG	5	17	2		0	2	3	
IIa	2	0		0.307[a]	0	0	0	1.000[a]
IIb	10	2			0	1	1	
III	1	2			0	1	1	
IV	4	1			0	0	1	
Symptom of OMG onset								
Sample size	21	34			11	4	6	
Ptosis	14	21		0.443	7	4	3	0.310
Diplopia	3	3			2	0	1	
Both	4	10			2	0	2	
Ptosis								
Sample size	14	21			7	4	3	
Left	3	2		0.133	2	1	0	0.323
Right	4	14			1	1	2	
Bilateral	7	5			4	2	1	

NA: not available, Both: concurrence of ptosis and diplopia, RMG: relapse of MG, NRMG: no relapse of MG, GMG: patients presenting with generalized symptoms at disease onset, OMG: patients presenting with pure ocular MG at disease onset, Time of recurrence (month): based on the duration between the time of relapse and the time of first symptom onset of MG

[a]Difference of MGFA grades between RMG and NRMG

[b]Age at onset was not divided into two groups (statistical analysis using correlation matrix)

[c]Age at onset was divided into two groups (statistical analysis using chi-square or fisher exact test)

statistically significant differences in above mentioned clinical features were observed among the three groups.

Predictors of OMG generalized to GMG.

Fifty nine OMG patients were included in this study, in which the second generalization information was available in 40 OMG patients. Among the 40 patients with initial pure ocular manifestations at disease onset, 6 (15%) remained pure OMG (OMG-R) during the first two years after disease onset, while 34 (85%) progressed to secondary generalized MG (SGMG). The age of disease onset was significantly older in the SGMG group in comparison to the OMG-R group (p = 0.021). Gender, first symptom of disease onset, thymus abnormality and other autoimmune diseases did not show statistically significant difference between the OMG-R and SGMG groups. The treatment outcome including glucocorticoid, pyridostigmine, thymectomy, IVIG, immunosuppressive drugs also showed no difference between the pure OMG and second generalized groups. The baseline clinical features are listed in Table 2.

Among the 34 patients with SGMG, 21 patients generalized within the first 6 months after symptom onset, 6 generalized within 7–24 months, whereas the generalization information was not available for the remaining 7 patients. Thymic hyperplasia was observed more frequently in the 6 months group than in the 7–24 months group (71.4% vs. 16.7%, p = 0.027, fisher exact test).

As the first onset symptom, either ptosis or diplopia was seen more frequently in 6 months group in comparison to 7–24 months group (71.4% vs. 16.7%), while concurrent ptosis and diplopia occurred more frequently in the 7–24 months group than in 6 months group (83.3% vs. 28.6%). First symptom of disease onset showed statistically significant differences between 6 months group and 7–24 months subgroup (p = 0.027, fisher exact test). Thymic abnormality and first symptom of OMG onset were useful features for predicting the development time of secondary generalization. However, there was no significant difference in gender, age of symptom occurrence and other autoimmune diseases between the two subgroups.

Furthermore, except 7 SGMG patients whose first symptom of generalization information was not available, other 27 SGMG patients were divided into three subgroups according to the appearance of first symptom of generalization. These three groups were limb group, bulbar group and concurrence of bulbar and limb group. The baseline characteristics of the patients in these three subgroups did not show statistical difference.

Discussion

The purpose of this study is to identify risk factors that would be able to predict MG relapse and OMG second generalization. The analysis showed that only 33.8% of MG patients relapsed and 85.0% of patients with OMG onset progressed to SGMG. Concomitant autoimmune disease is observed more commonly in RMG patients (73.3%) than in NRMG patients (18.6%). The presence of concomitant autoimmune disease was identified to be a significant risk factor for MG relapse. Late age of OMG patients (>40 years) at disease onset can predict the development of SGMG. Thymus hyperplasia and initial symptom ptosis or diplopia could serve as indicators for the generalization in the first six months. Concurrence of ptosis and diplopia was a useful predictor for generalization in 7-24 months after OMG onset.

Previously many studies have addressed the predictor of relapse in MG patients. Shigeaki Suzuki et al. reported that MG patients with anti-Kv1.4 antibodies experienced frequent MG relapses in comparison to those without anti-Kv1.4 antibodies [8]. Nobuo Wakata et al. found that thymus hyperplasia occurred more commonly in relapsed cases, and early thymectomy or administration of prednisolone can lead to a reduced relapse rate in MG patients [7]. However, the limitations of these studies were that only GMG patients were included and only reappearance of ocular symptoms was considered as the relapsed symptoms. In addition, these previous studies ignored the role of autoimmune diseases in MG relapse. Our result demonstrated strong evidence that other autoimmune diseases can be used to accurately predict the occurrence of MG relapse.

In the present study, 85% of OMG patients developed second generalization. The generalization rate was higher than that in the cases of other studies reported previously [1], [2], [14]. This discrepancy may be related to the late thymectomy or other immunosuppression treatment in our study. Late age of disease onset was found to be the only factor that can accurately predict OMG second generalization. Several studies reported that immunotherapy reduced the risk of generalization and AChR antibody, thymoma were predictive of the development of secondary generalization [1, 2, 14]. Our study also demonstrated that thymoma and autoimmune diseases occurred more frequently in SGMG patients than in OMG-R patients. However, the difference was not statistically significant. This may be due to the limited number of our MG patients. In addition, our results also showed that different clinical phenotype and thymus hyperplasia predicated the time when OMG developed second generalization. To the best of our knowledge, it is the first time that the relationship of ptosis and diplopia with the time of OMG generalization was investigated.

The mechanism underlying MG relapse and second generalization of OMG remain unclear. It may be related to the modification of immune system by β2 adrenergic receptor (β2-AR) [15, 16]. β2-AR is a G protein coupled

Table 2 Secondary generalization of ocular myasthenia gravis

	OMG-R	SGMG	NA	*P*-value	Time of generalization (month) ≤6	7–24	NA	*P*-value	First symptom of generalization Limb	bulbar	both	NA	*P*-value
Sample size	6	34	19		21	6	7		8	13	6	7	
Age of onset(year)[c]	6	34	19	0.017	21	6	7	0.588	8	13	6	7	0.329
Age of onset(year)[d]													
≤ 40	5	10		0.021	7	1	2	0.406	2	2	3	3	0.277
> 40	1	24			14	5	5		6	11	3	4	
Sex													
Male	2	14		0.544	8	4	2	0.219	4	5	3	2	0.834
Female	4	20			13	2	5		4	8	3	5	
Thymus													
Normal	2	3		0.058	1	1		0.027[a]	2	0	0	1	0.152
Thymic hyperplasia	2	20			15	1			5	9	3	3	
Thymoma	0	10			5	4			1	3	3	3	
NA	2	1			0	0			0	1	0	0	
Other autoimmune disease													
No	6	21		0.077	14	3	4	0.387	6	6	4	5	0.390
Yes	0	13			7	3	3		2	7	2	2	
Symptom of OMG onset													
Sample size	6	34				34				34			
Ptosis	5	20		0.487	12	1	7	0.027[b]	4	8	2	6	0.376
Diplopia	0	3			3	0	0		2	0	1	0	
Both	1	11			6	5	0		2	5	3	1	
Ptosis													
Sample size	5	20				20			20				
Left	1	2		0.404	1	1	0	0.400	0	1	0	1	1.000
Right	1	8			6	0	2		1	4	1	2	
Bilateral	0	5			2	0	3		1	2	0	2	
NA	3	5			5				5				

NA: not available; OMG-R: patients presenting with pure ocular MG and remaining with only ocular manifestations during the first two years after disease onset; SGMG: patients presenting with pure ocular MG at disease onset and developed secondary generalized symptoms and signs during the first two years after onset; Both: concurrence of ptosis and diplopia as the first onset symptom of OMG generalization

[a]: compared between thymic hyperplasia and other thymus histology (including normal thymus and thymoma)

[b]: compared between concurrence and not concurrence of ptosis and diplopia

[c] Age at onset was not divided into two groups (statistical analysis using correlation matrix)

[d] Age at onset was divided into two groups (statistical analysis using chi-square or Fisher exact test)

receptor with seven transmembrane domains. Our previous study implied that homozygosity for Arg16 of β2-AR gene could confer susceptibility to MG [17]. In addition, Arg16Gly was found to be more common in MG patients who also suffered other autoimmune diseases than in those without concomitant of other autoimmune diseases [18]. Results of our current study suggested that concomitant autoimmune disease was a significant risk factor for MG relapse [19]. Therefore, β2-AR gene polymorphism could contribute to MG relapse.

Moreover, β2-AR also plays a role in the prognosis of OMG. Our previous study showed that homozygosity for Arg16 mainly connected with the pathogenesis of late onset MG.[17] We also found that different genotypes at position 27 of β2-AR were related with the different thymus pathology of MG [20]. Our results suggested that late age of disease onset and thymus hyperplasia could predict the secondary generalization and the generalization time of OMG. Therefore, we speculated that β2-AR gene polymorphism might lead to the second generalization of OMG. Further studies should be conducted to address these issues in the future.

It should be pointed out that this study was a retrospective analysis done in one hospital and only examined the clinical factors that could cause MG relapse and OMG second generalization. Although treatment effect such as glucocorticoid, immunosuppressive drugs, pyridostigmine, thymectomy and IVIG between the groups showed no significant difference, future studies need further focus on the treatment including thymectomy as well as immunosuppression therapies and laboratory results such as different serum antibodies on the prognosis of MG for elucidating the pathogenesis of MG prognosis.

Conclusions

In summary, our study demonstrated that other autoimmune diseases were risk factors that could contribute to MG relapse. Age of disease onset is a significant predictor of OMG generalization. Thymus hyperplasia and ptosis or diplopia could predict early generalization of OMG.

Abbreviations

MG: Myasthenia gravis;; AChR-Ab: Anti-acetylcholine receptor antibody;; OMG: ocular myasthenia gravis;; SGMG: secondary generalized myasthenia gravis;; AChR: anti-acetylcholine receptor;; SFEMG: single-fiber electromyography;; MGFA: Myasthenia Gravis Foundation of America;; ACR: American College of Rheumatology

Acknowledgements

Not applicable.

Funding

Not applicable.

Authors' contribution

Study concept and design, drafting of manuscript: LW. Acquisition of data, or analysis of data: LW, YZ. Revision of manuscript for important intellectual content: MLH. All authors have read and approve of the final version of the manuscript.

Competing interests

The authors declare that they have no competing interests.

References

1. Hong YH, Kwon SB, Kim BJ, Kim BJ, Kim SH, Kim JK, et al. Prognosis of ocular myasthenia in Korea: a retrospective multicenter analysis of 202 patients. J Neurol Sci. 2008;273:10–4.
2. Allen JA, Scala S, Jones HR. Ocular myasthenia gravis in senior population: diagnosis, therapy, and prognosis. Muscle Nerve. 2010;41:379–84.
3. Papapetropoulous TH, Ellul J, Tsibri E. Development of generalized myasthenia gravis in patients with ocular myasthenia. Arch Neurol. 2003;60:1491–2.
4. Mee J, Paine M, Byrne E, King J, Reardon K, O'Day J. Immunotherapy of ocular myasthenia gravis reduces conversion to generalized myasthenia gravis. J Neuro opthalmol. 2003;23:251–5.
5. Kupersmith MJ, Latkany R, Homel P. Development of generalized disease at 2 years in patients with ocular myasthenia gravis. Arch Neurol. 2003;60:243–8.
6. Monsul NT, Patwa HS, Knorr AM, Lesser RL, Goldstein JM. The effect of prednisone on the progression from ocular to generalized myasthenia gravis. J Neurol Sci. 2004;217:131–3.
7. Wakata N, Iguchi H, Sugimoto H, Nomoto N, Kurihara T. Relapse of ocular symptoms after remission of myasthenia gravis-a comparison of relapsed and complete remission cases. Clin Neurol Neurosurg. 2003;105:75–7.
8. Suzuki S, Nishimoto T, Kohno M, Utsugisawa K, Nagane Y, Kuwana M, Suzuki N. Clinical and immunological predictors of prognosis for Japanese patients with thymoma-associated myasthenia gravis. J Neuroimmunol. 2013;258:61–6.
9. Mao ZF, Mo XA, Qin C, Lai YR, Olde Hartman TC. Course and prognosis of myasthenia gravis: a systematic review. Eur J Neurol. 2010;17:913–21.
10. Sieb JP. Myasthenia gravis. An update for the clinician. Clin Exp Immunol. 2014;175:408–18.
11. Hsu HS, Huang CS, Huang BS, Lee HC, Kao KP, Hsu WH, et al. Thymoma is associated with relapse of symptoms after transsternal thymectomy for myasthenia gravis. Interact Cardiovasc Thorac Surg. 2006;5:42–6.
12. Men LN, Liu WB, Chen ZG, He XT, Zhang Y, Huang R. Prognostic factors related to recurrence after extended thymectomy in patients with myasthenia gravis. Chin J Neurol. 2008;88:1446–9.
13. Jaretzki 3rd A, Barohn RJ, Ernstoff RM, Kaminski HJ, Keesey JC, Penn AS, et al. Myasthenia gravis: recommendations for clinical research standards. Task force of the Medical scientific advisory Board of the Myasthenia Gravis Foundation of America. Neurology. 2000;55:16–23.
14. Yu HY, Sun ZW, Qin B, Gong T, Zeng XY, Sun YC. Predictors and influencing factors on prognosis of ocular myasthenia gravis. Chin J Neuroimmunol& Neuro. 2010;17:107–9.
15. Nakai A, Hayano Y, Furuta F, Noda M, Suzuki K. Control of lymphocyte egress from lymph nodes through β2-adrenergic receptors. J Exp Med. 2014; 211:2583–98.
16. Guereschi MG, Araujo LP, Maricato JT, Takenaka MC, Nascimento VM, Vivanco BC, et al. Beta2-adrenergic receptor signaling in CD4+ Foxp3+ regulatory T cells enhances their suppressive function in a PKA-dependent manner. Eur J Immunol. 2013;43:1001–12.
17. Wang LL, Xie YC, Hou SF, Feng K, Yin J, Xu XH. Role of β2-adrenergic receptor polymorphisms in pathogenesis of myasthenia gravis. Chin J Neurol. 2009;42: 828–32.
18. Wang LL, Zhang Y, He ML. Role of β2-adrenergic receptor polymorphisms in prognosis of myasthenia gravis with other autoimmune diseases. Chin J Neurol. 2015; 48:390–4.
19. Wang LL, Zhang Y, He ML. Clinical characteristics of patients with myasthenia gravis associated with other autoimmune diseases. Chin J Contemp Neurol Neurosurg. 2014;14:873–7.
20. Wang LL, Zhang Y, He ML. Study of the association of β2-adrenergic receptor gene polymorphism with myasthenia gravis associated with thymus abnormality. Natl Med J China 2015; 95:1518–21.

6

Effect of tendon vibration during wide-pulse neuromuscular electrical stimulation (NMES) on the decline and recovery of muscle force

Vanesa Bochkezanian[1,2*], Robert U. Newton[1,2,3], Gabriel S. Trajano[4], Amilton Vieira[5], Timothy S. Pulverenti[2] and Anthony J. Blazevich[2]

Abstract

Background: Neuromuscular electrical stimulation (NMES) is commonly used to activate skeletal muscles and reverse muscle atrophy in clinical populations. Clinical recommendations for NMES suggest the use of short pulse widths (100–200 μs) and low-to-moderate pulse frequencies (30–50 Hz). However, this type of NMES causes rapid muscle fatigue due to the (non-physiological) high stimulation intensities and non-orderly recruitment of motor units. The use of both wide pulse widths (1000 μs) and tendon vibration might optimize motor unit activation through spinal reflex pathways and thus delay the onset of muscle fatigue, increasing muscle force and mass. Thus, the objective of this study was to examine the acute effects of patellar tendon vibration superimposed onto wide-pulse width (1000 μs) knee extensor electrical stimulation (NMES, 30 Hz) on peak muscle force, total impulse before "muscle fatigue", and the post-exercise recovery of muscle function.

Methods: Tendon vibration (Vib), NMES (STIM) or NMES superimposed onto vibration (STIM + Vib) were applied in separate sessions to 16 healthy adults. Total torque-time integral (TTI), maximal voluntary contraction torque (MVIC) and indirect measures of muscle damage were tested before, immediately after, 1 h and 48 h after each stimulus.

Results: TTI increased (145.0 ± 127.7%) in STIM only for "positive responders" to the tendon vibration (8/16 subjects), but decreased in "negative responders" (−43.5 ± 25.7%). MVIC (−8.7%) and rectus femoris electromyography (RF EMG) (−16.7%) decreased after STIM (group effect) for at least 1 h, but not after STIM + Vib. No changes were detected in indirect markers of muscle damage in any condition.

Conclusions: Tendon vibration superimposed onto wide-pulse width NMES increased TTI only in 8 of 16 subjects, but reduced voluntary force loss (fatigue) ubiquitously. Negative responders to tendon vibration may derive greater benefit from wide-pulse width NMES alone.

Keywords: Muscle stimulation, Muscle strength, Muscle function, Muscle fatigue, Muscle damage, Meuro-rehabilitation

* Correspondence: v.bochkezanian@ecu.edu.au; vanesaboch@gmail.com
[1]Exercise Medicine Research Institute, Edith Cowan University, Perth, Australia
[2]Centre for Sports and Exercise Science, School of Medical and Health Sciences, Edith Cowan University, Joondalup 270 Joondalup Drive, Joondalup, WA 6027, Australia
Full list of author information is available at the end of the article

Background

Muscular strength is a major predictor of mortality in clinical populations, and this appears to be partly explicable by the quantity (i.e. absolute muscle volume) and quality (i.e. muscle/intra-muscular adipose content) of limb muscle mass [1, 2]. Improvements in muscle mass are also observed to be beneficial for functional mobility and quality of life as well as preventing functional decline, cardiovascular disease and hospitalization [3]. Strength training is commonly used to stimulate gains in muscle strength and has been proven to enhance longevity and quality of life in a variety of clinical populations [4–7]. However, strength training poses an increasing challenge for people with a neurological condition, such as people with spinal cord injury (SCI) who have limited ability, or are unable, to voluntarily activate their muscles.

Due to this limitation, neuromuscular electrical stimulation (NMES) has been conventionally used in clinical practice, particularly in the form of functional electrical stimulation (FES), i.e. a continuous, prolonged stimulation at low-to-moderate frequencies (30–50 Hz) paired simultaneously or intermittently with a functional task (e.g. cycling) [8]. FES exercise has been shown to slow muscle weakening or even increase muscle strength as well as reduce the rate of skeletal muscle atrophy and weakness and improve physical health in people with a SCI [9–12]. However, such interventions evoke only low relative muscle forces [9, 13] and therefore may not optimally stimulate neuromuscular strength and mass increases [14]. Instead the imposition of a higher load on the muscle with intermittent rest periods to allow continuous higher force output would be preferable [15].

Possible reasons for the lack of clinical use of high-intensity, intermittent NMES protocols include a lack of scientific exploration of its efficacy and long term functional effect [16], and their propensity to elicit rapid muscle fatigue and (possibly) muscle damage [11, 12, 17, 18]. Whilst, muscle damaging effects can be reduced with repeated exposures (i.e. repeated bout effect), the rapid muscle fatigue induced by NMES is an ongoing issue [18–21]. This rapid fatigue partly results from the use of short-pulse widths (< 300 μs), which activate muscle fibres largely through depolarization of motor axons, and which typically leads to a random motor unit recruitment pattern and therefore a substantial recruitment of fast-fatiguing type II motor units. Fatigue may also result the use of non-physiologically high stimulation frequencies (e.g. ≥ 80 Hz) [19, 22–25] and the simultaneous activation of the same motor units in repeated contractions [24, 26–28]. Therefore, the intensity and duration of stimulation that can be applied to muscles in an exercise session are reduced, thus limiting the potential for muscle force capacity, muscle mass and musculoskeletal function adaptations [29–32].

To overcome some of these problems, wide-pulse width NMES (i.e. ≥ 1000 μs) appears to be a promising tool for use in clinical populations as it appears to recruit motor units through central (i.e. indirect) pathways [33–38]. Wide-pulse width NMES can elicit asynchronous motor unit activation through the reflexive recruitment of motor neurones [39], identified by the presence of spinal H-reflexes, or asynchronous motor unit activation through the triggering of persistent inward currents (PIC) via repetitive activation of Ia afferents or post-activation potentiation of neurotransmitter release [39–41]. However, the contribution of wide-pulse width NMES to asynchronous motor unit activation through central recruitment is shown mostly during higher frequencies of stimulation (>80 Hz) and appears to have minimal effect at lower frequencies (i.e. ≤ 20 Hz), which may preclude its use in a clinical context [42]. Also, when used at higher stimulation intensities the contribution of H-reflexes to muscle activation may be minimized by orthodromic-antidromic collision, and indeed recent evidence has indicated that wide-pulse width NMES may exacerbate muscle fatigue at the higher frequencies of stimulation that may be required to elicit higher levels of muscle force [43, 44]. Thus, there is a need to consider different strategies of activating motor units in a more physiological manner for future clinical applications.

One promising method is the application of tendon vibration during muscle stimulation. Tendon vibration evokes a tonic vibration reflex through both spinal and supraspinal pathways via repetitive activation of Ia afferent fibres and possibly triggers the development of persistent inward currents at the motor neuron level [45–47]. Tendon vibration could amplify and prolong synaptic input and create a sustained depolarization leading to an increased physiological recruitment of motor units, and thus increasing muscle force output [48]. Since tendon vibration can excite only low-threshold motor units (fatigue-resistant) [49], an additional excitation of the fatigue-resistant motor units may be elicited if it is coupled with wide-pulse width NMES, and thus may result in an additional increase in muscle force output [47, 50–52]. Moreover, in some functionally important muscles, such as the quadriceps femoris, the use of wide-pulse width NMES alone may not be effective in recruiting motor units through "central pathways" [39], so the addition of tendon vibration might help to recruit Ia afferent fibres and thus increase muscle force production. Such a phenomenon has already been demonstrated in healthy people in the plantar flexors [53].

Importantly, antidromic activation of motor neurons does not occur during tendon vibration [54] as it might during electrical stimulation. Therefore, superimposing tendon vibration onto wide-pulse width NMES at low-to-moderate frequencies (e.g. 30 Hz) may induce motor neuron discharge in synchrony with the stimulus. However, it is still uncertain whether the imposition of tendon vibration onto wide-pulse width NMES could increase the peak force production and reduce the rate of muscle fatigue for a given intensity of NMES. It is also not known whether tendon vibration might increase potential muscle damaging effects due to the higher evoked forces, or instead reduce the risk by eliciting a more normal physiological excitation of the motor neuron pool.

In the present study, therefore, the hypothesis was tested that the use of tendon vibration imposed during wide- pulse width NMES (1000 μs) at a low-to-moderate frequency (30 Hz) would enhance peak muscle force, impulse performed before "fatigue", and the post-exercise recovery of muscle function when compared to wide-pulse width NMES applied without tendon vibration in healthy individuals. These individuals also provided feedback about pain and comfort levels during the NMES protocols, so that these types of interventions might be better understood before their use in clinical populations in future research studies.

Methods

Participants

Sixteen healthy participants (6 women, 10 men) with no neurological or musculoskeletal disorders volunteered for the study (mean ± SD, age: 28.6 ± 7.5 y; height: 165.1 ± 27.8 cm; body mass: 77.4 ± 24.5 kg; BMI: 24.1 ± 2.2 kg/m^2). The subjects were physically active individuals who typically performed structured physical activity 2 to 4 times a week (i.e. recreationally trained). We chose to study the effects of our interventions in healthy individuals who can provide feedback regarding the pain and discomfort experienced, because such stimuli may trigger spasticity in clinical populations such as people with spinal cord injury, stroke, brain damage or other neurological disorders [55]. Prior to the study, the participants were given detailed information about the procedures and risks of participation and they all signed an informed consent document. The participants completed the Physical Activity Readiness Questionnaire (PAR-Q) to ensure safe exercise participation and refrained from vigorous exercise (48 h) and alcohol (24 h) and stimulant consumption (e.g. caffeine, energy drinks, 6 h) prior to testing. Twelve of the 16 participants were also measured at 1 h and 48 h after the intervention to assess muscle force recovery and markers of muscle damage (details on section Muscle fatigue and muscle damage). This study was approved by the University's Human Ethics Committee.

Study design: quasi-randomised cross-over design.

Setting of the study: Edith Cowan University. Joondalup campus. Perth. Western Australia.

Procedures

All participants attended the laboratory on four occasions at the same time of day with a minimum of 7 days between sessions. One week prior to the first experimental session, participants attended a full familiarization session where each participant received patellar tendon vibration as well as NMES with and without patellar tendon vibration, and performed maximal voluntary isometric contractions (MVIC) of the knee extensors to ensure they could tolerate the protocols. All participants tolerated the NMES and tendon vibration protocols well. The subsequent three sessions were used to complete the following three experimental protocols in a random order without replication: 1) NMES only (STIM); 2) NMES superimposed onto tendon vibration (STIM + Vib); and 3) Vibration only (Vib). All participants (n = 16) were tested immediately before (PRE), immediately after (POST) and a subset of participants (n = 12; four participants were unable to attend all follow-up testing) were also tested one hour (1H) and 48 h (48H) after each experimental session. A standardized warm-up protocol was performed at the beginning of every session, which consisted of six consecutive concentric knee extension contractions with resistance provided by the inertia of an isokinetic dynamometer (Biodex System 3 Pro Ronkonkoma, NY) and then one repetition of isometric knee extensions at 30%, 50%, 70% and 90% of perceived maximal effort before performing a series of knee extension MVICs.

In experimental sessions, three MVICs were performed at each time point (PRE, POST, 1H and 24H) separated by 1 min of rest, with a fourth completed if a difference in peak torque of ≥3% was observed between the best two attempts. The participants were seated with hip and knee joint angles of 85° and 90°, respectively (0° = full knee extension), with the thigh and trunk secured to the dynamometer chair and the knee joint was aligned with the centre of rotation of the dynamometer. Peak isometric knee extension torque was quantified during MVIC. Participants were instructed to produce a force against the dynamometer arm by extending the knee as fast and hard as possible for 3 s. Verbal encouragement and visual feedback was provided during all MVICs.

Neuromuscular electrical stimulation (NMES) and tendon vibration protocols

Following the MVICs, and to habituate participants to the electrical stimulations, two electrical square-wave stimuli (two 1000 μs square-wave pulses separated by 5 ms) were delivered to the dominant (stronger leg) every 20 s while the stimulation current was increased from 30 to 99 mA in 10-mA increments until a plateau in the maximum peak twitch torque was observed. Subsequently, trains of NMES were delivered by a high-voltage constant-current electrical stimulator (400 V, DS7A, Digitimer Ltd., Welwyn Garden City, UK) through four self-adhesive stimulation electrodes (Axelgaard, PALS, USA) placed over the rectus femoris (RF), vastus lateralis (VL), and vastus medialis (VM). Two 5 × 10 cm electrodes were placed over RF and one 5 × 5 electrode was placed on each of the VM and VL approximately at their motor points. The electrodes were placed to elicit the greatest twitch response with a low stimulation intensity, as determined in the familiarization session, and were marked with indelible ink on the skin to ensure identical electrode placement at subsequent sessions. The NMES protocol consisted of repeated 30-Hz trains of 58 wide-pulse width (1000 μs) symmetric biphasic pulses (0.033-s inter-pulse interval). A single train duration was 2-s and the inter-train interval was 2-s (i.e. 2-s on and 2-s off). 2-s contractions were used because extensive pilot testing revealed that shorter-duration contractions (i.e. 1 s) failed to evoke a torque plateau (i.e. maximal activation) during each train of stimulation, and that longer-duration contractions (i.e. ≥3 s) tended to elicit a rapid muscular fatigue. Symmetric biphasic NMES, which employed currents with balanced positive and negative phases (polarity), was used due to its superior efficacy (in contrast to monophasic) to produce tetanic contractions and its demonstrated therapeutic benefits in clinical practice [56, 57]. The intensity of NMES was chosen to elicit 20% of the best MVIC recorded during PRE measurements for each experimental session (henceforth referred to as the 'target torque') by delivering three single trains of the NMES protocol with increasing stimulation intensity separated by one minute. Whilst the contribution of afferent pathways to motor unit activation occurs mainly at a high frequency (i.e. >80 Hz) and at low stimulation force levels (i.e. 10% MVC) [40–42, 53], a higher force level (i.e. ≥ 20% MVIC) and low-to-moderate frequencies (20–30 Hz) (i.e. standard clinical conditions) were chosen to elicit higher forces that should stimulate significant changes in muscle force and mass in training interventions in clinical populations. Moreover, the use of 20% MVC has been previously investigated in the plantarflexors with a clear recruitment of motor units through the reflex arc during bouts of tendon vibration [47].

Patellar tendon vibration was applied with a vibration device (Deep Muscle Stimulator, Las Vegas, NV, USA) to mechanically vibrate the tendon at 55 Hz and amplitude of 7 mm (determined by direct measurement using high-speed video capture). The tip of the vibration device was maintained at a steady pressure in a fixed position on the tendon immediately distal to the inferior border of the patella. This position was marked on the skin, and covered by a thin (1 mm thickness) soft pad to minimize pain or abrasion (refer to Fig. 1).

The three experimental interventions were:

STIM: electrically-evoked muscle contractions were elicited by delivering the NMES protocol until the torque was reduced to ≤60% of the target torque (i.e. 20% MVIC) in one electrically-evoked contraction, which was defined as 'target fatigue'.

STIM ±Vib: electrically-evoked contractions delivered as in STIM, but were superimposed with patellar tendon vibration which was applied for at least 5 s before NMES and after target fatigue was reached.

Vib: continuous patellar tendon vibration for one minute.

Data collection and analysis

Peak torque, impulse, fatigue index and number of contractions

The peak voluntary isometric knee extensor torque assessed during the MVIC was used to normalize the torque elicited by NMES during the sessions. Peak voluntary isometric knee extensor torque was defined as the maximum torque produced over a 500-ms window and included the plateau phase after at least a 250 ms rise time above baseline. The torque-time integral (TTI) was used to provide a measure of the total exercise stimulus received by the muscle in each condition (Fig. 2). TTI was calculated as the product of torque and time calculated from the onset of the first stimulation train (STIM) or vibration onset (STIM + Vib) to the end of the final evoked contraction at the point of target fatigue (defined on section Neuromuscular electrical stimulation (NMES) and tendon vibration protocols). Peak evoked torque was defined as the highest torque value obtained after the onset of the first stimulation train for both STIM and STIM + Vib. TTI and peak evoked torque were compared between STIM and STIM + Vib. However, some participants responded with a greater TTI after STIM + Vib (positive responders to tendon vibration) whilst others showed a lower TTI after STIM + Vib (negative responders to tendon vibration), thus a second analysis was performed after separating participants into positive and negative responder to tendon vibration groups (described on section Results). Total number of contractions was measured as the number of contractions performed from the beginning of the first evoked contraction (i.e. not including up to 3 contractions used to establish the current that elicited the target torque) reaching the target torque until the last contraction before reaching the target fatigue (defined on section Neuromuscular electrical stimulation (NMES) and tendon vibration protocols).

Muscle activity (EMG)

Vastus lateralis (VL), vastus medialis (VM) and rectus femoris (RF) electromyograms (EMG) were recorded using bipolar electrode configurations sampled at analogue-to-digital conversion rate of 2000-Hz (bandwidth 25–450 Hz)

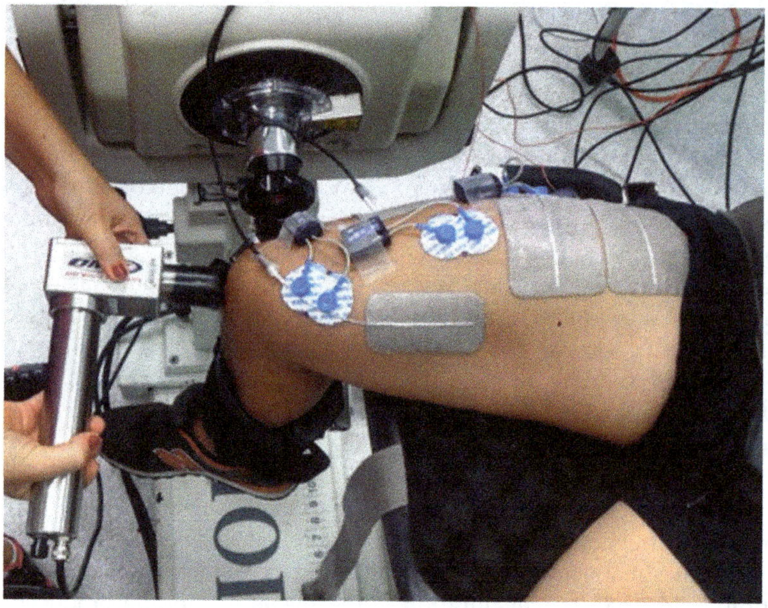

Fig. 1 Picture showing the electrodes position on the thigh muscles and the placement of tendon vibration during one of the sessions. Patellar tendon vibration was applied with a vibration device (Deep Muscle Stimulator, Las Vegas, NV, USA) to mechanically vibrate the tendon. The tip of the vibration device was maintained at a steady pressure in a fixed position on the tendon immediately distal to the inferior border of the patella. This position was marked on the skin, and covered by a thin (1 mm thickness) soft pad to minimize pain or abrasion

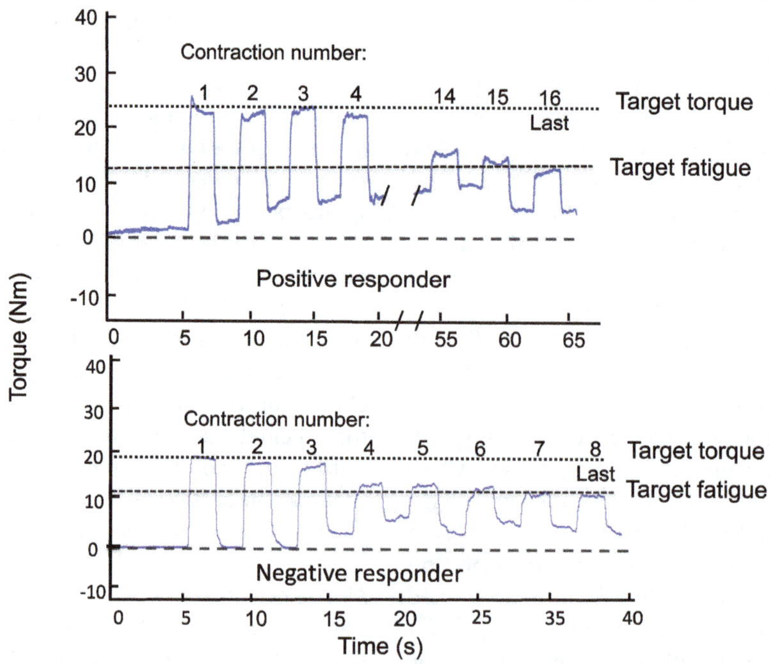

Fig. 2 Torque production (Nm) for a positive and a negative responder during STIM + Vib. Last: last contraction before target fatigue. Target torque = 20% MVIC. Target Fatigue = 60% of target torque

using a Wave wireless EMG system (Cometa Systems, Bareggio, Italy). The skin was carefully prepared by shaving, gently abrading and cleaning with alcohol prior to electrode placement. A bipolar electrode set (DE-2.1 single differential surface EMG sensor) with a 1-cm inter-electrode distance was attached to the skin over the belly of each muscle parallel to the predicted direction of muscle fibres, following the SENIAM recommendations [58]. Muscle activity was expressed as the root mean square of the EMG amplitude (applying a symmetric moving average with filter window = 500 ms) over the same time as the torque measurements, and the peak EMG was retained for analysis. Torque and EMG data were simultaneously recorded using LabChart version 8.0.2 Software (PowerLab System, ADInstruments Pty. Ltd., NSW, Australia) at the same analog-digital conversion rate.

Muscle fatigue and muscle damage

Muscle fatigue was determined immediately post-intervention (POST) in all participants and at 1 (1H) and 48 h (48H) in a subset of 12 participants. Muscle fatigue was calculated as the percent decrement in MVIC torque. To determine whether muscle damage may have been elicited and thus contributed to the fatigue, indirect muscle damage markers were assessed POST, 1H and 48H after the intervention. Ultrasound imaging of RF and VI muscle thickness, defined as the distance between the subcutaneous fat layer and deep muscle border were measured using B-mode axial-plane imaging (Aloka SSD-α10, Aloka Co., Ltd., Tokyo, Japan) [59]. Muscle thickness changes are considered to be an indicator of the osmotic fluid shift that results in muscle swelling subsequent to muscle damage [59]. The participants were seated on a plinth with hip and knees at 90°. The same examiner obtained images at the 50% distance between the anterior superior iliac spine and superior border of the patella. The probe was placed in a marked area in a perpendicular position using a spirit level attached to the probe. The mean of three images of the RF and VI muscle thickness measurements at the same level was obtained for each condition and time. Perception of muscle soreness was assessed using the visual analogue scale and palpation. Participants were asked to rate on a line from 0 to 100 mm (with "no pain" at 0 mm and "unbearable pain" at 100 mm) the soreness of the muscle after performing three bodyweight squats to approximately a 90° knee angle. The palpation assessment of muscle soreness consisted of the application of digital pressure using three fingers for approximately 3 s against the middle part of RF [60]. These tests have been extensively used in previous research studies evaluating indirect markers of muscle damage [60, 61].

Pain and comfort levels were also measured immediately after the completion of each NMES protocol (STIM and STIM + Vib). Subjects indicated the rate of perceived pain and comfort on a 1–10 scale based on how comfortable and painful the different protocols were perceived to be, with 1 being "comfortable and pain free" and 10 being "unbearable and extremely painful".

Statistical analysis

Two-way repeated measures analysis of variance (ANOVA) was used to compare changes in all variables between conditions (STIM, STIM + Vib and Vib) over time (PRE, POST, 1H and 48H) in the subset of 12 participants. A second two-way repeated measures ANOVA was used to compare STIM, STIM + Vib and Vib between PRE and POST in the full participant sample (N = 16). Repeated measures ANOVAs were used to compare EMG amplitude (RMS) in all individual muscles (RF, VM and VL) for STIM and STIM + Vib for PRE, POST, 1H and 48H. Pairwise t-tests were performed when significant interaction effects were found. Pearson's product moment coefficients were computed to quantify the linear association between torque-time integral (TTI), peak torque and total number of contractions during STIM condition, and a binomial logistic regression analysis was performed to ascertain the ability of the torque-time integral (TTI) and total number of contractions in STIM to predict positive and negative responders to tendon vibration (i.e. TTI difference between STIM and STIM + Vib). Statistical significance was set at an alpha level of 0.05 and values were reported as mean ± SD.

We certify that all applicable institutional and governmental regulations concerning the ethical use of human volunteers were followed during the course of this research.

Results

No significant changes were observed in any measure after Vib, thus the subsequent analysis focused on the changes in response to STIM and STIM + Vib conditions. Mean values for MVIC peak torque and surface EMG amplitudes for the Vib condition are presented in Table 1.

Torque-time integral (TTI), peak evoked torque and total number of contractions

No statistical differences in peak evoked torque (p = 0.94), TTI (p = 0.56) or total number of contractions (p = 0.49) were observed between STIM and STIM + Vib. Nonetheless (as described in Section 2 and shown in Fig. 2) the response to STIM + Vib was clearly greater in eight participants (50% of sample) but lesser (i.e. negative) in the other eight. Thus, a positive versus negative responder to tendon vibration analysis was undertaken where positive responders to tendon vibration were defined as participants who responded with a greater TTI after STIM + Vib and negative responders to tendon vibration as participants who showed

Table 1 MVIC peak torque and surface EMG amplitudes. (Mean (± SD, 95% CI)) at PRE, POST (n: 16), 1H and 48H (n: 12) for STIM, STIM + Vib and Vib conditions

Measure	PRE		POST		1H		48H	
	Mean ± SD	95% CI	Mean ± SD	95% CI	Mean ± SD	95% CI	Mean ± SD	95% CI
MVIC PT (N)								
STIM	237.8 ± 90.2	189.7–285.8	219.1 ± 90.0*	171.1–267.0	216 ± 72.0*	170.1–261.4	228.7 ± 72.2	182.8–274.6
STIM + Vib	229.3 ± 82.0	185.6–273.0	222.9 ± 84.8	177.7–268.0	222.1 ± 77.3	173.0–271.3	233.4 ± 67.2	190.6–276.0
Vib	214.2 ± 63.4	174.0–254.5	212 .8 ± 59.0	175.4–250.5	224.6 ± 73.8	177.7–271.5	230.5 ± 68.1	187.2–273.8
QUAD EMG (mV)								
STIM	1.27 ± 0.60	0.94–1.61	1.14 ± 0.48	0.88–1.40	1.20 ± 0.53	0.90–1.51	1.19 ± 0.48	0.85–1.52
STIM + Vib	1.32 ± 0.51	1.05–1.60	1.29 ± 0.52	1.01–1.56	1.38 ± 0.54	1.03–1.72	1.4 ± 0.49	1.09–1.71
Vib	1.14 ± 0.62	0.75–1.54	1.16 ± 0.60	0.78–1.54	1.16 ± 0.52	0.83–1.50	1.23 ± 0.64	0.82–1.63
RF EMG (mV)								
STIM	0.39 ± 0.16	0.30–0.48	0.32 ± 0.14 *	0.25–0.40	0.35 ± 0.19	0.23–0.47	0.33 ± 0.17	0.22–0.44
STIM + Vib	0.38 ± 0.17	0.29–0.47	0.38 ± 0.19	0.28–0.49	0.39 ± 0.23	0.25–0.53	0.39 ± 0.15	0.29–0.48
Vib	0.32 ± 0.2	0.20–0.45	0.33 ± 0.19	0.21–0.45	0.33 ± 0.17	0.22–0.44	0.37 ± 0.22	0.23–0.51
VM EMG (mV)								
STIM	0.50 ± 0.44	0.27–0.74	0.48 ± 0.38	0.28–0.68	0.51 ± 0.39	0.26–0.76	0.52 ± 0.37	0.28–0.75
STIM + Vib	0.47 ± 0.33	0.29–0.64	0.46 ± 0.34	0.28–0.64	0.51 ± 0.38	0.27–0.75	0.61 ± 0.43	0.34–0.88
Vib	0.35 ± 0.34	0.14–0.57	0.35 ± 0.33	0.14–0.56	0.34 ± 0.30	0.15–0.53	0.34 ± 0.33	0.13–0.56
VL EMG (mV)								
STIM	0.38 ± 0.22	0.26–0.50	0.33 ± 0.19	0.23–0.43	0.34 ± 0.24	0.19–0.50	0.35 ± 0.30	0.16–0.54
STIM + Vib	0.48 ± 0.30	0.32–0.64	0.45 ± 0.28	0.30–0.60	0.47 ± 0.36	0.24–0.70	0.40 ± 0.27	0.23–0.57
Vib	0.46 ± 0.37	0.23–0.69	0.48 ± 0.38	0.24–0.72	0.49 ± 0.36	0.26–0.72	0.51 ± 0.42	0.25–0.78
% from PRE (baseline MVIC PT)								
STIM	–	–	-8.72 ± 5.79 *	−11.80 - ¯5.64	−6.79 ± 7.26	−11.40 - ¯2.17	−0.67 ± 11.39	−7.91 - 6.57
STIM + Vib	–	–	−3.28 ± 6.44	−6.71 - 0.15	−1.61 ± 6.61	−5.80 - 2.59	4.52 ± 4.86	1.43–7.60
Vib	–	–	0.05 ± 5.76	−3.61- 3.71	4.42 ± 11.61	−2.95 - 11.80	7.93 ± 12.56	−0.06 -15.91

MVI maximal voluntary isometric contraction, *PT* peak torque, *VM* vastus medialis muscle, *VL* vastus lateralis muscle, *RF* rectus femoris muscle, EMG_{RMS} root mean square EMG amplitude, *SD* standard deviation, *95% CI* 95% Confidence Interval
*Significant difference from PRE ($P < 0.05$)

lower TTI after STIM + Vib compared to STIM (TTI: positive responders: STIM: 1201.1 ± 321.0 Nm·s; STIM + Vib: 2757.2 ± 1329.7 Nm·s; negative responders: STIM: 2402.6 ± 497.7 Nm·s; STIM + Vib: 1344.0 ± 674.6 Nm·s). This analysis revealed a group × condition interaction effect ($p = 0.00$) indicating a significant 145.0 ± 127.7% increase in TTI in STIM + Vib compared to STIM for positive responders to tendon vibration ($p = 0.014$) (see Fig. 3a), indicating an increase in the total cumulative force produced by the muscle in STIM + Vib. A significant decrease in TTI (−43.5 ± 25.7%) was observed in STIM + Vib ($p = 0.002$) in the negative responders to tendon vibration (see Fig. 3b). The mean peak evoked torques for the positive responders to tendon vibration for STIM and STIM + Vib were 49.3 ± 16.8 Nm and 52.1 ± 15.0 Nm for STIM + Vib, whilst for negative responders they were 51.7 ± 20.5 Nm and 48.1 ± 21.9 Nm. The mean total number of contractions for positive responders to tendon vibration for STIM was 16.2 ± 5.1 and for STIM + Vib was 29.1 ± 19.0, whilst the means for negative responders were 39.8 ± 25.0 for STIM and 17.1 ± 7.3 for STIM + Vib.

Subsequent analyses of participants' responses in STIM were undertaken to determine if the likelihood of having a positive or a negative response in STIM + Vib could be predicted. This involved examination of TTI, peak torque and total number of contractions evoked by STIM, as well as the difference in TTI between STIM and STIM + Vib. A strong and statistically significant negative correlation was observed between TTI measured in STIM ($r = -0.72$, CI 90%: -0.44 to −0.88) and the difference between the TTI measured in STIM versus STIM + Vib. Also, a correlation of −0.45 (CI 90%: -0.03 to −0.74) between TTI in STIM and the difference between STIM and STIM + Vib for the total number of contractions was observed, whilst for peak torque a correlation of −0.27 was found (CI 90%: 0.18

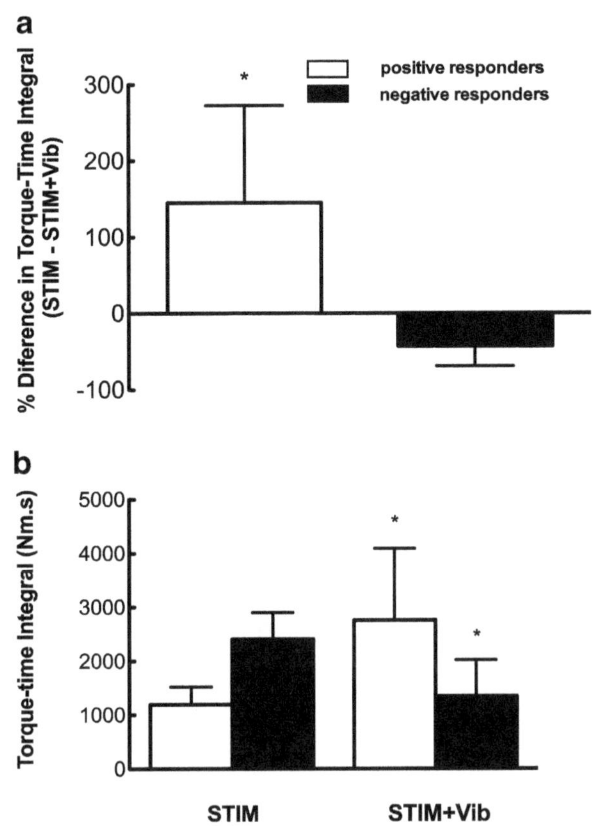

Fig. 3 a Percentage difference between STIM and STIM + Vib in torque-time integral (Nm·s) for positive and negative responders (145.0 ± 127.7% and −43.5 ± 25.7%). **b** Mean torque-time integral (TTI; Nm·s) for positive responders and negative responders for STIM (1201.2 ± 321.9 Nm·s and 2402.6 ± 497.7 Nm·s) and STIM + Vib (2757.2 ± 1329.8 Nm·s and 1344.0 ± 674.6 Nm·s). *Significant difference from STIM ($P < 0.05$)

to −0.62). Given the strong negative relationships observed between the difference in TTI in STIM + Vib and both TTI and total number of contractions in STIM, a binomial logistic regression analysis was performed to predict the likelihood of having a positive or a negative response to STIM + Vib. The logistic regression model was statistically significant for torque-time integral ($\chi^2 = 17.845$, $p < 0.0005$), explaining 89% (Nagelkerke R^2) and predicting 87.5%. For the total number of contractions ($\chi^2 = 10.515$, $p < 0.0005$) the model explained 64% (Nagelkerke R^2) and predicted 81.3% of positive and negative responders to tendon vibration. Based on these results, torque-time integral and total number of contractions in STIM can be used to determine whether an individual will be a positive or negative responder to STIM + Vib in 87.5% and 81.3% of cases. Under the conditions of the present study a positive responder to tendon vibration would perform ≤16 contractions whilst a negative responder to tendon vibration would perform >16 contractions until target fatigue. An example of the response of a positive responder to tendon vibration to STIM and STIM + Vib is shown in Fig. 4.

Peak voluntary isometric contraction (MVIC) torque

As shown in Fig. 5, a time × condition interaction effect ($p = 0.016$) was observed for MVIC with a significant decrease in STIM observed from PRE (237.8 ± 90.1 Nm) to POST (219.1 ± 90.0 Nm; $p = 0.001$) and from PRE to 1H (215.8 ± 7.0 Nm; $p = 0.007$), but no change in STIM + Vib at any point. MVIC peak torques for STIM, STIM + Vib are shown in Fig. 5. The percentage change in MVIC from PRE to POST was −8.7% for STIM and −3.3% for STIM + Vib, as shown inset of Fig. 5. However, a subgroup analysis for peak voluntary isometric contraction between positive and negative responders to tendon vibration did not reveal any statistically significant difference ($p = 0.30$ for condition × time × group interaction).

Muscle activity (EMG) during MVIC

An interaction effect ($p = 0.006$) was observed for RF EMG amplitude during MVIC, with a significant decrease (−16.7%) in the RF EMG amplitude after STIM from PRE (0.39 ± 0.16 mV) to POST (0.32 ± 0.14 mV; $p < 0.01$), but no differences for VM and VL EMG in STIM or any muscle in STIM + Vib. MVIC peak isometric torque and surface EMG amplitudes data during peak voluntary isometric torque at PRE, POST, 1H and 48H for STIM, STIM + Vib and Vib are presented in Table 1.

Indirect markers of muscle damage: muscle thickness and muscle soreness scales; pain and comfort scale

No changes were detected in combined RF and VI muscle thickness ($p = 0.66$) or muscle soreness scales either upon palpation ($p = 0.33$) or when performing bodyweight squats ($p = 0.37$). Thus, no indications of muscle damage or soreness were observed in any condition. No statistically significant differences were found in the pain and comfort scales between STIM and STIM +Vib conditions (STIM: 4.1 ± 2.1 STIM + Vib: 5.0 ± 2.3; $p = 0.21$). Thus, both protocols elicited only "light-to-moderate" levels of pain and discomfort.

Discussion

The main finding of the present study was that the torque-time integral (TTI) measured at the point of fatigue (i.e. 60% of initial evoked torque) was not statistically different between STIM and STIM + Vib. Based on these results, the tendon vibration superimposed onto the wide-pulse width NMES did not appear to provide any additional benefit that might not have been derived from stimulations alone under the

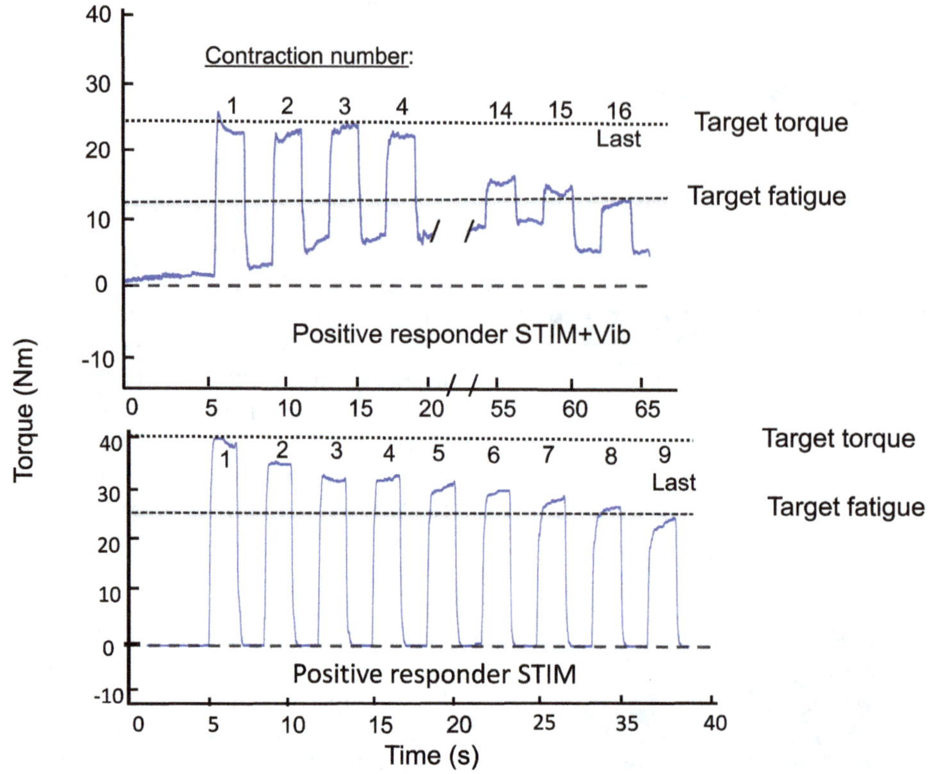

Fig. 4 Torque production (Nm) for a positive responder during STIM + Vib and STIM. Last: last contraction before target fatigue. Target torque = 20% MVIC. Target Fatigue = 60% of target torque

current conditions (30 Hz, 20% MVIC in quadriceps femoris muscle). However, a significantly greater TTI was observed in a subgroup (n = 8) of "positive responders" to tendon vibration. Thus, in 50% of the present participants, the addition of the tendon vibration allowed for a greater total muscular work to be performed, but this was not consistent among the participants.

Another notable, and practically relevant, finding was that a significant (−8.7%) reduction in maximal voluntary torque was evoked by STIM, which persisted for at least one hour and was associated with a reduction in RF EMG amplitude; thus, the wide-pulse width NMES elicited a notable fatigue response that persisted for at least 1 h after the session and which could affect post-training movement capacity. Nonetheless, reductions in voluntary force

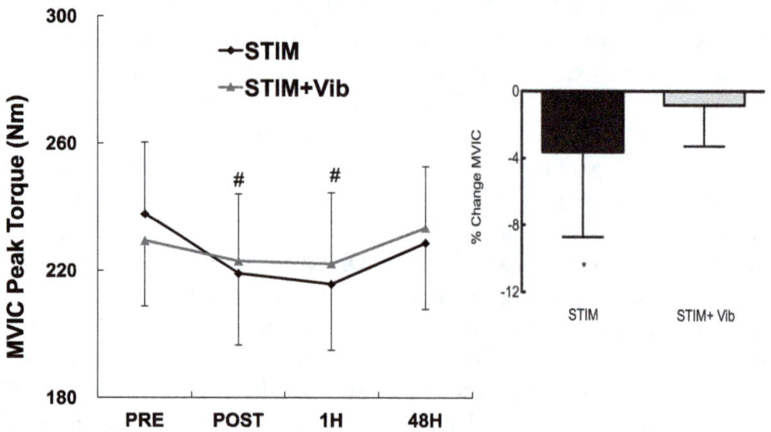

Fig. 5 Changes in peak isometric voluntary contraction torque (MVIC) across time (PRE, POST, 1H and 48H). #Significant difference from PRE ($P < 0.05$) for STIM. Mean values ± standard error (SE). *Inset*: Percentage change in MVIC from PRE to POST in STIM and STIM + Vib conditions. *Significant difference from PRE ($P < 0.05$). Mean change ± SD

and muscle activity were not observed when vibration was superimposed onto the NMES, even in negative responders to STIM + Vib. Therefore, the application of tendon vibration attenuated the fatigue response and allowed NMES to be used without a persisting voluntary muscle fatigue. These results are consistent with previous studies where the use of tendon vibration superimposed onto weak-to-moderate voluntary contractions was observed to attenuate the fatigue-induced decline in motor output, as assessed using standard surface EMG techniques during maximal voluntary contraction (e.G. *tibialis* anterior) [49]. Regarding the lack of effect of vibration alone (Vib) on the outcome variables, this was predictable as the vibration stimulation only recruits the lowest threshold motor units [62] and would not be sufficient to evoke strong muscle contractions, since larger, higher threshold motor units contribute more to higher force levels [63].

The finding of an increased torque-time integral being produced when tendon vibration was superimposed onto NMES in the positive responders to tendon vibration (8 of 16 participants; for example see Fig. 4) shows that an increase in total muscle contractile work was achieved. This could be considered advantageous in clinical practice as it would allow the muscle to produce a greater tension for longer, and thus may better evoke chronic increases in muscle strength and mass [64, 65] and potentially improve muscle performance in people with limited voluntary muscle activation capacity (e.g. stroke, spinal cord injury, brain injury) [66]. This result in positive responders was similar to previous observations of higher force levels (up to 50% maximal voluntary contraction) elicited by tendon vibration applied simultaneously with electrical stimulation in healthy participants [53]. These greater muscular forces might possibly be attributed to the development of persistent inward currents, which could amplify and prolong the synaptic input and generate a sustained depolarization of α-motor neurons leading to an increased recruitment of fatigue resistant motor units, maximizing the use of reflexive pathways and thus increasing muscle force production [35, 40, 41, 53, 67]. The augmented torque-time integral may also be attributed to the development of tonic vibration reflexes (TVR) occuring between muscle evoked contractions only when superimposed tendon vibration is applied (see Fig. 4).

Nonetheless, 8 of 16 participants (negative responders to tendon vibration) showed a decrease in their TTI when tendon vibration was superimposed onto the wide-pulse width NMES, indicating that tendon vibration may reduce the ability to produce force and decrease the total muscle contractile work during high-intensity NMES contractions, thus representing a disadvantage in this subgroup of participants. This negative response may speculatively have been caused by the stimulation of Golgi tendon organs by the low-to-moderate frequency (55 Hz) of vibration applied during the contraction [68]. Alternatively, the additional synaptic input provided by tendon vibration might have exacerbated fatigue mechanisms (e.g. ion channel function and neurotransmitter depletion), particularly for those individuals for whom the wide-pulse width NMES has already successfully recruited the lower threshold motor units.

In this case, we can infer that negative responders to tendon vibration might benefit from the sole application of (possibly wide-pulse width) NMES (STIM) based on the similar response in total amount of work (i.e. TTI) and total number of contractions performed under STIM in comparison to positive responders to tendon vibration under STIM + Vib (see Fig. 3b). So, if a lower TTI is found after STIM then the application of tendon vibration would likely improve performance to approximately equally to the "negative responders", whilst if a higher TTI is found after STIM then tendon vibration would likely reduce the TTI to similar levels to those found in "negative responders". Thus, it appears that negative responders to tendon vibration will show a decrease in total muscle contractile work if tendon vibration is added and in these cases tendon vibration superimposed onto wide-pulse width NMES may represent a disadvantage and thus, the use of NMES alone would be more beneficial to elicit a high muscle force production. Whether this group has derived *ben*efits from the wide-pulse width NMES as compared to standard (i.e. narrow pulse widths) remains to be explicitly investigated in future studies. The large inter-individual variability observed in our study is consistent with previous studies using wide-pulse width NMES, where substantial individual variability exists regarding its magnitude of effect [38, 44, 69, 70]. Due to this large inter-individual variability, clinicians may need to test individual responses to tendon vibration before its implementation in clinical practice.

Additionally, given that TTI and total number of contractions measured in STIM could be used to predict 87.5% and 81.3% of the positive and negative responders to tendon vibration, respectively, the measurement of TTI or the number of contractions during wide-pulse width NMES might be a clinically relevant method to predict whether a patient would benefit from superimposed tendon vibration (i.e. a positive response to tendon vibration). In that case, clinicians might determine whether to use tendon vibration on their patients based on their response to STIM alone. However, since measuring TTI in clinical practice may not be practically feasible in some cases, using total number of contractions, for example by visually counting until reaching a pre-determined torque level (representing muscle fatigue), might be used to identify patients who will benefit from additional tendon vibration.

A secondary finding of the present study was that a significant decrease in maximal voluntary force production was observed for at least 1 h in STIM but not STIM + Vib. It is important to note that these results were not influenced by the values obtained prior to the application of the electrical stimulation protocols (MVIC PRE), as these values were not statistically different ($p = 0.19$) and reliable between days (ICC = 0.95). This result showed an advantage of the superimposed tendon vibration that prevented the significant fatigue-induced decline in MVIC. Thus, in the clinical context, tendon vibration may provide a benefit of reduced voluntary muscle fatigue when compared to moderate-frequency, wide-pulse width NMES that could allow for further rehabilitation work or improved performance of activities of daily living and occupational tasks in the hours after a rehabilitation session. It is not clear from the present data how the vibration provided a fatigue-attenuation benefit. Speculatively, it may have reduced the synchrony of the motor unit activity during NMES, which may have then reduce the rate of muscle fatigue [45, 71]. This might occur if ongoing facilitation of fatigue-resistant motor units was provided due to the generation of trains of Ia afferent signals into the spinal cord, inducing an excitation of homonymous motor neurons through the development of persistent inward calcium (Ca^{2+}) or sodium (Na^{+}) currents (PIC) at their dendritic trees [45, 71]. Such a mechanism would evoke a tonic vibratory reflex influencing both spinal and supraspinal pathways [45, 71]. Tendon vibration-induced primary muscle spindle endings (i.e. Ia afferent activation) might also substitute for the fusimotor-driven Ia discharge and α-motor output decline that usually occurs during sustained voluntary contractions [49, 72]. This would have attenuated the muscle fatigue response observed in our study by continuing the Ia afferent activation response. Regardless of the potential mechanism, there seems to be a reversal of central drive failure when tendon vibration is superimposed onto wide-pulse width NMES, but further tests are needed to confirm this theory. However, the levels of muscle voluntary isometric fatigue observed in the present study (-8% after STIM) were somewhat smaller than the 22–30% reported by other studies [20, 73, 74]. This discrepancy may be attributed to the use of biphasic wide-pulse width NMES, the use of a lower stimulation frequency (30 vs. 75 Hz) or different duty cycle ratio (2–2 vs. 5–15 s), or that muscles were activated to only 20% of MVIC (with 'fatigue' being 60% of this value) in comparison to maximal tolerable levels of MVIC used by others [20, 74, 75]. Further explanation of these possibilities is required to accurately explain the differences in voluntary fatigue.

Another important finding was a reduced RF EMG amplitude observed during MVIC in STIM but not STIM + Vib, indicating that the loss of central drive to the muscle was minimized or eliminated with the application of tendon vibration. This selective decline in RF activation, but no other muscles, at POST may be attributed to the higher activity of RF during isometric knee extension at 90° of knee flexion [76] influencing the activation of the bi-articular RF over the vastii muscles (VM and VL) during STIM [77, 78] and the higher EMG fatigue experienced on RF due to its bi-articular nature [79]. It would be of interest to determine whether the decrease in EMG during MVIC and its "rescue" when tendon vibration is imposed onto NMES is observed in other skeletal muscles, or whether it is unique to RF or other biarticular muscles [79].

Of final note, no evidence for muscle damage or soreness was found in either condition at any time point, and levels of reported pain and comfort were "light-to-moderate" and not statistically different between conditions (mean for STIM = 4/10, STIM + Vib = 5/10). Therefore, the muscle stimulation and vibratory stimuli could be applied without concern for ongoing muscle fatigue or damage, and with reasonable levels of pain and comfort, at least in healthy individuals. The muscle damaging effects of electrically evoked isometric contractions have been previously attributed to the disruption of the muscle fibres and their surrounding connective tissue [74, 80–82], which causes a prolonged loss of muscle force generating capacity. The lack of damage in the present study might be explained by the fact that muscles were activated to only 20% of MVIC, whilst maximal tolerable levels of muscle contraction were evoked in previous studies [74, 80–82]. Moreover, being able to exercise regularly without ongoing soreness or force loss may have broad clinical relevance since pain can trigger life-threatening episodes in some clinical conditions such as autonomic dysreflexia in people with spinal cord injury [55]. Finally, since the levels of pain and discomfort were "light-to-moderate" and not different between the conditions, these NMES protocols can be considered safe for implementation in future clinical studies.

Limitations of this study are that our results are only pertinent under specific conditions of NMES (1000 μs, 30 Hz) at relatively higher torque levels than previously been investigated [40–42, 53]. Thus, a different response may result under different NMES conditions. Further studies using relatively higher intensities (i.e. 20% MVIC) and the same parameters of NMES as used in this study should be performed to confirm our results.

Conclusions

Based on the present results, the imposition of tendon vibration onto moderate-frequency wide-pulse width NMES may allow for a greater amount of muscular work to be performed, and thus for a more optimum training response to be achieved, in a proportion of participants who respond positively. However, a lesser response might be elicited in those individuals who respond negatively (50% of participants in the current study) and in these cases tendon vibration superimposed onto wide-pulse width NMES may represent a disadvantage and thus, the use of NMES alone would be more beneficial to elicit a high muscle force production. Nonetheless, the use of tendon vibration superimposed onto wide-pulse width NMES appeared to minimize the voluntary fatigue experienced after the training session and might therefore allow for additional rehabilitation work to be performed or for the trained muscle groups to be more effectively used for locomotion (i.e. crutches use) and activities of daily living after the session for both positive and negative responders to tendon vibration. Finally, since muscle damage and soreness were not observed, and levels of pain and discomfort were light-to-moderate after both NMES conditions, the application of these methods appear to be sufficiently safe to be used in clinical populations, such as in people with SCI. This is important as some clinical populations may be susceptible to high levels of muscle fatigue and muscle damage or might respond negatively to painful stimuli. Nonetheless, replication of these findings in a larger sample is encouraged before this type of NMES protocol is recommended in clinical practice.

Abbreviations

EMG: Electromyography; MVC: Maximal voluntary contraction; MVIC: Maximal voluntary isometric contraction; NMES: Neuromuscular electrical stimulation; RF: Rrectus femoris; SCI: Spinal cord injury; STIM: Neuromuscular electrical stimulation protocol; STIM + Vib: Neuromuscular electrical stimulation superimposed onto tendon vibration protocol; TTI: Total torque-time integral; Vib: Vibration only protocol; VL: Vastus lateralis; VM: Vastus medialis

Acknowledgements

This work was supported by a Spinal Cord Injuries Australia (SCIA) Collaborative Research Program grant to R.N.

Funding

Spinal Cord Injuries Australia (SCIA) Collaborative Research Program grant to Robert Newton. The funding body participated in the design of the study and collection, but no further participation existed for the analysis, and interpretation of data and in writing the manuscript.

Authors'contributions

VB, AB, RN, GT made substantial contributions to conception and design of this study. VB, AB, AV, GT, TP made substantial contributions to acquisition of data, analysis and interpretation of data. All authors participated in drafting the article or revising it critically for important intellectual content. All authors gave final approval of the version to be submitted and any revised version.

Competing interests

The authors declare that they have no competing interests.

Author details

[1]Exercise Medicine Research Institute, Edith Cowan University, Perth, Australia. [2]Centre for Sports and Exercise Science, School of Medical and Health Sciences, Edith Cowan University, Joondalup 270 Joondalup Drive, Joondalup, WA 6027, Australia. [3]UQ Centre for Clinical Research, University of Queensland, Brisbane, Australia. [4]School of Exercise and Nutrition Sciences, Queensland University of Technology, Brisbane, Australia. [5]UDF-University Centre, Brasilia, Brazil.

References

1. Schaap LA, Pluijm SM, Deeg DJ, Harris TB, Kritchevsky SB, Newman AB, et al. Higher inflammatory marker levels in older persons: associations with 5-year change in muscle mass and muscle strength. J Gerontol A Biol Sci Med Sci. 2009;64(11):1183–9.
2. Srikanthan P, Karlamangla AS. Muscle mass index as a predictor of longevity in older adults. Am J Med. 2014;127(6):547–53.
3. Solberg PA, Kvamme NH, Raastad T, Ommundsen Y, Tomten SE, Halvari H, et al. Effects of different types of exercise on muscle mass, strength, function and well-being in elderly. Eur J Sport Sci. 2013;13(1):112–25.
4. Caserotti P, Aagaard P, Larsen JB, Puggaard L. Explosive heavy-resistance training in old and very old adults: changes in rapid muscle force, strength and power. Scand J Med Sci Sports. 2008;18(6):773–82.
5. Andrade SD, da Silva JN. The effects of resistance training in osteoporosis: a systematic review. RBNE. 2015;9(50):144–9.
6. Clark JE, Goon DT. The role of resistance training for treatment of obesity related health issues and for changing health status of the individual who is overfat or obese: a review. J Sports Med Phys Fitness. 2015;55(3):205–22.
7. Orlando G, Balducci S, Bazzucchi I, Pugliese G, Sacchetti M. Neuromuscular dysfunction in type 2 diabetes: underlying mechanisms and effect of resistance training. Diab-Metabol Res Rev. 2016;32(1):40–50.
8. Thrasher TA, Ward JS, Fisher S. Strength and endurance adaptations to functional electrical stimulation leg cycle ergometry in spinal cord injury. NeuroRehabil. 2013;33(1):133–8.
9. Griffin L, Decker MJ, Hwang JY, Wang B, Kitchen K, Ding Z, et al. Functional electrical stimulation cycling improves body composition, metabolic and neural factors in persons with spinal cord injury. J Electromyogr Kinesiol. 2009;19(4):614–22.
10. Harvey LA, Fornusek C, Bowden JL, Pontifex N, Glinsky J, Middleton JW, et al. Electrical stimulation plus progressive resistance training for leg strength in spinal cord injury: A randomized controlled trial. Spinal Cord. 2010;48(7): 570–5.
11. Gregory CM, Bickel CS. Recruitment patterns in human skeletal muscle during electrical stimulation. Phys Ther. 2005;85(4):358–64.
12. Hillegass EA, Dudley GA. Surface electrical stimulation of skeletal muscle after spinal cord injury. Spinal Cord. 1999;37(4):251–7.
13. Gordon T, Mao J. Muscle atrophy and procedures for training after spinal-cord injury. Phys Ther. 1994;74(1):50–60.
14. Bersch I, Tesini S, Bersch U, Frotzler A. Functional electrical stimulation in spinal cord injury: clinical evidence versus daily practice. Artif Organs. 2015;39(10):849–54.
15. American College of Sports Medicine. Progression models in resistance training for healthy adults. Med Sci Sports Exerc. 2009;41(3):687–708.
16. Hortobagyi T, Maffiuletti NA. Neural adaptations to electrical stimulation strength training. Eur J Appl Physiol. 2011;111(10):2439–49.
17. Gorgey AS, Mahoney E, Kendall T, Dudley GA. Effects of neuromuscular electrical stimulation parameters on specific tension. Eur J Appl Physiol. 2006;97(6):737–44.
18. Ibitoye MO, Hamzaid NA, Hasnan N, Abdul Wahab AK, Davis GM. Strategies for rapid muscle fatigue reduction during fes exercise in individuals with spinal cord injury: a systematic review. PLoS One. 2016;11(2):e0149024.
19. Karu ZZ, Durfee WK, Barzilai AM. Reducing muscle fatigue in fes applications by stimulating with N-let pulse trains. IEEE Trans Biomed Eng. 1995;42(8):809–17.
20. Aldayel A, Jubeau M, McGuigan MR, Nosaka K. Less indication of muscle damage in the second than initial electrical muscle stimulation bout consisting of isometric contractions of the knee extensors. Eur J Appl Physiol. 2010;108(4):709–17.
21. Gorgey AS, Poarch HJ, Dolbow DR, Castillo T, Gater DR. Effect of adjusting pulse durations of functional electrical stimulation cycling on energy expenditure and fatigue after spinal cord injury. J Rehab Res Dev. 2014;51(9):1455–68.

22. Bigland-Ritchie B, Jones DA, Woods JJ. Excitation frequency and muscle fatigue: electrical responses during human voluntary and stimulated contractions. Exp Neurol. 1979;64(2):414–27.
23. Mizrahi J. Fatigue in functional electrical stimulation in spinal cord injury. J Electromyogr Kinesiol. 1997;7(1):1–2.
24. Bickel CS, Gregory CM, Dean JC. Motor unit recruitment during neuromuscular electrical stimulation: a critical appraisal. Eur J Appl Physiol. 2011;111(10):2399–407.
25. Fouré A, Nosaka K, Wegrzyk J, Duhamel G, Le Troter A, Boudinet H, et al. Time course of central and peripheral alterations after isometric neuromuscular electrical stimulation-induced muscle damage. PLoS One. 2014;9(9):e107298.
26. Adams GR, Harris RT, Woodard D, Dudley GA. Mapping of electrical muscle stimulation using MRI. J Appl Physiol. 1993;74(2):532–7.
27. Gorgey AS, Cho GM, Dolbow DR, Gater DR. Differences in current amplitude evoking leg extension in individuals with spinal cord injury. Neurorehabilitation. 2013;33(1):161–70.
28. Allen K, Goodman C. Using electrical stimulation: A guideline for allied health professionals. Sydney: Sydney Local Health District and Royal Rehabilitation Center; 2014.
29. Crameri RM, Weston A, Climstein M, Davis GM, Sutton JR. Effects of electrical stimulation-induced leg training on skeletal muscle adaptability in spinal cord injury. Scand J Med Sci Sports. 2002;12(5):316–22.
30. Black CD, McCully KK. Force per active area and muscle injury during electrically stimulated contractions. Med Sci Sports Exerc. 2008;40(9):1596–604.
31. Daussin FN, Zoll J, Ponsot E, Dufour SP, Doutreleau S, Lonsdorfer E, et al. Training at high exercise intensity promotes qualitative adaptations of mitochondrial function in human skeletal muscle. J Appl Physiol. 2008;104(5):1436–41.
32. Bouchard DR, Heroux M, Janssen I. Association between muscle mass, leg strength, and fat mass with physical function in older adults: influence of age and sex. J Aging Health. 2011;23(2):313–28.
33. Collins DF. Central contributions to contractions evoked by tetanic neuromuscular electrical stimulation. Exerc Sport Sci Rev. 2007;35(3):102–9.
34. Lagerquist O, Collins DF. Influence of stimulus pulse width on M-waves, H-reflexes, and torque during tetanic low-intensity neuromuscular stimulation. Muscle Nerve. 2010;42(6):886–93.
35. Bergquist AJ, Clair JM, Lagerquist O, Mang CS, Okuma Y, Collins DF. Neuromuscular electrical stimulation: implications of the electrically evoked sensory volley. Eur J Appl Physiol. 2011;111(10):2409–26.
36. Bergquist AJ, Wiest MJ, Okuma Y, Collins DF. H-reflexes reduce fatigue of evoked contractions after spinal cord injury. Muscle Nerve. 2014;50(2):224–34.
37. Clair-Auger JM, Collins DF, Dewald JPA. The effects of wide pulse neuromuscular electrical stimulation on elbow flexion torque in individuals with chronic hemiparetic stroke. Clin Neurophysiol. 2012;123(11):2247–55.
38. Neyroud D, Armand S, De Coulon G, Da Silva SRD, Wegrzyk J, Gondin J, et al. Wide-pulse-high-frequency neuromuscular electrical stimulation in cerebral palsy. Clin Neurophysiol. 2016;127(2):1530–9.
39. Bergquist AJ, Wiest MJ, Collins DF. Motor unit recruitment when neuromuscular electrical stimulation is applied over a nerve trunk compared with a muscle belly: quadriceps femoris. J Appl Physiol. 2012;113(1):78–89.
40. Collins DF, Burke D, Gandevia SC. Large involuntary forces consistent with plateau-like behavior of human motoneurons. J Neurosci. 2001;21(11):4059–65.
41. Collins DF, Burke D, Gandevia SC. Sustained contractions produced by plateau-like behaviour in human motoneurones. J Physiol. 2002;538(1):289–301.
42. Dean JC, Clair-Auger JM, Lagerquist O, Collins DF. Asynchronous recruitment of low-threshold motor units during repetitive, low-current stimulation of the human tibial nerve. Front Hum Neurosci. 2014;8:1002.
43. Clair-Auger JM, Lagerquist O, Collins DF. Depression and recovery of reflex amplitude during electrical stimulation after spinal cord injury. Clin Neurophysiol. 2013;124(4):723–31.
44. Neyroud D, Dodd D, Gondin J, Maffiuletti NA, Kayser B, Place N. Wide-pulse-high-frequency neuromuscular stimulation of triceps surae induces greater muscle fatigue compared with conventional stimulation. J Appl Physiol. 2014;116(10):1281–9.
45. Ribot-Ciscar E, Butler JE, Thomas CK. Facilitation of triceps brachii muscle contraction by tendon vibration after chronic cervical spinal cord injury. J Appl Physiol. 2003;94(6):2358–67.
46. Cotey D, Hornby TG, Gordon KE, Schmit BD. Increases in muscle activity produced by vibration of the thigh muscles during locomotion in chronic human spinal cord injury. Exp Brain Res. 2009;196(3):361–74.
47. Trajano GS, Seitz LB, Nosaka K, Blazevich AJ. Can passive stretch inhibit motoneuron facilitation in the human plantar flexors? J Appl Physiol. 2014;117(12):1486–92.
48. McPherson JG, Ellis MD, Heckman CJ, Dewald JP. Evidence for increased activation of persistent inward currents in individuals with chronic hemiparetic stroke. J Neurophysiol. 2008;100(6):3236–43.
49. Bongiovanni LG, Hagbarth KE. Tonic vibration reflexes elicited during fatigue from maximal voluntary contractions in man. J Physiol. 1990;423:1–14.
50. Behrman AL, Bowden MG, Nair PM. Neuroplasticity after spinal cord injury and training: an emerging paradigm shift in rehabilitation and walking recovery. Phys Ther. 2006;86(10):1406–25.
51. Edgerton VR, Roy RR. Activity-dependent plasticity of spinal locomotion: implications for sensory processing. Exerc Sport Sci Rev. 2009;37(4):171–8.
52. Magalhães FH, de Toledo DR, Kohn AF. Plantar flexion force induced by amplitude-modulated tendon vibration and associated soleus V/F-waves as an evidence of a centrally-mediated mechanism contributing to extra torque generation in humans. J NeuroEng Rehabil. 2013;10(1):32.
53. Magalhaes FH, Kohn AF. Vibration-induced extra torque during electrically-evoked contractions of the human calf muscles. J Neuroeng Rehabil. 2010;7. doi:10.1186/1743-0003-7-26.
54. Burke D, Schiller HH. Discharge pattern of single motor units in the tonic vibration reflex of human triceps surae. J Neurol Neurosurg Psychiatry. 1976;39(8):729–41.
55. Rabchevsky AG, Kitzman PH. Latest approaches for the treatment of spasticity and autonomic dysreflexia in chronic spinal cord injury. Neurotherapeutics. 2011;8(2):274–82.
56. Laufer Y, Ries JD, Leininger PM, Alon G. Quadriceps femoris muscle torques and fatigue generated by neuromuscular electrical stimulation with three different waveforms. Phys Ther. 2001;81(7):1307–16.
57. Field-Fote EC, Anderson B, Robertson VJ, Spielholz NI. Monophasic and biphasic stimulation evoke different responses. Muscle Nerve. 2003;28(2):239–41.
58. Hermens HJ, Freriks B, Disselhorst-Klug C, Rau G. Development of recommendations for SEMG sensors and sensor placement procedures. J Electromyogr Kinesiol. 2000;10(5):361–74.
59. Nosaka K, Clarkson PM. Muscle damage following repeated bouts of high force eccentric exercise. Med Sci Sports Exerc. 1995;27(9):1263–9.
60. Ohrbach R, Gale EN. Pressure pain thresholds, clinical assessment, and differential diagnosis, reliability and validity in patients with myogenic pain. Pain. 1989;39(2):157–69.
61. Nosaka K, Clarkson PM. Changes in indicators of inflammation after eccentric exercise of the elbow flexors. Med Sci Sports Exerc. 1996;28(8):953–61.
62. Kanda K, Burke RE, Walmsley B. Differential control of fast and slow twitch motor units in the decerebrate cat. Exp Brain Res. 1977;29(1):57–74.
63. Henneman E, Somjen G, Carpenter DO. Functional significance of cell size in spinal motoneurons. J Neurophysiol. 1965;28(3):560–80.
64. Ahtiainen JP, Pakarinen A, Alen M, Kraemer WJ, Hakkinen K. Muscle hypertrophy, hormonal adaptations and strength development during strength training in strength-trained and untrained men. Eur J Appl Physiol. 2003;89(6):555–63.
65. Bax L, Staes F, Verhagen A. Does neuromuscular electrical stimulation strengthen the quadriceps femoris? A systematic review of randomised controlled trials. Sports Med. 2005;35(3):191–212.
66. Smith GV, Alon G, Roys SR, Gullapalli RP. Functional MRI determination of a dose-response relationship to lower extremity neuromuscular electrical stimulation in healthy subjects. Exp Brain Res. 2003;150(1):33–9.
67. Dean JC, Yates LM, Collins DF. Turning on the central contribution to contractions evoked by neuromuscular electrical stimulation. J Appl Physiol. 2007;103(1):170–6.
68. Fallon JB, Macefield VG. Vibration sensitivity of human muscle spindles and Golgi tendon organs. Muscle Nerve. 2007;36(1):21–9.
69. Regina Dias Da Silva S, Neyroud D, Maffiuletti NA, Gondin J, Place N. Twitch potentiation induced by two different modalities of neuromuscular electrical stimulation: implications for motor unit recruitment. Muscle Nerve. 2015;51(3):412–8.
70. Wegrzyk J, Foure A, Le Fur Y, Maffiuletti NA, Vilmen C, Guye M, et al. Responders to wide-pulse, high-frequency neuromuscular electrical stimulation show reduced metabolic demand: a 31P-MRS study in humans. PLoS One. 2015;10(11):e0143972.

71. Ribot-Ciscar E, Rossi-Durand C, Roll JP. Muscle spindle activity following muscle tendon vibration in man. Neurosci Lett. 1998;258(3):147–50.
72. Macefield G, Hagbarth KE, Gorman R, Gandevia SC, Burke D. Decline in spindle support to alpha-motoneurones during sustained voluntary contractions. J Physiol. 1991;440:497–512.
73. Jubeau M, Sartorio A, Marinone PG, Agosti F, Van Hoecke J, Nosaka K, et al. Comparison between voluntary and stimulated contractions of the quadriceps femoris for growth hormone response and muscle damage. J Appl Physiol. 2008;104(1):75–81.
74. Nosaka K, Aldayel A, Jubeau M, Chen TC. Muscle damage induced by electrical stimulation. Eur J Appl Physiol. 2011;111(10):2427–37.
75. Jubeau M, Muthalib M, Millet GY, Maffiuletti NA, Nosaka K. Comparison in muscle damage between maximal voluntary and electrically evoked isometric contractions of the elbow flexors. Eur J Appl Physiol. 2012;112(2):429–38.
76. Watanabe K, Akima H. Normalized EMG to normalized torque relationship of vastus intermedius muscle during isometric knee extension. Eur J Appl Physiol. 2009;106(5):665–73.
77. Maffiuletti NA, Lepers R. Quadriceps femoris torque and EMG activity in seated versus supine position. Med Sci Sports Exerc. 2003;35(9):1511–6.
78. Matta TT, Nascimento FX, Trajano GS, Simao R, Willardson JM, Oliveira LF. Selective hypertrophy of the quadriceps musculature after 14 weeks of isokinetic and conventional resistance training. Clin Physiol Funct Imaging 2015. doi:10.1111/cpf.12277.
79. Ebenbichler G, Kollmitzer J, Quittan M, Uhl F, Kirtley C, Fialka V. EMG fatigue patterns accompanying isometric fatiguing knee-extensions are different in mono- and bi-articular muscles. Electroencephalogr Clin Neurophysiol. 1998;109(3):256–62.
80. Mackey AL, Bojsen-Moller J, Qvortrup K, Langberg H, Suetta C, Kalliokoski KK, et al. Evidence of skeletal muscle damage following electrically stimulated isometric muscle contractions in humans. J Appl Physiol. 2008;105(5):1620–7.
81. Aldayel A, Jubeau M, McGuigan M, Nosaka K. Comparison between alternating and pulsed current electrical muscle stimulation for muscle and systemic acute responses. J Appl Physiol. 2010;109(3):735–44.
82. Mackey AL, Brandstetter S, Schjerling P, Bojsen-Moller J, Qvortrup K, Pedersen MM, et al. Sequenced response of extracellular matrix deadhesion and fibrotic regulators after muscle damage is involved in protection against future injury in human skeletal muscle. FASEB J. 2011;25(6):1943–59.

7

A case of neuropsychiatric lupus Erythematosus characterized by the Owl's eye sign

Bolin Hu[1], Pengcheng Wu[1], Yibiao Zhou[2], Yan Peng[1], Xiaoping Tang[3], Weijiang Ding[1], Ming Zhang[1] and Xueliang Qi[1*]

Abstract

Background: Systemic lupus erythematosus (SLE) is an autoimmune inflammatory disorder characterized by multiple affected systems. More than half of SLE patients will suffer from neuropsychiatric lupus erythematosus (NPSLE) during the course of their disease. Although nearly half of the NPSLE patients have normal MRI manifestations, the abnormalities found in the remainder can be located anywhere in the brain, and especially in the subcortical white matter of the frontal and temporal lobe. However, NPSLE involving the medulla oblongata and spinal cord which presents as the "owl's eye" sign has to our best knowledge not been reported to date.

Case presentation: A 19-year-old girl presented at our hospital with a 7-day history of fever and headache since a one day's exertion, accompanied by 2 days of weakness. The patient had slurred speech. Neurological examination revealed the presence of horizontal nystagmus and a limitation of bilateral eye movement when looking up and down. At the same time, she showed difficulty in raising the jaw, accompanied by a weak pharyngeal reflex. Muscle strength was remarkably decreased in all four extremities: the MRCS grade of the upper limbs was 4/5, while in the lower limbs it was 0/5. Hypotonia was apparent in the lower extremities. Regarding subjective sensation, the patient appeared to be experiencing an increased sense of pain in the whole body, and especially in the cervical region, abdomen, and feet. An examination of shallow reflex documented the reinforcement of the abdominal reflex. Deep tendon reflexes were symmetric: absent in lower, normal in upper extremities. The patient also had a stiff neck with a positive Kernig's sign. The laboratory examination showed elevated C - reactive protein and rheumatoid factor, as well as complement components 3 and 4. Symptomatic treatments were applied, but she did not respond well, after which we did immunological laboratory examinations. The results showed the presence of anti-nRNP/Sm, anti-dsDNA and anti-AMA M2 antibodies. An MRI scan and enhancement of the cervical and thoracic regions displayed abnormal signs in the medulla and bilateral anterior horn of the lower thoracic spine. Following the exclusion of other possible diseases, neuropsychiatric lupus was diagnosed. High-dose intravenous gamma-globulin combined with methylprednisolone gradually improved her condition.

Conclusion: We report the first case of NPSLE presenting with medulla oblongata and spinal cord involvement, manifesting as the "owl's eye" sign in MRI.

Keywords: Neuropsychiatric lupus, Magnetic resonance imaging, Owl' eye sign, Case report

* Correspondence: qixueliang766@163.com
[1]Department of Neurology, The Second Affiliated Hospital of Nanchang University, No. 1, Minde Road, Nanchang, Jiangxi 330006, People's Republic of China
Full list of author information is available at the end of the article

Background

Systemic lupus erythematosus (SLE) is an autoimmune inflammatory disorder characterized by multiple affected systems [1]. More than half of SLE patients will suffer from neuropsychiatric lupus erythematosus (NPSLE) during the course of their disease [2, 3]. An exact definition of NPSLE is challenging because of the broad spectrum of its manifestations. In 1999 NPSLE was classified by the American College of Rheumatology (ACR), which identified 19 neuropsychiatric syndromes including 12 central nervous system (CNS) forms and 7 peripheral nervous system forms [4]. Even though nearly half of all NPSLE patients have a normal MRI presentation [5], the abnormalities in the other patients can be found anywhere in the brain, and especially in the subcortical white matter of the frontal and temporal lobe [6]. However, NPSLE with medulla oblongata and spinal cord involvement which presents as the "owl's eye" sign has to our best knowledge not been reported before. We therefore report the first case of NPSLE with medulla oblongata and spinal cord involvement, manifesting as the "owl's eye" sign in MRI.

Case presentation

A 19-year-old girl was admitted to our hospital with a 7-day history of fever and headache since an episode of one day's exertion, and two days of weakness. Seven days before clinical presentation, the girl had developed a headache, sore throat, bucking, vomiting and fever after one day's hard work. Consequently, she went to the local hospital, and after several days of symptomatic treatment, only the temperature dropped slightly. She therefore came to our hospital for further diagnosis and treatment. The patient had a history of recurring joint swelling, chilblains and alopecia. Her personal history was unremarkable, and no similar symptoms were found in her family. When she was transferred to our hospital, she was in a state of sleepiness, dysarthria, dysphagia and fever, with a body temperature of 37.8 °C, while an examination of the heart, lungs and abdomen revealed that they were normal. A neurological examination revealed a horizontal nystagmus and a limitation of bilateral eye movement when looking up and down. She also showed difficulty in raising the jaw, accompanied by a weak pharyngeal reflex. Muscle strength was remarkably decreased in all four extremities, with upper limbs having an MRCS grade of 4/5, while it was 0/5 in the lower limbs. Hypotonia was apparent in the lower extremities. Regarding the patient's subjective sensation, she appeared to exhibit an increased sense of pain in the whole body, and especially in the cervical region, abdomen, and feet. An examination of shallow reflex documented a reinforcement of the abdominal reflex. Deep tendon reflexes were symmetric: absent in the lower, normal in the upper extremities. The patient also had a stiff neck with a positive Kernig's sign.

Laboratory examination revealed elevated inflammatory indicators, with a white blood cell count of 8.41 × 10^9/L(normal range 4–10 × 10^9/L), NE% of 87.8%(normal range 50–70%), erythrocyte sedimentation rate of 72 mm/h(normal range 0-20 mm/h), and C-reactive protein concentration of 44.50 mg/L(normal range 0–8 mg/L). Quantitative serum analysis revealed the presence of 676.21 IU/ml of anti-dsDNA antibodies (normally < 100 IU/ml), with a titer of 1:40. Furthermore, the results for the anti-nRNP/Sm, anti-dsDNA, anti-ANuA, anti-AMA M2 antibody and IgM antiphospholipid antibody were all positive (normal being negative). The titer of the speckled anti-nuclear antibody was 1:640. The results of quantitative analysis for serum complement components 3 and 4 were 0.47 g/L and 40.05 g/L, respectively (normal range 0.9–1.8 g/L and 0.1–0.4 g/L, respectively). Simultaneously, rheumatoid factors were present at 23.70 IU/m (normally < 20 IU/m). Lumbar puncture revealed a cerebrospinal fluid pressure of 220mmH_2O (normal range 80–180 mmH_2O), with elevated protein at 775.79 mg/L (normal range 150-450 mg/L), IgG at 224.00 mg/L (normal range 0–34 mg/L), and a leukocyte number of 110 × 10^6/L (normal range 1.5–4.0 × 10^9/L). By contrast, tests for tumor cells and bacterial, viral, or fungal infection of CSF were all negative. Other indicators, including anti-aquaporin 4 antibody, the serum IgG oligoclonal band, and antibodies related to paraneoplastic symptoms of CSF were negative (normal). The EEG documented a significant amount of bilateral hemispheric slow waves with a moderate amplitude. The MRI comprising coronal T2 flair magnetic resonance and axial T2 weighted imaging showed diffuse swelling and high signal intensities involving the medulla oblongata (Fig. 1a and b. On sagittal T2 weighted imaging, high intensity signals were found in the medulla oblongata and thoracic spinal cord (Fig. 2a and b). In addition, axial T2 weighted imaging and the magnified image of the thoracic spinal cord revealed a small rough high signal in the bilateral anterior horn showing an"owl's eye" sign (Fig. 3. At the same time, CT angiography from the cervical region to the skull base was normal. According to the clinical features, laboratory examination and imaging results, SLE was confirmed, and after ruling out other possible diseases, NPSLE was finally diagnosed. Intravenous immunoglobulin (400 mg/kg, Qd, for 5 days), methylprednisolone (1000 mg/day for 3 days, followed by 500 mg/day for another 3 days, and 250 mg/day for another 3 days), cyclophosphamide (400 mg weekly), and aspirin (100 mg/day) were administered for therapy. The patient's eye movement, dysarthria and dysphagia recovered obviously within a week. The mobility of the soft palate normalized completely and the muscle strength of the lower limbs improved to grade 2/5 within 22 days. At the 3-month follow-up, the patient's neurological deficit was completely resolved with weekly i.v. pulsed cyclophosphamide (400 mg/week)

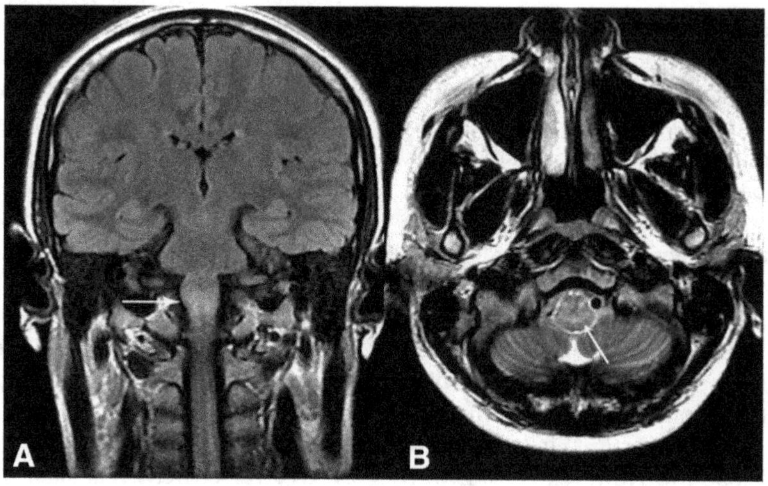

Fig. 1 a and **b** coronal T2 flair magnetic resonance and axial T2 weighted imaging showing diffuse swelling and high signal intensity involving the medulla oblongata

and prednisolone (20 mg/day). From then on, the patient was able to walk independently.

Discussion

NPSLE encompasses a number of neurological or psychiatric symptoms in which the SLE involves the central or peripheral nervous system. When NPSLE is considered, SLE should be diagnosed primarily, and possible non-NPSLE diseases such as the side-effects of medicines, mental or functional conditions should be excluded. In various studies, about 28% to 40% of adult SLE patients were found to develop NPSLE before or during the diagnosis of SLE, and about 63% developed NPSLE within one year after the diagnosis of SLE [6]. Several imaging modalities can be used to investigate NPSLE. Owing to its sensitivity, availability, and ability to exclude various similar conditions, MRI is the method of choice for the evaluation of NPSLE [5, 7]. Both longitudinal and transverse myelitis have been reported in SLE, and they represent well-characterized neurological manifestations of the disorder [8, 9]. However, NPSLE with medulla oblongata and spinal cord involvement which presents as the "owl's eye" sign has to our best knowledge not been reported to date.

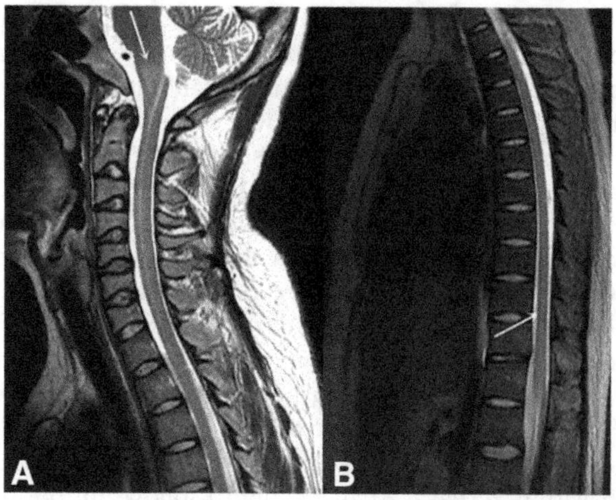

Fig. 2 a and **b** sagittal T2 weighted imaging showing high signal intensity involving the medulla oblongata and thoracic spinal cord

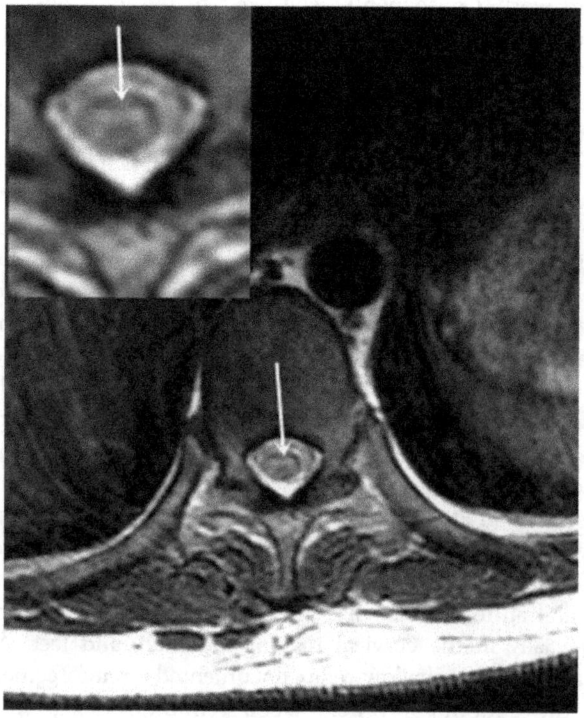

Fig. 3 Axial T2 weighted imaging and magnified image of thoracic spinal cord, showing a small rough high signal appearing in the bilateral anterior horn presenting as the "owl's eye" sign

The main pathophysiological changes found in NPSLE are vascular lesions characterized by hyaline degeneration, proliferation of endothelial cells and gliosis around vessels [10]. However, the underlying pathophysiological mechanisms of NPSLE remain unknown. Nevertheless, it is known that a disruption of the function of the blood-brain barrier may play a role in the development of NPSLE [11], and autoantibodies complement components, and cytokines are integral to the pathogenesis pathways, with more than 20 autoantibodies reported to be linked to NPSLE [12]. Furthermore, several studies have shown that cerebrovascular diseases and transverse myelitis in SLE are strongly related to the antiphospholipid antibodies, which accelerate atherosclerosis and thrombosis [13–15]. Regrettably, the presence of autoantibodies was not analyzed in this patient.

Medulla oblongata and spinal cord involvement has been reported in several cases. Neuman-Andersen et al. found swelling and signal changes in the medulla oblongata and the entire spinal cord, especially in the lower thoracic cord and conus [16]. Kimura et al. discovered a longitudinal lesion spanning the region from the medulla oblongata, C6 and Th12, reaching to the conus [17]. Mimenza-Alvarado et al. also found brain stem disorders in SLE patients [18]. Although medulla and/or spinal cord involvement was found in said cases, the changes included neither diffuse swelling nor increased signal density in the sagittal and/or axial MRI. Luckily, we have the honor of having discovered a unique change in neuropsychiatric lupus erythematosus, which presented as the "owl's eye" sign in the MRI.

The "owl's eye" sign, or alternatively "snake-eye" sign, is a specific finding in neuroimaging characterized by bilaterally symmetrical high signal intensity in the anterior horn of the spinal cord in axial T2-weighted MR imaging, which evokes the eyes of an owl or snake [19]. It has been reported in a number of diseases, such as complex cervical spondylosis, Hirayama disease, poliomyelitis, encephalitis caused by HIV infection, spinal cord infarction, neuromyelitis optica, paraneoplastic neurological syndrome and flail arm syndrome [20, 21]. Neuroimaging-documented appearance of the "owl's eye" sign may reflect cystic necrosis in the central gray matter near the ventrolateral posterior column, and is consequently regarded as an unfavorable prognostic factor for the recovery of upper-extremity motor weakness, due to the destruction of gray matter accompanied by significant neuronal loss in the anterior horn [22].

After the initial 7-day history of fever and headache, our patient quickly developed catastrophic flaccid paralysis of the legs, accompanied by areflexia, disordered eye movement, dysarthria, and dysphagia within 24 h. This case is characterized by involvement of both medulla oblongata and spinal cord, which presented as the "owl's eye" sign. In contrast to spinal cord infarction and similar diseases, which also lead to an "owl's eye" sign, the prognosis of NPSLE is good with timely treatment. It is therefore necessary to consider a diagnosis of NPSLE early if the patient does not respond well to the non-NPSLE treatment.

Conclusions

In summary, the case reported here presented with typical medulla oblongata and spinal cord involvement, which is rare in NPSLE patients. It therefore illustrates that NPSLE may involve the medulla oblongata and spinal cord, manifesting as the "owl's eye" sign in MRI. The owl's eye sign can thus be present in yet another disease, in addition to the many known examples such as complex cervical spondylosis, Hirayama disease, poliomyelitis, encephalitis caused by HIV infection, spinal cord infarction, neuromyelitis optica, paraneoplastic neurological syndrome and flail arm syndrome.

Abbreviations

CRP: C-reactive protein; CSF: Cerebrospinal fluid; CT: Computed tomography; EEG: Electroencephalogram; IgG: Immunoglobulin G; IgM: Immunoglobulin M; MRI: Magnetic resonance imaging; NPSLE: Neuropsychiatric systemic lupus erythematosus; SLE: Systemic lupus erythematosus

Acknowledgments

We thank the patient for cooperation.

Authors' contributions

BH: neurological evaluation of the patient and manuscript composition; PW, YZ, YP, WD and MZ: neurological evaluation of the patient and suggestions regarding manuscript composition; XT: image collection, processing and suggestions regarding manuscript composition; XQ: neurological evaluation of the patient, manuscript composition, corresponding author. All authors read and approved the final manuscript.

Competing interests

The authors declare that they have no competing interests.

Author details

[1]Department of Neurology, The Second Affiliated Hospital of Nanchang University, No. 1, Minde Road, Nanchang, Jiangxi 330006, People's Republic of China. [2]Department of Orthopedics, The First Affiliated Hospital of Nanchang University, Nanchang, Jiangxi 330006, People's Republic of China. [3]Department of MRI, The Second Affiliated Hospital of Nanchang University, Nanchang, Jiangxi 330006, People's Republic of China.

References

1. Brey RL. Neuropsychiatric lupus, clinical and imaging aspects. Bullet NYU Hosp Jt Dis. 2007;65:194–9.
2. Yu CH, Lee MB, Tseng MM, Liao SC. Obsessive compulsive symptoms as a manifestation of neuropsychiatric systemic lupus erythematosus. J Formus Med Assoc. 2008;107:68–72.

3. Harel L, Sandborg C, Lee T, von Scheven E. Neuropsychiatric manifestation in paediatric SLE and association with antiphospholipid antibodies. J Rheumatol. 2006;33:1873–7.
4. The American College of Rheumatology nomenclature and case definitions for neuropsychiatric lupus syndromes. Arthritis Rheum. 1999;42:599–608.
5. Toledano P, Sarbu N, Espinosa G, Bargallo N, Cervera R. Neuropsychiatric systemic lupus erythematosus: magnetic resonance imaging findings and correlation with clinical and immunological features. Autoimmun Rev. 2013; 12:1166–70.
6. Hanly JG. Diagnosis and management of neuropsychiatric SLE. Nat Rev Rheumatol. 2014;10:338–47.
7. Kivity S, Agmon-Levin N, Zandman-Goddard G, Chapman J, Shoenfeld Y. Neuropsychiatric lupus: a mosaic of clinical presentations. BMC Med. 2015;13:43.
8. Jennekens FG, Kater L. The central nervous system in systemic lupus erythematosus. Part 1. Clinical syndromes: a literature investigation. Rheumatology (Oxford). 2002;41:605–18.
9. Heinlein AC, Gertner E. Marked inflammation in catastrophic longitudinal myelitis associated with systemic lupus erythematosus. Lupus. 2007;16:823–6.
10. Rhiannon JJ. Systemic lupus erythematosus involving the nervous system: presentation, pathogenesis, and management. Clin Rev Allergy Immunol. 2008;34:356–60.
11. Abbott NJ, Mendonca LL, Dolman DE. The blood-brain barrier in systemic lupus erythematosus. Lupus. 2003;12:908–15.
12. Zandman-Goddard G, Chapman J, Shoenfeld Y. Autoantibodies involved in neuropsychiatric SLE and antiphospholipid syndrome. Semin Arthriris Rheum. 2007;36:297–315.
13. Petri M, Orbai AM, Alarcon GS, Gordon C, Merrill JT, Fortin PR, et al. Derivation and validation of the Systemic Lupus International Collaborating Clinics classification criteria for systemic lupus erythematosus. Arthritis Rheum. 2012;64:2677–86.
14. Kovacs B. LaaffertyTL, BrentLH, DeHoratius RJ. Transverse myelopathy in systemic lupus erythematosus: an analysisi of 14 cases and review of the literature. Ann Rheum Dis. 2000;59:120–4.
15. Matsuura E, Hughes GR, Khamashta MA. Oxidation of LDL and its clinical implication. Autoimmun Rev. 2008;7:558–66.
16. Neuman-Andersen G, Lindgren S. Involvement of the entire spinal cord and medulla oblongata in acute catastrophic-onset transverse myelitis in SLE. Clin Rheumatol. 2000;19:156–60.
17. Kimura KY, Seino Y, Hirayama Y, Aramaki T, Yamaguchi H, Amano H, et al. Systemic lupus Erythematosus related transverse myelitis presenting longitudinal involvement of the spinal cord. Intern Med. 2002;41:156–60.
18. Mimenza-Alvarado AJ, Tellez-Zenteno JF, Cantu-Brito C, Garcia-Ramos G. Systemic lupus erythematosus with affection to brainstem: report of three cases. Rev Neurol. 2002;35:128–31.
19. Faiss JH, Schroth G, Grodd W, Koenig E, Will B, Thron A. Central spinal cord lesions in stenosis of the cervical canal. Neuroradiology. 1990;32:117–23.
20. Lebouteux MV, Franques J, Guillevin R, Delmont E, Lenglet T, Bede P, et al. Revisiting the spectrum of lower motorneuron diseases with snake eyes appearance on magnetic resonance imaging. Eur J Neurol. 2014;21:1233–41.
21. Kumar S, Mehta VK, Shukla R. Owl's eye sign: a rare neuroimaging finding in flail armsyndrome. Neurology. 2015;84:1500.
22. Mizuno J, Nakagawa H, Inoue T, Hashizume Y. Clinicopathological study of "snake-eye appearance" in compressive myelopathy of the cervical spinal cord. J Neurosurg. 2003;99:162–8.

8

Intracranial lesion as onset symptom in a patient with early undifferentiated connective tissue disease

Ying Du†, Chuan Li†, Dai-di Zhao, Jia-rui Lu, Wei Zhang* and Zhu-yi Li*

Abstract

Background: Undifferentiated connective tissue disease (UCTD) is widely considered to be a distinct clinical entity, and now divided into two subgroups: stable UCTD and early UCTD. The most frequent onset symptoms of UCTD include arthralgias, arthritis, Raynaud's phenomenon, mucocutaneous involvement, and sicca symptoms. However, Neurologic involvement is rare, and intracranial lesion as onset symptom in a patient with early UCTD has not yet been reported.

Case presentation: A 51-year-old Chinese female experienced progressive left leg weakness for 14 days before hospitalizing in our department. The lesion on right parietal lobe was initially detected by brain magnetic resonance imaging. Although the patient declined a cerebral biopsy, the possibility of stroke, cerebral venous sinus thrombosis, NMOSD, MS, autoimmune encephalitis, intracranial infections, and malignant tumors as cause of the lesion was excluded by intracranial angiogram, CSF study, MRI enhancement and MRS examination. Moreover, immunologic studies showed high titer of antinuclear antibody, increased erythrocyte sedimentation rate and C-reactive protein. These results led to a diagnosis of early UCTD with central nerve system (CNS) involvement. After low dose corticosteroid and azathioprine therapy, the patient's symptoms, abnormalities in immunologic tests and cerebral radiologic examinations were all greatly improved within a short duration.

Conclusions: This is the first report of intracranial lesion as onset symptom in a patient with early UCTD. Our case suggested that central nerve system (CNS) involvement could be the onset symptom in early UCTD, and should be recognized quickly with exclusion of other causative factors in the differential diagnosis. Prompt and adequate treatment with low-dose steroid and immunosuppressive drugs could improve the prognosis of both early UCTD and CNS involvement.

Keywords: Intracranial lesion, Undifferentiated connective tissue disease

Background

The term undifferentiated connective tissue disease (UCTD) refers to unclassifiable systemic autoimmune diseases, which share some clinical and serological manifestations with definite connective tissue diseases (CTDs) but not fulfilling any of the existing classification criteria for certain CTDs, such as systemic lupus erythematosus (SLE), systemic sclerosis (SSc), Sjögren syndrome (SS), dermatomyositis/polymyositis (DM/PM), mixed connective tissue diseases (MCTD) and rheumatoid arthritis (RA) [1]. It is now widely accepted that UCTD represent a distinct clinical entity including two subgroups: stable UCTD and early UCTD. Among these UCTD patients, severe organ involvements (such as heart, renal or neurological manifestations) are rarely reported [2–4]. Here, we firstly described a female early UCTD patient with intracranial lesions as the onset and main clinical manifestations in order to improve the diagnosis and treatment of the disease.

Case presentation

A 51-year-old Chinese female experienced progressive left leg weakness for 14 days before hospitalizing in our department. At the onset of the symptom, the patient

* Correspondence: zw711711@hotmail.com; lizhuyi@fmmu.edu.cn
†Equal contributors
Department of Neurology, Tangdu Hospital, Fourth Military Medical University, Xi'an City, Shaanxi Province 710038, China

presented dizziness and left lower limb weakness, and the symptom was still progressive, even after treatment as brain ischemia. Then the patient was transferred to our department. On admission, the physical examinations were all normal, and neurologic examination disclosed that proximal and distal muscle strength of left lower limb was 3/5 by manual muscles testing (MTT). The superficial and deep sensory examinations were completed by cotton swab, tuning fork and pinprick, and all sensory modalities and tendon reflexes were normal, and pathologic reflexes were negative. Cranial nerve function and the mental examination were normal. No family history of neurological disease and metabolic-related disorders had been previously documented, according to her medical records.

Blood analysis showed erythrocyte sedimentation rate of 40 mm/h (normal <20 mm/h) and C-reactive protein of 55.1 mg/L (normal <3.0 mg/L). In the tests for autoantibody, the antinuclear antibody (ANA) was positive, and the titer was greatly elevated to 1:10,000. But, antibodies to double stranded DNA, Sm, Ro, La, Scl-7, Jo-1, ACA, ribonucleoprotein, nucleosomes, and histone were negative. Rheumatoid factor, anti-CCP antibody, and ANCA were also negative. The values for blood glucose, liver function, renal function, electrolytes, serum folate, vitamin B12, homocysteine, lactic acid, tumor markers, thyroid function and associated antibodies, C3, and C4 were their normal ranges. Tests for virus, syphilis, HIV, NMOSD, MS (Additional file 1) and autoimmune encephalitis were all negative.

Lumbar puncture was performed and showed a normal intracranial pressure; the biochemical and hematologic tests of the cerebrospinal fluid (CSF) revealed a normal glucose, chloride and protein level; the white cell count was elevated 27 × 106/L with increasing percentage of lymphocyte 77.8%; and the CSF cultures for bacteria, viruses, and fungi were all negative.

Intracranial angiogram was normal (Fig. 1). Brain magnetic resonance imaging (MRI) revealed a lesion on right parietal lobe that was hypointensity on T1-weighted, hyperintensity on T2-weighted images, and high signal on FLAIR. There was slim contrast enhancement along the surface of swollen gyrus lesion after Gd-DTPA injection (10 mL/kg of body weight). MRS showed slightly decreased NAA and increased Cr and Cho peak on the right parietal lobe lesion compared to same region on normal left side (Fig. 2). Chest CT showed normal. The patient declined a cerebral biopsy.

Based on a series of examination, the patient was diagnosed as having early undifferentiated connective tissue disease (UCTD). From the 5th hospital day, 10 mg of intravenous dexamethasone was administered for 14 days, and changed to oral prednisolone (30 mg/day) with gradual tapering (5 mg/month). At the same time, the patient was placed on maintenance therapy with azathioprine (50 mg/day). After treatment for 2 weeks, the symptom of left lower limb weakness was almost recovered. The patient was discharged and came in for regular visits. Follow-up MRI, performed at 6 weeks after the initial glucocorticoid therapy, showed much regression of lesion and enhancement on right parietal lobe. MRS showed normal NAA, Cr and Cho peak of previous lesion on the right parietal lobe compared to same region on normal left side (Fig. 3). Blood analysis showed normal erythrocyte sedimentation rate of 7 mm/h and C-reactive protein of 1.57 mg/L. The titer of antinuclear antibody decreased to 1:1000. Lumbar puncture and tests of the CSF showed normal intracranial pressure, glucose, chloride and protein level; the white cell count (WBC) was 2 × 106/L with normal percentage of lymphocyte 64.1%. The patient was continuously administrated with a low dosage of azathioprine and gradually tapering prednisolone, and followed up regularly.

Discussion and conclusions

The concept of undifferentiated connective tissue disease (UCTD) was put forward for the first time by LeRoy in 1980, and considered to be the early stage of connective tissue disease (CTD), which could be developed into a

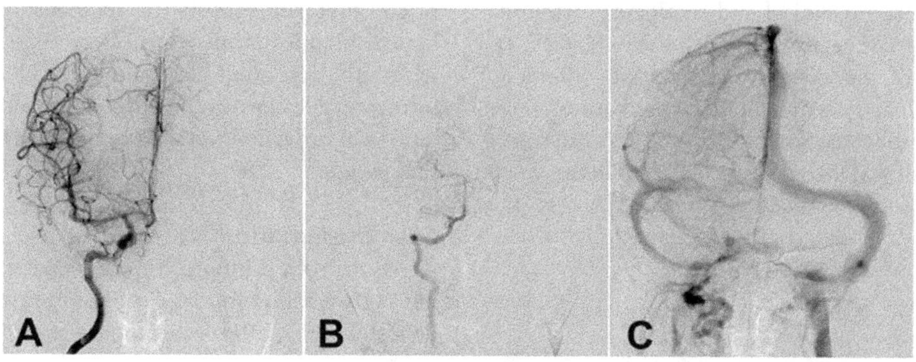

Fig. 1 Intracranial angiogram on 3rd hospital day before treatment showed that *right* internal carotid artery **a**, *right* vertebral artery and basilar artery **b**, and all venous sinuses **c** were normal

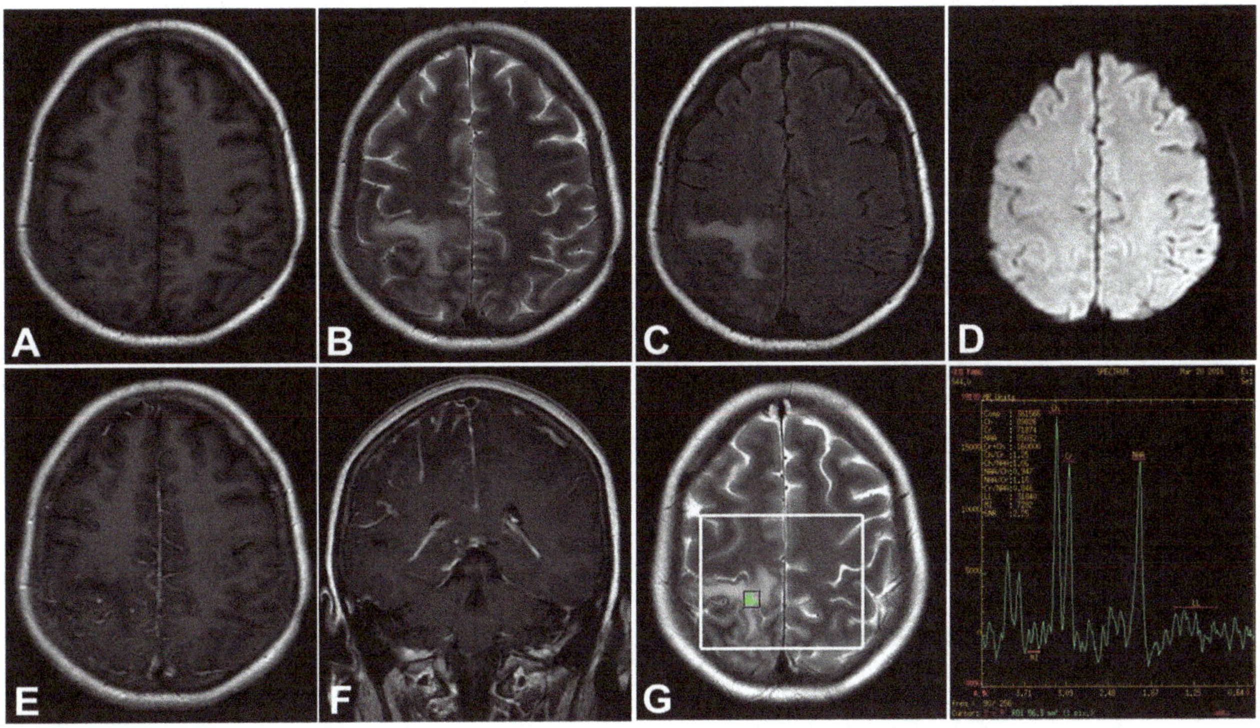

Fig. 2 MRI on the 1st hospital day showed a lesion on *right* parietal lobe that was hypointensity on T1-weighted (**a**), hyperintensity on T2-weighted images (**b**), high signal on FLAIR (**c**), and normal signal on DWI (**d**). MRI enhancement showed contrast enhancement along the surface of swollen gyrus lesion (**e**) and (**f**). MRS showed slightly decreased NAA and increased Cr and Cho peak on the lesion (**g**)

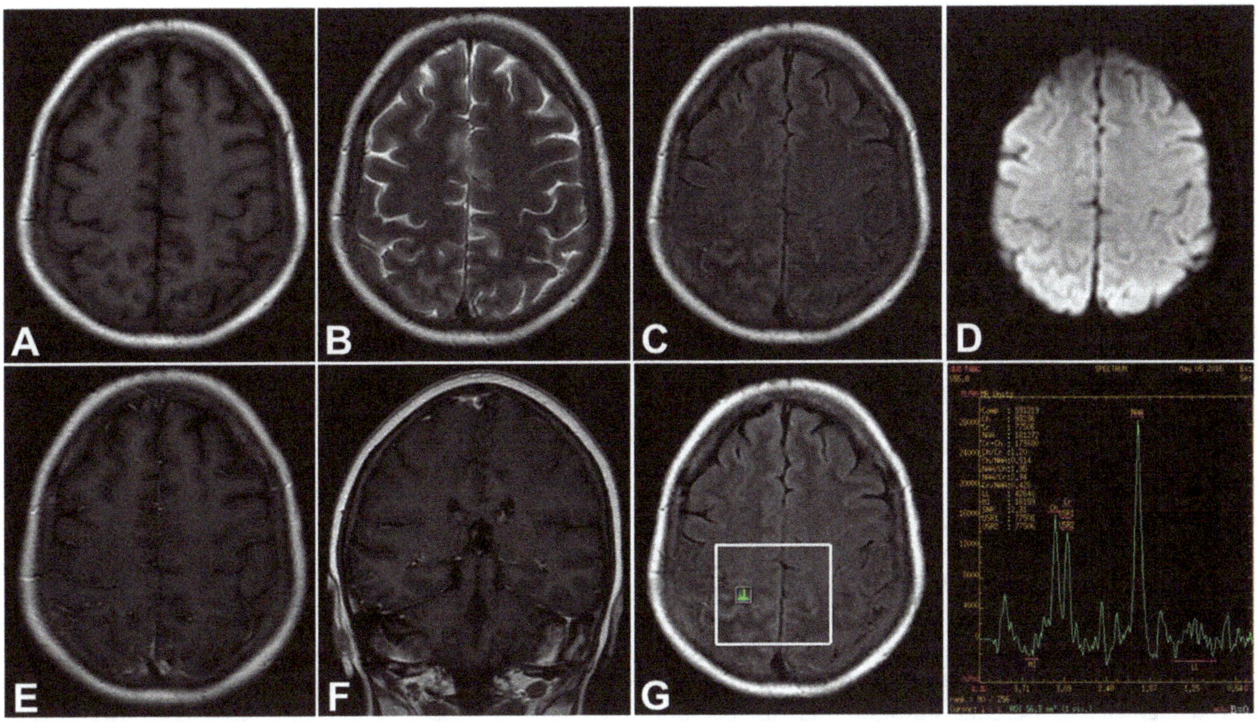

Fig. 3 After treatment for 6 weeks, follow-up MRI showed nearly complete regression of lesion on *right* parietal lobe on T1-weighted (**a**), T2-weighted images (**b**), FLAIR (**c**), and still normal signal on DWI (**d**). MRI enhancement showed that the previous slim contrast enhancement almost disappeared (**e**) and (**f**). MRS also showed normal NAA, Cr and Cho peak of previous lesion (**g**)

specific kind of CTD, or maintained in undifferentiated state without progression [5]. After a long-lasting scientific debate, it is widely accepted that UCTD represent a distinct clinical entity with peculiar clinical findings; the proposed preliminary classification criteria for UCTD include: (1) at least one clinical manifestation of CTDs, (2) positive ANA results, and (3) disease duration of at least three years. However, the criteria may have limitation in making diagnosis, directing treatment and estimating prognosis of those patients with short disease duration no more than 3 years. In fact, although epidemiological data are not available in the literature, up to 50% of the patients with an undifferentiated CTD of less than one year of duration have been reported [6]. Recently, researchers have distinguished two different conditions of UCTD with variable disease course and prognosis, "stable UCTD" and "early UCTD". Among the division, the so called "stable UCTD" refers to the condition that is up to the traditional criteria as described before and clinically stable over time only with necessarily mild therapeutic intervention. Moreover, the "early UCTD" refers to those patients with recent onset of symptoms and unclassifiable clinical picture which are very likely to progress into a definite CTD in the short time, and it has a crucial clinical importance in term of treatment decision making and disease monitoring [2].

Researches about stable UCTD have revealed that Raynaud's phenomenon, artralgias/arthritis, skin rash and mild cytopenias are the most frequent onset manifestations; the serological autoantibody profile frequently presents single specificity with ANA positivity highly ranging from 58–90% [1, 7–9]; and after low-dose corticosteroids and immunosuppressive drugs treatment, 70% stable UCTD patients will be maintained in undifferentiated state without progression [6]. Among these stable UCTD patients, severe organ involvements such as heart, renal or neurological manifestations were rarely reported. As far as we know, only 3 cases of CNS involvement in stable UCTD have been reported. Among these cases, two of them were hypertrophic cranial pachymeningitis (HCP), and the other one was reversible posterior leucoencephalopathy syndrome (RPLS). After symptomatic treatment, low-dose corticosteroid or immunosuppression treatment such as azathioprine or methotrexate, all the patients' symptoms and radiologic abnormalities of brain were improved [10–12]. However, up to now, there is still lack of definite researches about clinical course, prognosis and organ involvement of early UCTD.

In ours case, the increased erythrocyte sedimentation rate, C-reactive protein and titer of antinuclear antibody suggested an active systemic autoimmune disease, but the patient did not meet the existing classification criteria for a certain connective tissue disease, and the disease duration was no more than 3 years. Therefore, the patient was diagnosed as having early UCTD. The lesion on right parietal lobe, presenting hypointensity on MRI T1, hyperintensity on T2 and high signal on FLAIR, was responsible for the onset symptom of left lower limb weakness. The patient declined a cerebral biopsy, but according to the normal intracranial angiogram, the results of CSF study, MRI enhancement and MRS examination, we could exclude the possibility of stroke, cerebral venous sinus thrombosis, NMOSD, MS, autoimmune encephalitis, intracranial infections, and malignant tumors as cause of the lesion. Moreover, examinations in the CNS showed slightly elevated white cell count with increasing percentage of lymphocyte in CSF, and slim contrast enhancement along the surface of swollen gyrus lesion in MRI. Thus, we presumed CNS involvement in this early UCTD patient. After treatment of low-dose corticosteroid and azathioprine, the symptom of left lower limb weakness was almost recovered, abnormalities of immunologic tests and neuroimaging were also greatly improved within a short duration. To our knowledge, the case we described here is the first report of CNS involvement as onset manifestations in a patient with early UCTD.

In summary, CNS involvement may be the onset symptom in early UCTD, and must be recognized early in the presence of systemic blood exam alterations such as high ESR, CRP and ANA, because of good prognosis with prompt and adequate treatment. Diagnosis is difficult as all causative factors must be excluded, and cerebral biopsy is not always feasible. Low-dose steroid and immunosuppressive therapy seems to be effective to the CNS damages in early UCTD, and long-term follow-up is also necessary to investigate the prognosis of early UCTD and CNS involvement.

Abbreviations

ANA: Antinuclear antibody; CNS: Central nerve system; CSF: Cerebrospinal Fluid; CTD: Connective tissue disease; MRI: Magnetic resonance imaging; MS: Multiple sclerosis; NMOSD: Neuromyelitis optica spectrum disorder; UCTD: Undifferentiated connective tissue disease

Acknowledgments

We thank the patient and her son for their collaboration.

Funding

This work was supported by research grants from the National Natural Science Foundation of China (81371209), the Natural Science Foundation Research Project of Shaanxi Province (S2014JC9313), Tangdu hospital innovation development foundation (2016LYJ007).

Authors' contributions

Study concept and design: WZ, ZL. Acquisition of data: YD, CL, WZ, ZL. CSF analysis: DZ. Intracranial angiogram: JL. All authors read and approved the final manuscript.

Competing interests

The authors declare that they have no competing interests.

References

1. Mosca M, Neri R, Bombardieri S. Undifferentiated connective tissue diseases (UCTD): a review of the literature and a proposal for preliminary classification criteria. Clin Exp Rheumatol. 1999;17:615–20.
2. Mosca M, Tani C, Vagnani S, et al. The diagnosis and classification of undifferentiated connective tissue diseases. J Autoimmun. 2014;48–49:50–2.
3. Bodolay E, Csiki Z, Szekanecz Z, et al. Five-year follow-up of 665 Hungarian patients with undifferentiated connective tissue disease (UCTD). Clin Exp Rheumatol. 2003;21:313–20.
4. Mosca M, Tani C, Carli L, et al. Analysis of the evolution of UCTD to defined CTD after a long term follow-up. Clin Exp Rheumatol. 2013;31:471.
5. LeRoy EC, Maricq HR, Kahaleh MB. Undifferentiated connective tissue syndromes. Arthritis Rheum. 1980;23:341–3.
6. Mosca M, Tani C, Bombardieri S. A case of undifferentiated connective tissue disease: is it a distinct clinical entity? Nat Clin Pract Rheumatol. 2008; 4(6):328–32.
7. Mosca M, Tani C, Talarico R, et al. Undifferentiated connective tissue diseases (UCTD): simplified systemic autoimmune diseases. Autoimmun Rev. 2011;10:256–8.
8. Mosca M, Tavoni A, Neri R, et al. Undifferentiated connective tissue diseases: the clinical and serological profiles in 91 patients followed for at least 1 year. Lupus. 1998;7:95–100.
9. Mosca M, Neri R, Bencivelli W, et al. Undifferentiated connective tissue disease: analysis of 83 patients with a minimum follow up of 5 years. J Rheumatol. 2002;29:2345–9.
10. Lampropoulos CE, Zain M, Jan W, et al. Hypertrophic pachymeningitis and undifferentiatedd connective tissue disease: a case report and review of the literature. Clin Rheumatol. 2006;25:399–401.
11. Kim JH, Joo YB, Kim J, et al. A case of hypertrophic cranial pachymeningitis presenting with scleritis in a patient withundifferentiated connective tissue disease. J Korean Med Sci. 2010;25:966–9.
12. Singh S, Balakrishnan C, Mangat G, et al. Reversible posterior leucoencephalopathy syndrome in a patient with undifferentiated connective tissue disease. Scand J Rheumatol. 2006;35:248–9.

Sex differences underlying orofacial varicella zoster associated pain in rats

Crystal Stinson[1†], Mohong Deng[3†], Michael B Yee[2], Larry L. Bellinger[1], Paul R. Kinchington[2] and Phillip R. Kramer[1*]

Abstract

Background: Most people are initially infected with varicella zoster virus (VZV) at a young age and this infection results in chickenpox. VZV then becomes latent and reactivates later in life resulting in herpes zoster (HZ) or "shingles". Often VZV infects neurons of the trigeminal ganglia to cause ocular problems, orofacial disease and occasionally a chronic pain condition termed post-herpetic neuralgia (PHN). To date, no model has been developed to study orofacial pain related to varicella zoster. Importantly, the incidence of zoster associated pain and PHN is known to be higher in women, although reasons for this sex difference remain unclear. Prior to this work, no animal model was available to study these sex-differences. Our goal was to develop an orofacial animal model for zoster associated pain which could be utilized to study the mechanisms contributing to this sex difference.

Methods: To develop this model VZV was injected into the whisker pad of rats resulting in IE62 protein expression in the trigeminal ganglia; IE62 is an immediate early gene in the VZV replication program.

Results: Similar to PHN patients, rats showed retraction of neurites after VZV infection. Treatment of rats with gabapentin, an agent often used to combat PHN, ameliorated the pain response after whisker pad injection. Aversive behavior was significantly greater for up to 7 weeks in VZV injected rats over control inoculated rats. Sex differences were also seen such that ovariectomized and intact female rats given the lower dose of VZV showed a longer affective response than male rats. The phase of the estrous cycle also affected the aversive response suggesting a role for sex steroids in modulating VZV pain.

Conclusions: These results suggest that this rat model can be utilized to study the mechanisms of 1) orofacial zoster associated pain and 2) the sex differences underlying zoster associated pain.

Keywords: Post-herpetic neuralgia, Shingles, Chickenpox, Trigeminal ganglia, Orofacial

Background

Varicella zoster virus (VZV) is a human herpesvirus that infects a majority of the unvaccinated population worldwide. While recovery from varicella "chickenpox" occurs with lifelong immunity the virus persists in a latent state in the nuclei of neurons within sensory and autonomic ganglia across the entire neuro-axis. VZV chromatin remains in the infected cells (extrachromosomal) but viral protein expression and virus production remain repressed [1–4]. However, reactivation from latency occurs in about one third of VZV positive individuals to cause herpes zoster (HZ), with the incidence of HZ increasing with age and declining immune status. The skin rash of HZ is often large but geographically restricted to a dermatome infiltrated by one or two specific ganglia. Reactivation is accompanied by extensive intra-ganglionic spread, infection of multiple neurons and numerous inflammatory and physiological processes that contribute to the development of pain. Almost all HZ is associated with acute pain, with up to 90% of HZ patients seeking prescription level pain relief [5]. However, some 30% of HZ patients report a chronic pain state termed post herpetic neuralgia (PHN), defined as pain lasting more than 3 months after the resolution of the skin lesions [6–8]. A fraction of PHN patients may suffer pain more than one year after other disease symptoms dissipate [9].

* Correspondence: pkramer@tamhsc.edu
†Equal contributors
[1]Department of Biomedical Sciences, Texas A&M University College of Dentistry, 3302 Gaston Avenue, Dallas, TX 75246, USA
Full list of author information is available at the end of the article

PHN is debilitating, difficult to treat, and can have secondary long term consequences that can greatly affect quality of life. In the absence of the current HZ vaccine approximately 1 million people annually in the US and about 5% of the total population will suffer from PHN [9–11]. The majority of HZ sufferers are age 60 years or older [12, 13]. Given that the number of people 60 years of age or older is one of the fastest growing and is expected to double in the next 50 years [9], HZ and the associated pain will be an ever increasing problem in the future. While the HZ vaccine reduces the incidence of HZ by 51% and PHN by 68%, the vaccine remains to be widely used largely due to cost/reimbursement issues, reluctance to vaccination, and ignorance of both the target population and their physicians. [11]. Even if every candidate receives the vaccine (which is far from being achieved) the US would still have some half million HZ cases each year with many suffering from PHN. As such, better prevention and therapy for both zoster and PHN are an unmet need.

It has been difficult to model HZ and PHN because no animal model shows reactivation of latent VZV. In general, VZV is considered human specific, for reasons not yet clear. However it has been shown that VZV injected into the footpad of either Wistar or Sprague Dawley rats results in measurable hypersensitivity that is similar to that in humans with PHN [14–20]. The footpad animal model has been developed as a platform for one, mechanistic studies of chronic pain after VZV infection of dorsal root ganglia and two, for drug evaluation focused on HZ associated pain relief [20, 21]. Treatment of these animals with antivirals, opioids or NSAIDS mirrors HZ patients treated with these same drugs, in that, zoster associated pain does not respond to antivirals, but does respond to treatment with gabapentin or sodium channel blockers [16, 17, 20, 21].

Given that the rat footpad model has been used to study the mechanism by which VZV associated pain develops and can be used for pre-clinical screening of analgesic drugs [17, 21] we considered whether the model can be extended to orofacial pain that follows VZV reactivation in the trigeminal ganglia. Extension of the model to the orofacial region would be significant because the trigeminal ganglia of human cadavers have the highest latent VZV load, and up to 1 in 5 HZ cases occurs in the orofacial or naso-ocular region [22, 23]. Importantly, females report HZ associated pain 3.75 times more often than men, and HZ associated pain has been reported to be 36% higher in females [24, 25]. The basis for this disparity is not understood. Currently, neither the orofacial effects nor the sex differences have been determined in any zoster associated pain model. In this report, an animal model for zoster associated orofacial pain was characterized that could be utilized first, to study the mechanisms of HZ associated pain in the orofacial region and second, to study the mechanisms resulting in women reporting HZ pain more often than men.

Methods

Cells and viruses

VZV Parent of Oka (pOka), a varicella isolate that was the parent strain used to derive the current VZV vaccine strain, was used in all this work. pOka VZV was previously shown to induce chronic pain indices in the rat model [15]. Virus was used at less than 12 passes beyond receipt from M. Takahashi (Osaka University, Japan) and propagated as detailed previously [26, 27] on the VZV permissive MeWo human cell line (ATCC, Manassas, VA). Cells and virus were grown in Minimal Essential Media (MEM) supplemented with 10% fetal bovine serum (FBS) and antibiotic and antimycotic mixture (Sigma, St. Louis, MO). VZV was prepared to high titer as previously detailed [15] on confluent monolayers of MeWo cells infected at ~0.1 plaque forming units (pfu)/cell. Virus infected cells incubated at 35 °C for 48–72 h post infection were harvested by trypsin digestion, and optimal VZV cell viability was maintained by slow freezing aliquots in MEM containing 20% FBS and 10% dimethyl sulfoxide (Sigma, St. Louis, MO), followed by storage under liquid nitrogen. Virus titers of frozen stocks were assessed by an infectious center assay. Uninfected cell equivalents were prepared using similar treatments. All virus and cellular stocks were provided by Dr. Kinchington's laboratory.

Animal studies

All work with animals was approved by the Texas A&M University College of Dentistry Institutional Animal Care and Use Committee. Male and female Sprague-Dawley or Long Evans rats (280–300 g) were purchased from Envigo (Indianapolis, IN) and kept on a 14:10 light/dark cycle. The rats were given food and water ad libitum. After a 4 day acclimation period, experiments were carried out in accordance with NIH regulations on animal use. Vaginal smears were performed daily on female rats to determine the stage of the estrous cycle. The body weights were recorded weekly. Six experiments using different batches of rats (see Table 1) were completed to measure behavior after injection of a high (1900 pfu/μl) or low (650 or 360 pfu/μl) dose of VZV (pOka strain). Male Sprague-Dawley rats were used in the experiments unless otherwise indicated.

Training for thermal and mechanical hypersensitivity assay

In the first experiment the animals were trained to obtain reward using the orofacial test chamber from Ugo Basile (Italy) [28–30]. The reward was a sweetened condensed milk mixture, 100 ml milk and 200 ml water. Drinking time was measured by using an infrared beam

Table 1 Experiments completed for each study (i.e. set of animals)

Study	Experiment	Groups	Number of animals (male Sprague Dawley rats unless otherwise indicated)
Study #1	Thermal and mechanical hypersensitivity assay (Figure 3). Neurite retraction study using PGP 9.5 (*n* = 3/group randomly selected, Figure 2).	Mewo (control) Poka (VZV)	*n* = 10 *n* = 10
Study #2	Place escape/avoidance paradigm (Figure 4). VZV infection detected with IE62 marker (Figure 1).	PBS (vehicle) Mewo (control) Poka (VZV virus)	*n* = 6 *n* = 6 *n* = 6
Study #3	Gabapentin assay (Figure 5).	Mewo/vehicle Mewo/gabapentin Poka/vehicle Poka/gabapentin	*n* = 5 *n* = 5 *n* = 5 *n* = 5
Study #4	Sex differences study comparing males and females (Figure 6).	Mewo/female Mewo/male Poka/female Poka/male	*n* = 24 *n* = 7–15 *n* = 25 *n* = 7–15
Study #5	OVX females as compared to males (Sprague Dawley and Long Evans, Figure 7). VZV infection detected with IE62 marker (Sprague-Dawley rats, no figure).	Mewo/male Mewo/female Mewo/OVX female Poka/male Poka/female Poka/OVX female	*n* = 5 *n* = 4 *n* = 4 *n* = 7 *n* = 6 *n* = 6 *n* = 5 (Long Evans) for all treatment groups
Study #6	Female estrous cycle study (Figure 8).	Mewo diestrus Mewo proestrus/estrus Poka diestrus Poka proestrus/estrus	$n \geq 8$ $n \geq 8$ $n \geq 8$ $n \geq 8$

that detects when the animal has placed their nose into the spigot area to access the drinking supply. No thermal testing or filament testing was performed during the initial one week training period where the animals were placed in the chambers daily for 10 min to obtain a reward. No filaments or thermal coils were present in the training period. Next, the pre-testing training period continued another two weeks and included a daily 12 h fast followed by 10 min of familiarization with the chamber environment with the reward inaccessible and 10 min of active testing with the reward accessible. Training was successful when animals consistently drank milk for 300 ± 50 s out of a 600 s testing period with thermal coils or filaments in place at the spigot opening. All testing was done in the beginning of the dark phase with red lights.

To measure thermal and mechanical hypersensitivity induced by VZV the animals were anesthetized briefly with 2% isoflurane using a 2 l per minute flow of air, the whisker pad of Sprague Dawley rats were then inoculated with uninfected MeWo cells, or the same number of MeWo cells infected with (1900 pfu/μl) VZV by injecting a 100 μl volume subcutaneously. The animals were mobile within 5 min of the injection. The whisker pad was chosen as the injection site because it has a large number of sensory terminals that would allow for infection of VZV. Testing was completed either before the injection (pre-injection) or one week after injection. Testing continued once every seven days thereafter. For the thermal test the coils of the test chamber were set to 45 degrees Celsius. For the filament test, twelve nickel/titanium/chromium wires 0.16 mm (0.006″) in diameter were placed evenly around a circular opening 3.5 cm in diameter. Each wire projected 1.5 cm into the center of the opening. The weekly test schedule assessed baseline responses without either a thermal coil or a filament on the first day of each week, followed by thermal testing the following day and filament testing on the next day. Testing was done for a 6 week period.

Place escape/avoidance paradigm (PEAP) testing in male rats

In a second experiment behavioral responses were measured using the PEAP test. Testing was completed by a tester blinded to the treatment. For this experiment the whisker pad of a second group of male rats was injected with a high dose of VZV (1900 pfu/μl), or equivalent control MeWo cells or PBS (100 μl volume). Rats were anesthetized as described previously for the injection. At 7 days post inoculation the animals were placed in a 30 cm X 30 cm X 30 cm acrylic box in which half the box was covered in black cloth. This test chamber was modeled from the PEAP test performed and detailed by the Fuchs lab [31]. PEAP testing has been used in inflammatory and neuropathic pain models, used in both sexes and various strains and ages of rats as a means of measuring affective aspects of pain [31–37]. Each individual rat was placed into the chamber; rodents being nocturnal prefer the dark side of the chamber. The study was then initiated by stimulating the face with a 60 g filament every 15 s; rats on the dark side of the chamber receive a stimulus at the injected side, whereas rats with their head on the clear side of the chamber were stimulated on the contralateral non-injected side. The region receiving the stimulus was in the region below the eye and caudal to the whisker pad, which is innervated by the second branch of the trigeminal ganglia. Because sensory neurons of the second branch also innervate the whisker pad, we expected sensitivity of the face around the eye [38]. The time spent on the dark side of the box was recorded in 5 min bins and testing was performed for a total of 30 min on the test day. Testing was performed one day a week and continued for 8 weeks.

VZV injection in male rats to investigate analgesia efficacy

A third group of male rats were injected at the whisker pad with either a low dose of VZV (360 pfu/μl) or control MeWo cells. One week after VZV injection the rats were given a 3.5 ml gavage of either 0.9% saline, or 50 mg/ml gabapentin (Amneal Pharmaceuticals, Branchburg, NJ). PEAP testing was performed 30 min after gavage. The effect of analgesics can be undetectable "swamped out" if the nociceptive response is too great thus, the lowest dose of VZV known to elicit a behavioral response was implemented before administration of gabapentin.

Sex differences in VZV induced aversive behavior

In a fourth set of studies intact male and intact female rats were injected with 650 pfu/μl of VZV or equivalent control MeWo cells. PEAP testing was performed once a week over a six week period.

Compare VZV induced aversive behavior of ovariectomized females to intact males

Female rats were ovariectomized to simulate menopause because a majority of women with HZ pain will be in a post-menopausal state and post-menopausal women report HZ associated pain more than older men. In this fifth study intact male, intact female and OVX females from two strains of rat were utilized (Sprague Dawley and Long Evans rats). Sprague Dawley rats were inoculated with 650 pfu/μl of VZV and Long Evans rats were inoculated with 360 pfu/μl of VZV. PEAP testing was performed 7 days after injection and continued once a week for 2 weeks. Long Evans rats were reported by Envigo to be less docile than Sprague Dawley rats and thus, the Long Evans rats were injected with a lower dose of VZV as compared to the Sprague Dawley rats in Study #5. This lower dose was expected to compensate for the greater inherent activity of Long Evans rats during the behavioral testing.

Ovariectomy surgery

Animals were anesthetized with 2% isoflurane using a 2 l per minute flow of air. The anesthetized female was placed in ventral recumbency with their tail toward the surgeon. The dorsal surgical area was shaved and swabbed with surgical scrub. A short dorsal midline skin incision was made halfway between the caudal edge of the ribcage and the base of the tail. An abdominal muscle wall incision was made lateral to the spine to provide access to the peritoneal cavity. The ovary and the oviduct were exteriorized through the muscle wall incision. A sterile silk ligature was placed around the oviduct. Each ovary and part of the oviduct was removed with a single cut through the oviduct near the ovary. The remaining tissue was replaced into the peritoneal cavity and the opening sutured. The ovary on the contralateral side was removed in a similar manner and the animal was given a 2 mg/kg dose of nalbuphine.

Compare VZV induced aversive behavioral response over estrous cycle

In a sixth set of studies vaginal smears were taken immediately after PEAP testing each week using the intact females from the fourth study. The groups were then divided based on the phase of the estrous cycle.

Immuno-fluorescent staining

After testing for hypersensitivity or aversive behavior the rats were sacrificed and perfused for immunohistochemistry. Whisker pad tissue was collected from the first study and trigeminal ganglia were collected from the second study and fifth study (see Table 1). Because VZV infection, as determined by the presence of IE62, showed greater levels of IE62 at 1 month and 18 months post infection versus one week post infection [39]. Thus, we expected greater VZV infection and neurite retraction in the first and second studies that were of longer duration. Tissue in study five was analyzed to determine if the sex differences were due to differences in VZV infection.

After administering 100 mg/kg ketamine/10 mg/kg xylazine the rats were perfused with 9% sucrose followed by 4% paraformaldehyde. Fixed tissues were stored in 25% sucrose, frozen, cryo-sectioned and the 20 μm sections placed on Histobond slides (VWR international, Radnor, PA). The tissue was then blocked with a PBS solution containing 5% normal goat serum and 0.3% Triton-X 100 for 2 h at room temperature. The slides were incubated in a primary antibody solution overnight at 4 °C. Primary antibodies consisted of a 1:200 dilution of the mouse monoclonal IE62 antibody (Acris Antibodies Inc., San Diego, CA) and a 1:250 dilution of the rabbit monoclonal NeuN antibody (Abcam, San Francisco, CA); or a 1:500 dilution of the rabbit polyclonal PGP9.5 antibody (BioRad, Raleigh, NC). Primary antibodies were diluted with PBS, 5% BSA and 0.3% Triton X-100. After incubation in primary antibody the slides were rinsed three times in PBS and Triton-X 100 for a total of 45 min and placed for 2 h in a 1:500 dilution of secondary antibody in PBS and 0.3% Triton X-100. Secondary antibodies included a mixture of goat anti-mouse 568 and goat anti-rabbit 488 1:500 dilution (Invitrogen, Carlsbad, CA). For the PGP9.5 antibody staining a 1:500 dilution of a goat anti-rabbit 568 secondary was used. After rinsing the slides three times in PBS for a total of 45 min, the slides were then mounted with Fluoromount-G mounting medium containing Hoechst 33,342 stain (Electron Microscopy Sciences, Hatfield, PA). The fluorescent signal was imaged using a Nikon fluorescent microscope and NIS-Elements imaging software and a Photometrics CoolSnap K4 CCD camera (Roper Scientific, Inc., Duluth, GA).

Cell counting

Quantitation of IE62 staining was completed by a blinded reviewer counting the number of IE62 and NeuN positive cells within a randomly chosen 0.5 mm circular field near either the V3 branch or the V1/V2 branches. The neurons were primarily circular in shape and were divided into small C-fibers (<23 μm diameter), A-δ medium-sized (23–32 μm diameter) and A-α/β large neurons (32 > μm diameter) based on findings from the dorsal root ganglia [40]. Or the counts for all NeuN positive cells were combined. Three randomly chosen trigeminal ganglia sections were analyzed for each animal. Three animals were randomly chosen from each treatment group.

Measurement of neurite infiltration was performed as recently detailed [15]. Sections were counted for PGP9.5 positive neurites in coronal whisker pad sections, and were determined by a reviewer blinded to the treatment group. All PGP9.5 positive filaments that crossed the stratum basale/dermis border terminating between the surface of the skin and this border were counted; counts were determined along each mm of skin in the section. Neurite counts were completed by choosing a single random field ~5 mm in length along the stratum basale/dermis border on 10 randomly chosen sections taken from three randomly chosen animals from each treatment group. The number of filaments counted per mm of skin for each section was reported.

Statistical analysis

Data was analyzed with ANOVA and each time point was considered a replication. Dependent variables included the hypersensitivity measurements, PEAP data or cell counts and the independent variables were treatment, sex, cell size and trigeminal ganglia branch. When a significant effect was observed Bonferroni post-hoc tests were completed (Prism 5.04, GraphPad Software, La Jolla, CA, or Abstat, Anderson Bell Corp, Arvada CO). When two groups were being compared a two-tailed Mann-Whitney t-test was performed. The number of animals per group is outlined in Table 1.

Results

VZV accesses the trigeminal ganglia after whisker pad inoculation

In the virus injected group NeuN positive cells co-localize with IE62 within the trigeminal ganglia (Fig. 1a and b). IE62 is one of the first proteins translated from the VZV genome after infection. IE62 is an essential intermediate early gene that regulates expression of most VZV genes and the production of VZV localizes to both the nucleus and cytoplasm [41]. From the image the majority of IE62 was in the neuronal cell population but an analysis of other cell types was not completed. In these male rats IE62 staining was in neurons of all sizes (Fig. 1c) but there was a significantly greater percent of IE62 in the smaller neurons, $F(2, 68) = 8.02$, $p < 0.001$ and this staining was significantly greater in the region innervated by the V1/V2 branch, $F(1, 68) = 17.09$, $p < 0.001$ (Fig. 1d). Note that the whisker pad injection site is innervated by the V2 branch of the trigeminal ganglia. No IE62 stain was observed in the MeWo or PBS groups (data not shown).

As in humans virus infection induces neurite retraction

Skin biopsies of zoster patients suffering PHN have reduced peripheral innervation of the skin in comparison to zoster patients not suffering from PHN [42, 43]. This was also recently found in the rat footpad PHN model [44]. We therefore examined peripheral innervation of neurites at the whisker pad, using PGP9.5 staining to identify and visualize neurites (Fig. 2a, b). Rats showing hypersensitivity due to VZV injection (pOka strain) had a significantly reduced peripheral innervation of the whisker pad skin (Fig. 2c).

Development of pain behaviors after VZV inoculation of the whisker pad

Whisker pad injection of MeWo cells infected with VZV (pOka strain) revealed the development of some facial thermal hypersensitivity $F(1170) = 7.1$, $p < 0.01$ as compared to control uninfected cells (Fig. 3a). There was no significant interaction of treatment and time $F(1170) = 0.63$, $p = 7.2$. Testing for mechanical hypersensitivity showed a significant response over the 51 day testing period $F(1170) = 16.3$, $p < 0.0001$ with no significant interaction between treatment and time $F(1170) = 1.7$, $p = 0.1$ (Fig. 3b). Post-hoc

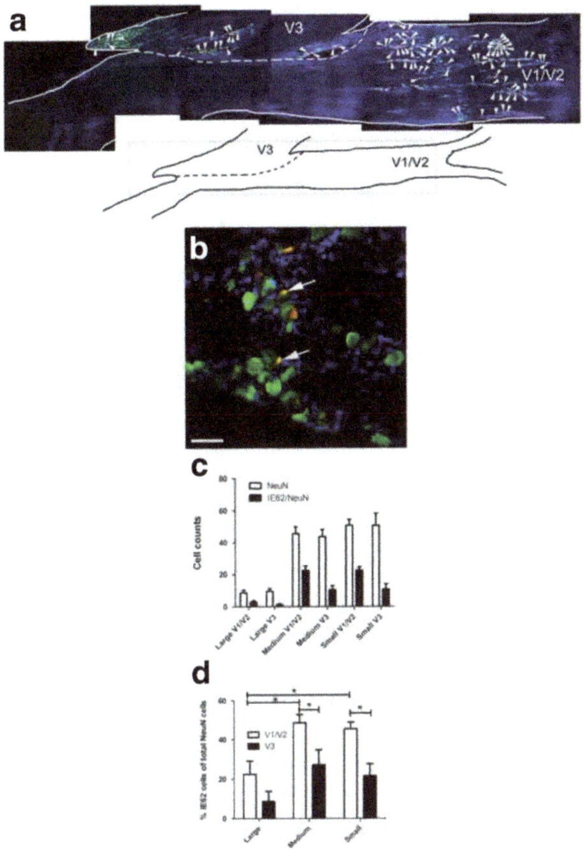

Fig. 1 The VZV marker IE62 was expressed in neurons of the trigeminal ganglia after injecting the whisker pad with virus. Sprague Dawley rats from the second study were injected with 100 μl of 1900 pfu/ μl VZV and tissues were collected 8 weeks following injection. Immunofluorescent detection of IE62 (*red*) and the neuronal marker NeuN (*green*) was completed on fixed frozen sections. *Blue* was nuclear Hoeschst stain. A sagittal section of the trigeminal ganglia is shown in panel **a** (low magnification) and in **b** (high magnification). In panel **a** the boxed area within the cartoon shows the stained region of the trigeminal ganglia. *Yellow cells* co-labeled with IE62 and NeuN in panel **a** are indicated by arrowheads. The branches of the trigeminal ganglia are labeled V1, V2 and V3. The V3 border is represented by a *dotted line*. In panel **b**, co-localization of NeuN and IE62 was shown in *yellow* and cells were indicated by *arrows*. Bar equals 50 μm. Panel **c** shows the total number of NeuN and double stained NeuN and IE62 positive cells in the trigeminal ganglia. Panel **d**, the percent of NeuN/IE62 double labeled cells in the total NeuN positive population was calculated for the neurons in different regions of the trigeminal ganglia. Small neurons were <23 μm in diameter, medium-sized neurons were 23–32 μm in diameter and large neurons were >32 μm in diameter. An asterisk indicates $p < 0.05$, $n = 6$. Values shown are the mean and SEM

testing revealed a significant difference between the pOka and MeWo treatment groups at days 15 and 23 (Fig. 3b).

In addition to measuring thermal and mechanical hypersensitivity a PEAP test was completed after whisker pad injection. In this assay, reduced time on the dark side during the stimulation phase indicates a greater affective pain response [31]. The response to VZV injection showed a remarkable difference that was significant for 7 weeks in comparison to control (Fig. 4). Significance was observed in week one, $F(2,75) = 19.9$, $p < 0.001$ (Fig. 4a); week two $F(2,75) = 196.1$, $p < 0.001$ (Fig. 4b); week three $F(2,75) = 31.3$, $p < 0.001$ (Fig 4c); week four $F(2,75) = 14.7$, $p < 0.001$ (Fig. 4d); week five $F(2,75) = 20.1$, $p < 0.001$ (Fig. 4e); week six $F(2,75) = 5.2$, $p < 0.05$ (Fig. 4f); and week seven $F(2,75) = 6.4$, $p < 0.01$ (Fig. 4g). The effect of virus in week eight was no longer significant, $F(2,75) = 2.4$, $p = 0.12$ (Fig, 4h). A significant interaction between the PBS, MeWo and virus pOka groups was observed in weeks two $F(10,75) = 5.8$, $p < 0.001$ (Fig. 4b) and three $F(10,75) = 2.5$, $p < 0.05$ (Fig. 4b). No significant interaction was observed in the other weeks (data not shown). Post hoc testing demonstrated a difference between the VZV and control groups for 7 out of the 8 weeks (Fig. 4a-g) but after eight weeks, there was no significant difference (Fig. 4h). These results strongly suggest the development of a virus specific pain response that did not develop after injecting uninfected cells or PBS. The PEAP assay was found to be more indicative and sensitive to changes resulting from virus injection and thus, the PEAP assay was continued throughout the rest of the following studies. During the first 5 min there was no significant difference in the time spent on the light side of the box when comparing groups in the first week to following weeks. This data suggests the animals do not recall the events of previous week when the 30 min testing periods are separated by a 7 day period of no testing.

VZV induced orofacial pain responds to gabapentin.

Seven days after injecting the whisker pad (360 pfu/μl VZV), gabapentin was administered by oral gavage. Injection of virus induced a pain response $F(2, 171)$, 13.41, $p < 0.01$ (Fig. 5), however gabapentin significantly $F(2, 171) = 6.75$, $p < 0.01$ reduced this response 30 min after administrating gabapentin. Post-hoc testing demonstrated that gabapentin significantly reduced the response at the 15, 20, 25 and 30 min testing periods (Fig. 5). A significant virus/drug interaction was observed $F(2, 171) = 7.77$, $p < 0.01$. No significant differences were observed between the MeWo/vehicle and MeWo/gabapentin treatment groups.

Sex based differences in the development of VZV induced pain at the whisker pad.

We carried out a comparison of the pain response in male and female rats to determine if sex differences exist in this virus model. One week after VZV injection, the PEAP response significantly increased in the virus versus MeWo control group $F(1, 395) = 19.1$, $p < 0.001$ (Fig. 6a) in both sexes of rats, and there was no significant difference between the sexes $F(1, 395) = 0.03$, $p = 0.85$. In contrast, two weeks $F(1, 443) = 12.1$, $p < 0.001$ and three weeks after

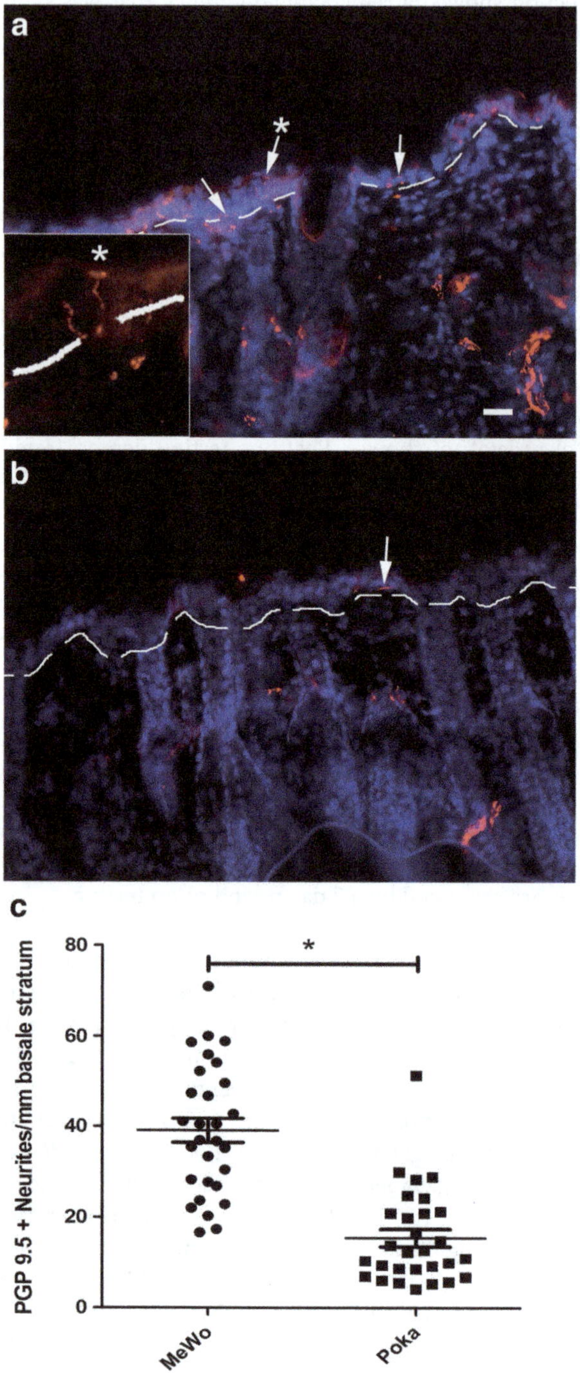

Fig. 2 VZV induced peripheral retraction of PGP9.5 positive neurites in the skin of the whisker pad. At six weeks after whisker pad injection with either MeWo cells (**a**) or MeWo cells containing VZV (**b**) male Sprague Dawley rats from the first study were sacrificed and the whisker pad skin processed for analyses. Ten 20 μm coronal sections were cut from each injected whisker pad. Representative images for MeWo injected (**a**) and pOka injected (**b**) rats are shown after staining with the PGP9.5 antibody (*red*), cell nuclei are stained *blue*. The border between the stratum basale and dermis is shown as a white dotted *line*. *Arrows* point to PGP9.5 positive filaments. Asterisk above the *arrow* indicates enlarged region within box. Bar = 50 μm. In panel **c**, each data point on the histogram shows the average number of PGP9.5 positive neurites per mm that terminate above or cross the basale/dermis border for each section. There were ten sections per rat and three rats per treatment group. An asterisk indicates $p < 0.05$. Mean and SEM are shown

injection $F(1, 473) = 11.0$, $p < 0.01$ there was a significantly greater pain response in the virus versus control group for the females but not the males (Fig. 6b and c). Moreover, the difference between male and female virus groups was significant in week two $F(1443) = 16.6$, $p < 0.001$ (Fig. 6b), three $F(1, 473) = 15.4$, $p < 0.001$ (Fig. 6c), four $F(1, 473) = 10.6$, $p < 0.01$ (Fig. 6d) and five $F(1, 473) = 8.4$, $p < 0.01$ (Fig. 6e). This sex difference was no longer significant in week 6 (Fig. 6f). No significant interaction between sex and virus was observed in week one and five but in week two, three and four a significant interaction was observed $F(1443) = 4.9$, $p < 0.05$, $F(1, 473) = 16.8$, $p < 0.001$, $F(1, 473) = 11.0$, $p < 0.01$, respectively.

Our data also show that a dose response to VZV occurred, in that a lower responses was detected after injecting a lower VZV dose of 650 pfu/ml (Fig 6) contrasted to the more significance responses seen with the higher VZV dose in Fig. 4 (1900 pfu/ μl). With the lower VZV dose, significant behavioral responses were much shorter in male rats, lasting for only one week (Fig. 6), while the pain response to a higher dose lasted for seven weeks (Fig. 4).

Pain was reduced in male rats versus female rats in a post-menopausal state

Because a majority of females suffering from PHN are post-menopausal and have low levels of plasma estradiol the pain response of ovariectomized females was compared to males. Sprague Dawley rats injected with virus (650 pfu/μl) showed a significant response $F(1, 144) = 117.0$, $p < 0.001$ in the first week but there was no significant sex difference (Fig. 7a). Two weeks after VZV infection the intact and OVX females showed significantly greater behavioral response than males (Fig. 7b). Long Evans rats also had a significant response to VZV infection (360 pfu/μl) in the first week $F(1, 144) = 74.5.0$, $p < 0.001$ and two weeks after VZV inoculation the intact female and OVX female rats had a significantly greater response than males (Fig. 7d).

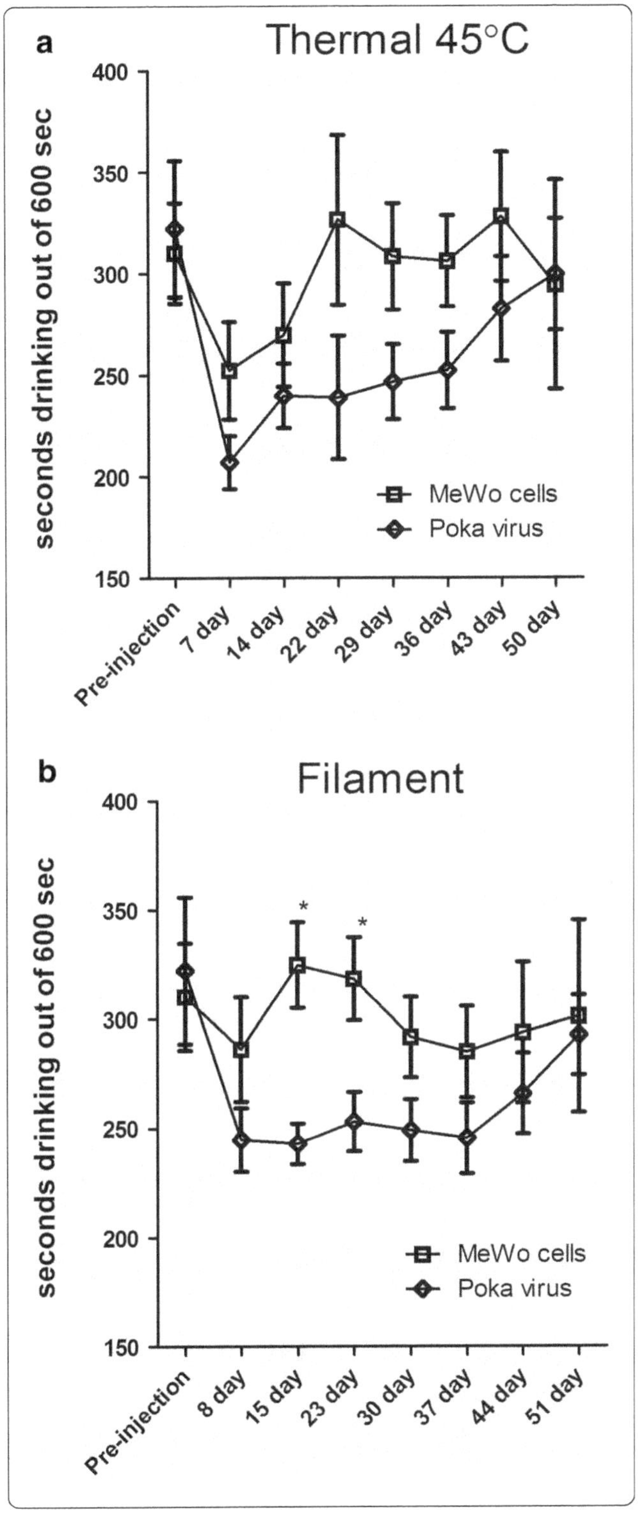

Fig. 3 Thermal and mechanical hypersensitivity increased after inoculating the whisker pad with VZV. Male Sprague Dawley rats were injected with either MeWo cells or MeWo cells infected with 1900 pfu/μl VZV. Testing was performed for 50–51 days post injection. Testing was completed using the orofacial test module from Ugo Basile. Thermal testing (panel **a**) was completed at 45 °C and filament testing (panel **b**) was performed with a custom circular opening containing 12 filaments. Fewer seconds drinking is an indicator of greater hyperalgesia or allodynia. Asterisk indicates a significant difference ($p < 0.05$) between the MeWo and VZV (pOka) treatment groups. There were 10 animals per treatment group and values are the mean and SEM

The increased pain response observed in female rats was not the result of greater viral infection

Two weeks of PEAP testing the animals were sacrificed and the ganglia isolated for immunostaining with the VZV marker IE62. The percentage of trigeminal ganglia neurons (NeuN positive) staining for the VZV marker IE62 was 16% ± 1.5 for the intact Sprague Dawley females, 10% ± 1.3 for the OVX females and 28% ± 3.7 for the males. The males had a significantly greater percentage of neurons staining for IE62 ($p > 0.05$) as compared to the females and there was no significant difference between the intact and OVX female groups.

Aversive behavioral response in cycling females after VZV injection

The behavioral response after VZV injection of the whisker pad was determined during the estrous cycle. In Fig. 8 the estrus and proestrus data were combined and the diestrus I and diestrus II (i.e., metestrus) data were combined because of their similar estradiol levels (data not shown). A significantly greater response was observed in rats with low estradiol (Diestrus pOka) versus the rats with higher plasma estradiol (Proestrus/estrus pOka) in week one $F(1, 281) = 5.8$, $p < 0.05$ (Fig. 8a, n≥8), two $F(1, 281)= 4.4$, $p<0.05$ (Fig. 8b), three $F(1, 281)= 61.6$, $p<0.001$ (Fig. 8c) and four $(1, 281)= 12.4$, $p<0.01$ (Fig. 8d). No significant cycle response was observed in weeks five and six (data not shown). During the first $F(1, 281)= 19.2$, $p<0.001$, second $F(1, 281)= 11.2$, $p<0.01$, third $F(1, 281)= 21.2$, $p<0.001$, fourth $F(1, 281)= 4.3$, $p<0.05$ week there was a significant virus effect. A significant interaction between cycle and virus treatment was observed in week two $F(1, 281)= 9.4$, $p<0.01$, three $F(1, 281)= 21.3$, $p<0.001$ and four $(1, 281)= 14.6$, $p<0.001$. Post-hoc testing indicated a significant decrease in the Diestrus pOka group versus the Diestrus MeWo group at the 15, 20, 25 and 30 min time points in weeks one, two, three, and four. No significant difference was observed in week five and six. These results indicate that the development of pain responses to VZV is influenced by the stage of the estrous cycle.

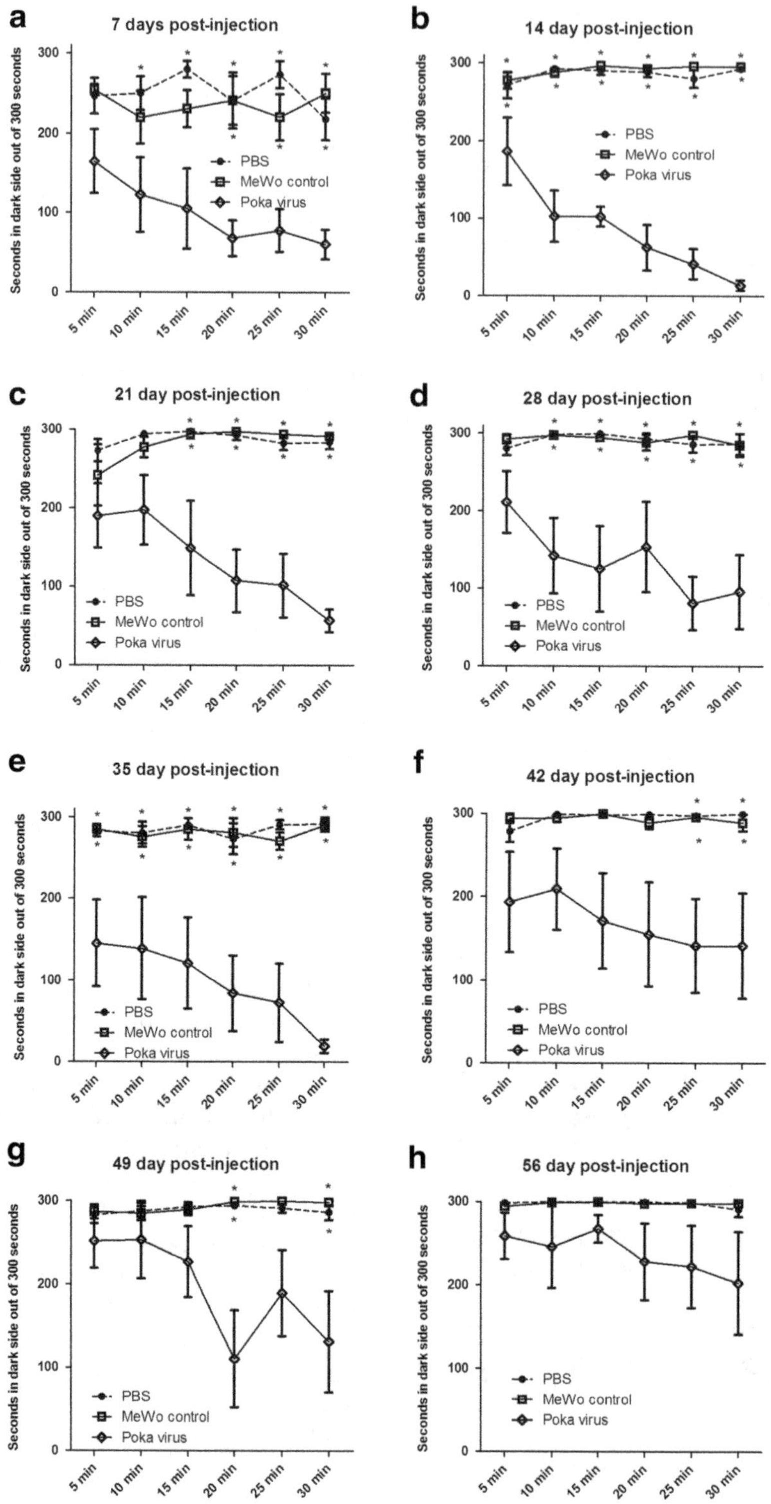

Fig. 4 VZV increased aversive behavior as measured by the Place Escape/Avoidance Paradigm (PEAP) test. PEAP was completed on males whose whisker pad was injected with either PBS (vehicle), MeWo cells or MeWo cells infected with VZV (1900 pfu/ μl). The PEAP test was performed for eight weeks and each panel shows the data for a different week; panel **a** shows week 1, panel **b** week 2, panel **c** week 3, panel **d** week 4, panel **e** week 5 and panel **f** week 6, panel **g** week 7 and panel **h** week 8. The upper row of asterisks indicate a significant difference ($p < 0.05$) between the PBS and pOka treatment groups. Asterisks on the lower row indicate a significant difference ($p < 0.05$) between MeWo and pOka treatment groups. There were 6 animals per treatment group

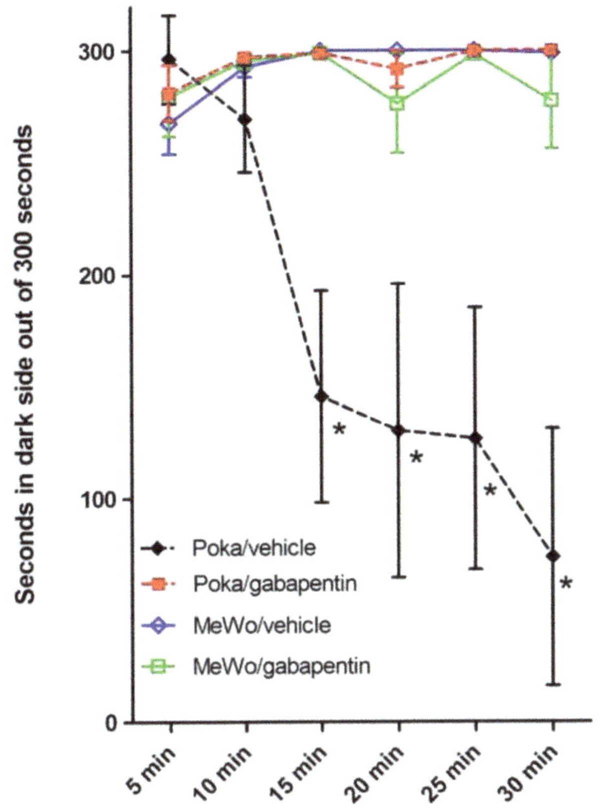

Fig. 5 Gabapentin relieves the VZV induced aversive response. The PEAP test was assessed at 7 days post infection in rats whose whisker pad was injected with either MeWo cells or MeWo cells infected with a low dose of VZV (360 pfu/ µl). An asterisk indicates a significant difference between the VZV pOka/vehicle group and the VZV pOka/gabapentin group, as well as, a significant difference between the Mewo/vehicle group and the pOka/vehicle group. There were 5 animals per treatment group

Discussion

Mechanical allodynia is the most common, most debilitating and the most difficult to treat component seen in PHN patents. Persistent mechanical allodynia and thermal hyperalgesia are present after VZV inoculation of the footpad [14–20]. The study here expands the footpad model to the orofacial region by demonstrating that VZV induces a significant behavioral response after stimulating the facial region [20, 21, 44]. These responses included thermal and mechanical hypersensitivity, as well as, an aversive response. Interestingly the aversive response, as measured by the PEAP assay [31], lasted several weeks longer than the hypersensitivity measured by Ugo Basile chambers. The longer PEAP response suggests that either the PEAP assay was more sensitive than the Ugo Basile chambers in measuring responses or that the affective component is present longer than the sensory component. In contrast to our results, previous studies injecting compete Freund's adjuvant into the paw showed that sensory responses (von Frey) and affective responses (PEAP test) lasted for similar times [31]. One explanation for this inconsistency would be that adjuvant induces pain through a different mechanism than VZV. Behavioral tests, such as the PEAP test, require supraspinal pain processing and would be useful in the drug development for patients [36, 37]. In one example of preclinical drug testing, gabapentin reduced the affective PEAP response in this rat model consistent with gabapentin being efficacious in treating patients with HZ associated pain [45]. It is interesting to note that anxiety-like behaviors were not reversed by gabapentin treatment in previous studies [20], but gabapentin does effect the PEAP measurement (reverse the aversive behavior), consistent with the idea that anxiety does not bias the PEAP measurement [36, 46].

Pain is reported 3.75 times more often in women than in men after HZ infection [25] but no model currently exists to study this sex difference. We show here that VZV induced pain was influenced by sex. VZV inoculated female rats experienced the same level of aversive behavior as the VZV injected males post-injection week 1, but by week 2 females clearly experienced a higher level of pain behavior, consistent with females experiencing more orofacial pain-related sensations [47–49]. One reason for the sex difference could be related to sex steroids. Of note is the fact that the males had a greater percentage of IE62 positive neurons but showed less aversive behavior suggesting that viral infection rates do not explain the sex difference. Moreover, our data support a role for sex steroids because during the estrous cycle there was a significantly greater PEAP response in diestrus rats (when estradiol is low) in comparison to proestrus/estrus rats (when estradiol is higher). This data is consistent with the nociceptive response in an inflammatory TMJ model where rats given a diestrus level of estradiol (low) had a greater nociceptive response in comparison to rats given a proestrus dose of estradiol (high) [50]. Mechanistically estradiol has been shown to alter the pain response through G-protein signaling [51]. Moreover, estradiol utilizes G-protein signaling to alter the nociceptive response by changing the responsiveness of N-methyl-D-aspartic acid (NMDA) receptors and by enhancing dendritic spine growth [52]. Although the mechanism is unclear as to why the nociceptive response was higher in females this animal model can be used to explore the mechanisms contributing to the observed sex difference.

Humans with HZ associated pain do not require continued replication of VZV because administration of the antiviral acyclovir (blocks viral replication) does not reduce the pain response [53]. Similarly, VZV induced pain was not ameliorated by antiviral agents in the rat footpad model [54]. As in humans, VZV induced hypersensitivity in rodents can be present without detectable

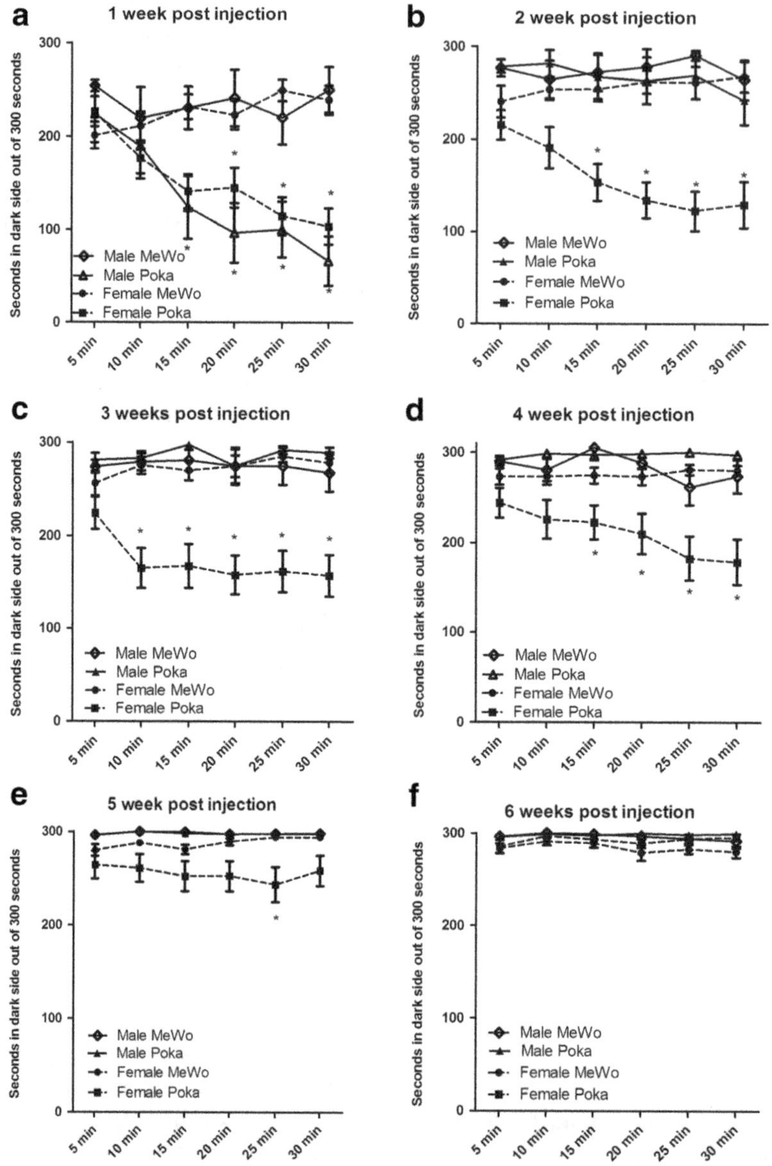

Fig. 6 Sex differences in VZV induced aversive response. Male and female whisker pads were injected with either MeWo cells or MeWo cells infected with 650 pfu/ µl VZV. PEAP testing was completed weekly over six weeks, each panel shows data for a different week. In panel **a** the upper row of asterisks indicate a significant difference between the Female MeWo and Female pOka treatment groups and the lower row of asterisks indicate a significant difference between the Male MeWo and Male pOka treatment groups. In panels **b-f** an asterisk indicates a significant difference ($p < 0.05$) between the Female MeWo and Female pOka treatment groups. There were 24 control and 25 virus infected females and the number of males in both the MeWo and pOka treatment groups was 7 for week one, 10 for week two and 15 for weeks three, four, five and six

viral replication [44, 55, 56]. Recent work has indicated that VZV goes through a partial replication cycle in animals resulting in translation of viral proteins that can induce pain [53]. Together the data suggests continued production of lytic virus and necrosis of neurons is not a mechanism for induction or maintenance of the pain response [57]. To date, no animal has supported VZV ganglionic reactivation [58], so PHN after reactivation cannot be studied. Interestingly, Dr. Kinchington's group has recently reported the first reliable experimental VZV reactivation in vitro using human neuron cultures [59] and proposed that both human PHN and pain in rats are the result of VZV gene expression without viral replication. Our studies add to this previous work by extending the pain response to the orofacial region which contributes to pain in up to 28% of herpes zoster patients [22, 23]. Using this novel model of VZV these pain mechanisms can be determined in the orofacial region.

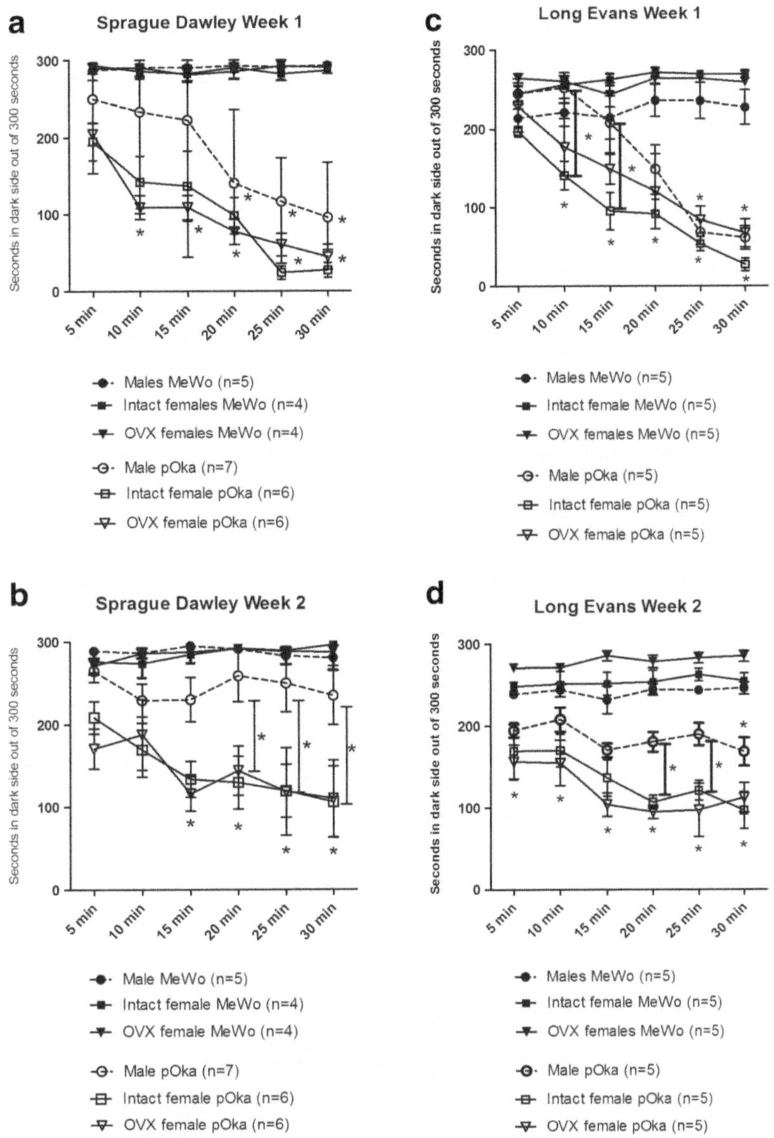

Fig. 7 OVX female rats show an increased VZV induced aversive response as compared to males. The whisker pads of male and intact or ovariectomized (OVX) female rats were injected with either MeWo cells or MeWo cells infected with 650 pfu/μl VZV (Sprague Dawley rats, panels **a** and **b**) or 360 pfu/μl VZV (Long Evans rats, panels **c** and **d**). PEAP testing was completed weekly over two weeks. The lower row of asterisks indicate a significant difference between the Female MeWo and Female pOka treatment groups (both intact and OVX) and the upper row of asterisks indicate a significant difference between the Male MeWo and Male pOka treatment groups. In panels **b** and **d** the bar with an asterisk indicates a significant difference ($p < 0.05$) between the Male pOka and the intact and OVX Female pOka treatment groups. In panel **c** the bar with an asterisk indicates a significant difference ($p < 0.05$) between the Male pOka and the intact Female POka treatment groups. The number of animals in each treatment group was pre-determined and is shown on the figure in parentheses

Zoster-associated pain may last 30–90 days during the acute phase however, about 20–30% of individuals develop chronic pain (>90 days) termed post-herpetic neuralgia (PHN), which may last months to years [6–8, 60, 61]. In males a VZV dose of 65,000 pfu/whisker pad resulted in a significant response for one week and a dose of 190,000 pfu/whisker pad resulted in a 7 week response. Assuming a linear relationship between dosage and response an injection of 300,000 pfu/whisker pad would result in a 12 week response. A 12 week or 90 day pain response is one of the diagnostic criteria for PHN [60]. Future studies investigating higher dosages could indicate that this model is applicable for studying the mechanisms resulting in the development of PHN.

VZV infection of the whisker pad resulted in IE62 staining within the V1/V2 and V3 regions of the trigeminal ganglia. Because the V1/V2 branch innervates the whisker pad it was not clear why some IE62 staining was

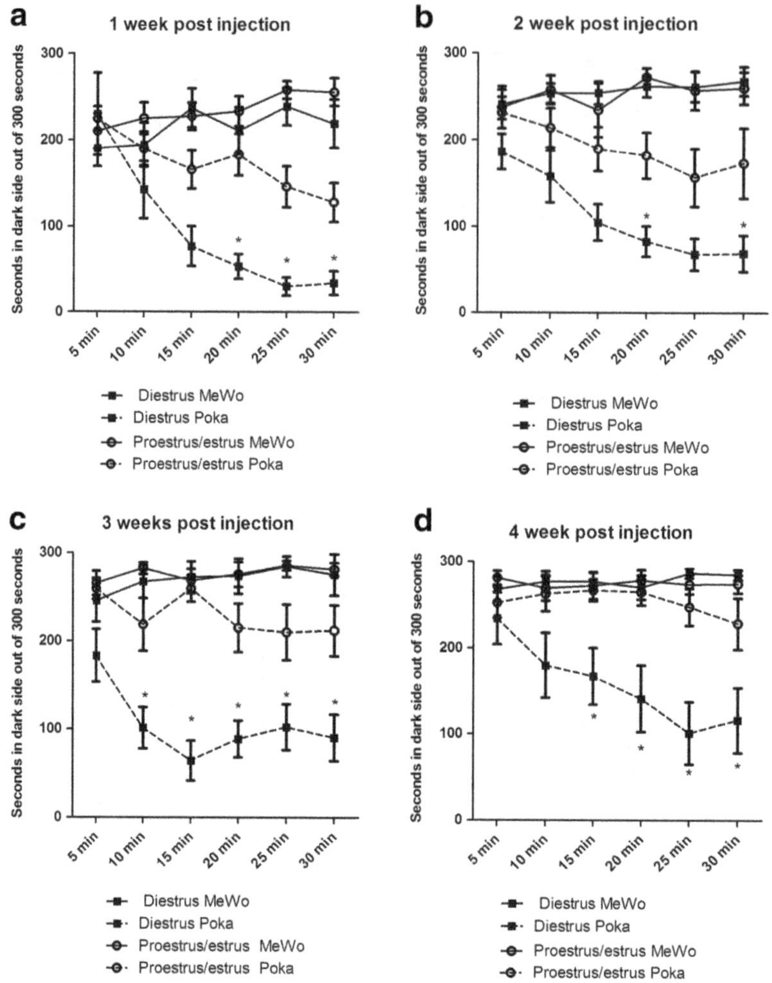

Fig. 8 VZV induced and aversive response that was affected by the estrous cycle. Weekly PEAP testing was completed on cycling female rats after VZV injection. A total of 24 rats whose whisker pad was injected with MeWo cells and a total of 25 rats whose whisker pad was injected with MeWo cells infected with 650 pfu/ µl VZV were included in this experiment. Smears were completed on each day of testing and the number of animals at each cycle phase (i.e., diestrus or proestrus/estrus) was a minimum of 8 rats but that number would vary from week to week depending on the estrous cycle. Testing was performed once a week for four weeks after whisker pad injection, in panel **a** testing was completed 1 week after injection, in panel **b** 2 weeks after injection, in panel **c** 3 weeks after injection and in panel **d** 4 weeks after injection. An asterisk indicates a significant difference ($p < 0.05$) between the Diestrus pOka group and the Proestrus/estrus pOka group

present within the V3 region. This is the first evidence for VZV infection of the trigeminal ganglia after injection into the rodent whisker pad but VZV is a human herpes virus, one of eight types of herpes viruses. Whisker pad injection of herpes simplex virus type 1 (one of the eight types of herpes viruses) resulted in a small amount of infection of the V3 region with a majority of the infection being present in the V1/V2 region [62], consistent with our results. Studies of the somatotopic organization of the trigeminal ganglia indicated that there was overlap in the ganglionic regions that contribute to the V1/V2 and V3 branches [63]. The results could be explained by this overlap; if some of the IE62 positive neurons in the V3 region actually project to the whisker pad then it would be expected that these neurons would become infected by VZV.

Conclusions

Our study uses behavioral testing to assess zoster associated orofacial pain in the rat model. For the first time a sex difference is shown after VZV injection, consistent with epidemiological evidence that women report PHN more than men [24, 25]. This model can be utilized to study one, the mechanisms of zoster-associated orofacial pain, two, test drug therapies to treat humans effectively and three, study the mechanisms contributing to the sex differences underlying zoster associated pain.

Abbreviations

VZV: Varicella zoster virus; HZ: Herpes zoster; PHN: Post-herpetic neuralgia; pOka: VZV Parent of Oka; MEM: Minimal Essential Media; FBS: Fetal bovine serum; PEAP: Place Escape/Avoidance Paradigm; Pfu: Plaque forming units

Acknowledgements

The authors wish to thank Xiaoju Zou, Priscilla Gillaspie-Hooks, Connie Tillberg and Gerald Hill for their excellent technical assistance. This study was supported by NIDCR grant DE022129 (PRKramer) and a grant from the 30, 300, 3000 Pain Research Challenge from the University of Pittsburgh Clinical and Translational Science Institute (PRKinchington). PRKinchington also acknowledges support from NEI core grant EY08098, a NINDS grant NS064022 and a grant from Research to prevent Blindness Inc. There are no conflicts of interest with this work.

Author contributions

CS and MD made substantial contributions to conception and design, or acquisition of data. MY made a substantial contributios to acquisition of data. CS, LLB, PRKinchington, PRKramer were involved in drafting the manuscript or revising it critically for important intellectual content. PRKramer conceived of the study, and participated in its design and coordination. All authors read and approved the final manuscript.

Competing interest

The authors declare that they have no competing interests.

Author details

[1]Department of Biomedical Sciences, Texas A&M University College of Dentistry, 3302 Gaston Avenue, Dallas, TX 75246, USA. [2]Dept Ophthalmology and of Molecular Microbiology and Genetics, 203 Lothrop St., Pittsburgh, PA 15213, USA. [3]Department of Oral and Maxillofacial Surgery, The State Key Laboratory Breeding Base of Basic Science of Stomatology & Key Laboratory of Oral Biomedicine Ministry of Education, School & Hospital of Stomatology, Wuhan University, Wuhan, People's Republic of China.

References

1. Mahalingam R, Wellish M, Wolf W, Dueland AN, Cohrs R, Vafai A, Gilden D. Latent varicella-zoster viral DNA in human trigeminal and thoracic ganglia. N Engl J Med. 1990;323(10):627–31.
2. Clarke P, Beer T, Cohrs R, Gilden DH. Configuration of latent varicella-zoster virus DNA. J Virol. 1995;69(12):8151–4.
3. Mahalingam R, Wellish M, Cohrs R, Debrus S, Piette J, Rentier B, Gilden DH. Expression of protein encoded by varicella-zoster virus open reading frame 63 in latently infected human ganglionic neurons. Proc Natl Acad Sci U S A. 1996;93(5):2122–4.
4. Lungu O, Panagiotidis CA, Annunziato PW, Gershon AA, Silverstein SJ. Aberrant intracellular localization of Varicella-zoster virus regulatory proteins during latency. Proc Natl Acad Sci U S A. 1998;95(12):7080–5.
5. Johnson RW, Bouhassira D, Kassianos G, Leplege A, Schmader KE, Weinke T. The impact of herpes zoster and post-herpetic neuralgia on quality-of-life. BMC Med. 2010;8:37.
6. Kinchington PR, Goins WF. Varicella zoster virus-induced pain and post-herpetic neuralgia in the human host and in rodent animal models. J Neurovirol. 2011; 17(6):590–9.
7. Dubinsky RM, Kabbani H, El-Chami Z, Boutwell C, Ali H. Practice parameter: treatment of postherpetic neuralgia: an evidence-based report of the quality standards Subcommittee of the American Academy of neurology. Neurology. 2004;63(6):959–65.
8. Mitchell BM, Bloom DC, Cohrs RJ, Gilden DH, Kennedy PG. Herpes simplex virus-1 and varicella-zoster virus latency in ganglia. J Neurovirol. 2003;9(2):194–204.
9. Kawai K, Gebremeskel BG, Acosta CJ. Systematic review of incidence and complications of herpes zoster: towards a global perspective. BMJ Open. 2014;4(6):e004833.
10. Yawn BP, Saddier P, Wollan PC, St Sauver JL, Kurland MJ, Sy LS. A population-based study of the incidence and complication rates of herpes zoster before zoster vaccine introduction. Mayo Clin Proc. 2007;82(11):1341–9.
11. Harpaz R, Ortega-Sanchez IR, Seward JF: Prevention of herpes zoster: recommendations of the advisory Committee on immunization practices (ACIP). MMWR Recomm Rep : Morbidity and mortality weekly report Recommendations and reports / Centers for Disease Control 2008, 57(RR-5): 1-30; quiz CE32-34.
12. Cruccu G, Biasiotta A, Galeotti F, Iannetti GD, Innocenti P, Romaniello A, Truini A. Diagnosis of trigeminal neuralgia: a new appraisal based on clinical and neurophysiological findings. Suppl Clin Neurophysiol. 2006;58:171–86.
13. Katusic S, Beard CM, Bergstralh E, Kurland LT. Incidence and clinical features of trigeminal neuralgia, Rochester, Minnesota, 1945-1984. Ann Neurol. 1990; 27(1):89–95.
14. Fleetwood-Walker SM, Quinn JP, Wallace C, Blackburn-Munro G, Kelly BG, Fiskerstrand CE, Nash AA, Dalziel RG. Behavioural changes in the rat following infection with varicella-zoster virus. J Gen Virol. 1999;80(Pt 9):2433–6.
15. Guedon JM, Zhang M, Glorioso JC, Goins WF, Kinchington PR. Relief of pain induced by varicella-zoster virus in a rat model of post-herpetic neuralgia using a herpes simplex virus vector expressing enkephalin. Gene Ther. 2014; 21(7):694–702.
16. Rowbotham MC, Fields HL. The relationship of pain, allodynia and thermal sensation in post-herpetic neuralgia. Brain. 1996;119(Pt 2):347–54.
17. Dalziel RG, Bingham S, Sutton D, Grant D, Champion JM, Dennis SA, Quinn JP, Bountra C, Mark MA. Allodynia in rats infected with varicella zoster virus–a small animal model for post-herpetic neuralgia. Brain Res Brain Res Rev. 2004;46(2):234–42.
18. Kennedy PG, Montague P, Scott F, Grinfeld E, Ashrafi GH, Breuer J, Rowan EG. Varicella-zoster viruses associated with post-herpetic neuralgia induce sodium current density increases in the ND7-23 Nav-1.8 neuroblastoma cell line. PLoS One. 2013;8(1):e51570.
19. Zhang GH, Lv MM, Wang S, Chen L, Qian NS, Tang Y, Zhang XD, Ren PC, Gao CJ, Sun XD, et al. Spinal astrocytic activation is involved in a virally-induced rat model of neuropathic pain. PLoS One. 2011;6(9):e23059.
20. Garry EM, Delaney A, Anderson HA, Sirinathsinghji EC, Clapp RH, Martin WJ, Kinchington PR, Krah DL, Abbadie C, Fleetwood-Walker SM. Varicella zoster virus induces neuropathic changes in rat dorsal root ganglia and behavioral reflex sensitisation that is attenuated by gabapentin or sodium channel blocking drugs. Pain. 2005;118(1–2):97–111.
21. Hasnie FS, Breuer J, Parker S, Wallace V, Blackbeard J, Lever I, Kinchington PR, Dickenson AH, Pheby T, Rice AS. Further characterization of a rat model of varicella zoster virus-associated pain: relationship between mechanical hypersensitivity and anxiety-related behavior, and the influence of analgesic drugs. Neuroscience. 2007;144(4):1495–508.
22. Goh CL, Khoo L. A retrospective study of the clinical presentation and outcome of herpes zoster in a tertiary dermatology outpatient referral clinic. Int J Dermatol. 1997;36(9):667–72.
23. Haanpaa M, Laippala P, Nurmikko T. Pain and somatosensory dysfunction in acute herpes zoster. Clin J Pain. 1999;15(2):78–84.
24. Alvarez FK, de Siqueira SR, Okada M, Teixeira MJ, de Siqueira JT: Evaluation of the sensation in patients with trigeminal post-herpetic neuralgia. J Oral Pathol Med : official publication of the International Association of Oral Pathologists and the American Academy of Oral Pathology 2007, 36(6):347–350.
25. Hillebrand K, Bricout H, Schulze-Rath R, Schink T, Garbe E. Incidence of herpes zoster and its complications in Germany. J Infect. 2015;70(2):178–86.
26. Eisfeld AJ, Yee MB, Erazo A, Abendroth A, Kinchington PR. Downregulation of class I major histocompatibility complex surface expression by varicella-zoster virus involves open reading frame 66 protein kinase-dependent and -independent mechanisms. J Virol. 2007;81(17):9034–49.
27. Erazo A, Yee MB, Osterrieder N, Kinchington PR. Varicella-zoster virus open reading frame 66 protein kinase is required for efficient viral growth in primary human corneal stromal fibroblast cells. J Virol. 2008;82(15):7653–65.
28. Prochazkova M, Terse A, Amin ND, Hall B, Utreras E, Pant HC, Kulkarni AB. Activation of cyclin-dependent kinase 5 mediates orofacial mechanical hyperalgesia. Mol Pain. 2013;9:66.
29. Abd-Elsayed AA, Ikeda R, Jia Z, Ling J, Zuo X, Li M, Gu JG. KCNQ channels in nociceptive cold-sensing trigeminal ganglion neurons as therapeutic targets for treating orofacial cold hyperalgesia. Mol Pain. 2015;11:45.

30. Cha M, Kohan KJ, Zuo X, Ling JX, Gu JG. Assessment of chronic trigeminal neuropathic pain by the orofacial operant test in rats. Behav Brain Res. 2012; 234(1):82–90.
31. LaBuda CJ, Fuchs PN. A behavioral test paradigm to measure the aversive quality of inflammatory and neuropathic pain in rats. Exp Neurol. 2000; 163(2):490–4.
32. Wilson HD, Uhelski ML, Fuchs PN. Examining the role of the medial thalamus in modulating the affective dimension of pain. Brain Res. 2008;1229:90–9.
33. Ansah OB, Bourbia N, Goncalves L, Almeida A, Pertovaara A. Influence of amygdaloid glutamatergic receptors on sensory and emotional pain-related behavior in the neuropathic rat. Behav Brain Res. 2010;209(1):174–8.
34. LaGraize SC, Labuda CJ, Rutledge MA, Jackson RL, Fuchs PN. Differential effect of anterior cingulate cortex lesion on mechanical hypersensitivity and escape/avoidance behavior in an animal model of neuropathic pain. Exp Neurol. 2004;188(1):139–48.
35. Baastrup C, Maersk-Moller CC, Nyengaard JR, Jensen TS, Finnerup NB. Spinal-, brainstem- and cerebrally mediated responses at- and below-level of a spinal cord contusion in rats: evaluation of pain-like behavior. Pain. 2010;151(3):670–9.
36. Baastrup C, Jensen TS, Finnerup NB. Pregabalin attenuates place escape/avoidance behavior in a rat model of spinal cord injury. Brain Res. 2011; 1370:129–35.
37. Uhelski ML, Morris-Bobzean SA, Dennis TS, Perrotti LI, Fuchs PN. Evaluating underlying neuronal activity associated with escape/avoidance behavior in response to noxious stimulation in adult rats. Brain Res. 2012;1433:56–61.
38. DaSilva AF, DosSantos MF. The role of sensory fiber demography in trigeminal and postherpetic neuralgias. J Dent Res. 2012;91(1):17–24.
39. Kennedy PG, Grinfeld E, Bontems S, Sadzot-Delvaux C. Varicella-zoster virus gene expression in latently infected rat dorsal root ganglia. Virology. 2001; 289(2):218–23.
40. Djouhri L, Fang X, Okuse K, Wood JN, Berry CM, Lawson SN. The TTX-resistant sodium channel Nav1.8 (SNS/PN3): expression and correlation with membrane properties in rat nociceptive primary afferent neurons. J Physiol. 2003;550(Pt 3):739–52.
41. Cilloniz C, Jackson W, Grose C, Czechowski D, Hay J, Ruyechan WT. The varicella-zoster virus (VZV) ORF9 protein interacts with the IE62 major VZV transactivator. J Virol. 2007;81(2):761–74.
42. Oaklander AL. The density of remaining nerve endings in human skin with and without postherpetic neuralgia after shingles. Pain. 2001;92(1–2):139–45.
43. Rowbotham MC, Yosipovitch G, Connolly MK, Finlay D, Forde G, Fields HL. Cutaneous innervation density in the allodynic form of postherpetic neuralgia. Neurobiol Dis. 1996;3(3):205–14.
44. Guedon JM, Yee MB, Zhang M, Harvey SA, Goins WF, Kinchington PR. Neuronal changes induced by Varicella zoster virus in a rat model of postherpetic neuralgia. Virology. 2015;482:167–80.
45. Hempenstall K, Nurmikko TJ, Johnson RW, A'Hern RP, Rice AS. Analgesic therapy in postherpetic neuralgia: a quantitative systematic review. PLoS Med. 2005;2(7):e164.
46. Wilson HD, Boyette-Davis J, Fuchs PN. The relationship between basal level of anxiety and the affective response to inflammation. Physiol Behav. 2007; 90(2–3):506–11.
47. Dao TT, LeResche L. Gender differences in pain. J Orofac Pain. 2000;14(3):169–84.
48. LeResche L, Mancl L, Sherman JJ, Gandara B, Dworkin SF. Changes in temporomandibular pain and other symptoms across the menstrual cycle. Pain. 2003;106(3):253–61.
49. Sherman JJ, LeResche L. Does experimental pain response vary across the menstrual cycle? A methodological review. Am J Physiol Regul Integr Comp Physiol. 2006;291(2):R245–56.
50. Kramer PR, Bellinger LL. The effects of cycling levels of 17beta-estradiol and progesterone on the magnitude of temporomandibular joint-induced nociception. Endocrinology. 2009;150(8):3680–9.
51. Zhang Y, Lu N, Zhao ZQ, Zhang YQ. Involvement of estrogen in rapid pain modulation in the rat spinal cord. Neurochem Res. 2012;37(12):2697–705.
52. Xiao X, Yang Y, Zhang Y, Zhang XM, Zhao ZQ, Zhang YQ. Estrogen in the Anterior Cingulate Cortex Contributes to Pain-Related Aversion. Cerebral cortex. 2013;23(9):2190–2203.
53. Gershon AA, Gershon MD. Pathogenesis and current approaches to control of varicella-zoster virus infections. Clin Microbiol Rev. 2013;26(4):728–43.
54. Delaney A, Colvin LA, Fallon MT, Dalziel RG, Mitchell R, Fleetwood-Walker SM: Postherpetic neuralgia: from preclinical models to the clinic. Neurotherapeutics : the journal of the American Society for Experimental NeuroTherapeutics 2009, 6(4):630-637.
55. Schaap-Nutt A, Sommer M, Che X, Zerboni L, Arvin AM. ORF66 protein kinase function is required for T-cell tropism of varicella-zoster virus in vivo. J Virol. 2006;80(23):11806–16.
56. Schaap A, Fortin JF, Sommer M, Zerboni L, Stamatis S, Ku CC, Nolan GP, Arvin AM. T-cell tropism and the role of ORF66 protein in pathogenesis of varicella-zoster virus infection. J Virol. 2005;79(20):12921–33.
57. Steain M, Sutherland JP, Rodriguez M, Cunningham AL, Slobedman B, Abendroth A. Analysis of T cell responses during active varicella-zoster virus reactivation in human ganglia. J Virol. 2014;88(5):2704–16.
58. Chen JJ, Gershon AA, Li Z, Cowles RA, Gershon MD. Varicella zoster virus (VZV) infects and establishes latency in enteric neurons. J Neurovirol. 2011; 17(6):578–89.
59. Markus A, Lebenthal-Loinger I, Yang IH, Kinchington PR, Goldstein RS. An in vitro model of latency and reactivation of varicella zoster virus in human stem cell-derived neurons. PLoS Pathog. 2015;11(6):e1004885.
60. Fashner J, Bell AL. Herpes zoster and postherpetic neuralgia: prevention and management. Am Fam Physician. 2011;83(12):1432–7.
61. Colon Y. Patient education and self-advocacy: questions and responses on pain management. J Pain Palliat Care Pharmacother. 2009;23(1):51–61.
62. Nicoll MP, Proenca JT, Connor V, Efstathiou S. Influence of herpes simplex virus 1 latency-associated transcripts on the establishment and maintenance of latency in the ROSA26R reporter mouse model. J Virol. 2012;86(16):8848–58.
63. Leiser SC, Moxon KA. Relationship between physiological response type (RA and SA) and vibrissal receptive field of neurons within the rat trigeminal ganglion. J Neurophysiol. 2006;95(5):3129–45.

10

Comparative assessment of clinical rating scales in Wilson's disease

Hanna M. Volpert[1], Jan Pfeiffenberger[1], Jan B. Gröner[3], Wolfgang Stremmel[1], Daniel N. Gotthardt[1], Mark Schäfer[1], Karl Heinz Weiss[1*†] and Markus Weiler[2*†]

Abstract

Background: Wilson's disease (WD) is an autosomal recessive disorder of copper metabolism resulting in multifaceted neurological, hepatic, and psychiatric symptoms. The objective of the study was to comparatively assess two clinical rating scales for WD, the Unified Wilson's Disease Rating Scale (UWDRS) and the Global Assessment Scale for Wilson's disease (GAS for WD), and to test the feasibility of the patient reported part of the UWDRS neurological subscale (termed the "minimal UWDRS").

Methods: In this prospective, monocentric, cross-sectional study, 65 patients (median age 35 [range: 15–62] years; 33 female, 32 male) with treated WD were scored according to the two rating scales.

Results: The UWDRS neurological subscore correlated with the GAS for WD Tier 2 score ($r = 0.80$; $p < 0.001$). Correlations of the UWDRS hepatic subscore and the GAS for WD Tier 1 score with both the Model for End Stage Liver Disease (MELD) score ($r = 0.44/r = 0.28$; $p < 0.001/p = 0.027$) and the Child-Pugh score ($r = 0.32/r = 0.12$; $p = 0.015/p = 0.376$) were weak. The "minimal UWDRS" score significantly correlated with the UWDRS total score ($r = 0.86$), the UWDRS neurological subscore ($r = 0.89$), and the GAS for WD Tier 2 score ($r = 0.86$).

Conclusions: The UWDRS neurological and psychiatric subscales and the GAS for WD Tier 2 score are valuable tools for the clinical assessment of WD patients. The "minimal UWDRS" is a practical prescreening tool outside scientific trials.

Keywords: Copper metabolism, German network of hereditary movement disorders (GeNeMove), Global assessment scale for Wilson's disease (GAS for WD), Unified Wilson's disease rating scale (UWDRS), Wilson disease

Background

Wilson's disease (WD) is an autosomal recessive disorder caused by mutations in the *ATP7B* gene leading to excessive copper overload, predominantly in the liver and the brain [1, 2]. The severity of the disease varies considerably between patients, and it remains unclear why some patients have hepatic symptoms while others develop neurological, psychiatric, or combined symptomatology [3–5]. Hepatic features range from asymptomatic patients with slightly elevated liver enzymes to liver cirrhosis or acute hepatic failure [6]. Neurological symptoms are usually characterized by multiple motor impairments characteristic for dysfunctions of the basal ganglia and the cerebellum. This results in various neurological symptoms including rigidity, tremor, dyskinesia, dystonia, ataxia, chorea, dysarthria, dysphagia, or excessive salivation [6–10]. Psychiatric symptoms are diverse and may include concentration difficulties, attention disorders, behavioral abnormalities with alterations of personality, depression, and psychosis [11–14]. The severity of the symptoms clearly determines the extent to which a patient is restricted in their activities of daily living (ADL).

To prevent progression of the disease and lethal outcomes, lifelong therapy pursuing a negative copper balance is imperative; hence, underlining the importance of an early diagnosis and an individually adapted therapy

* Correspondence: karl-heinz.weiss@med.uni-heidelberg.de; markus.weiler@med.uni-heidelberg.de
†Equal contributors
[1]Department of Internal Medicine IV, Heidelberg University Hospital, Im Neuenheimer Feld 410, Heidelberg, Germany
[2]Department of Neurology, Heidelberg University Hospital, Im Neuenheimer Feld 400, 69120 Heidelberg, Germany
Full list of author information is available at the end of the article

[15]. However, neurological worsening in WD patients following initiation of penicillamine standard therapy is a major concern [16]. Given the multifaceted symptomatology in WD, a comprehensive, standardized, and practical clinical rating scale is indispensable to monitor individual therapeutic effects and side effects in daily practice and to use as a valid end point in clinical trials testing therapies.

Currently, there are two clinical rating scales for WD: the Unified Wilson's Disease Rating Scale (UWDRS) and the Global Assessment Scale for Wilson's Disease (GAS for WD). The UWDRS has neurological, hepatic, and psychiatric subscales. The neurological subscale of the UWDRS was developed in collaboration with the European Network, EuroWilson, and the German Network of Hereditary Movement Disorders (GeNeMove). The first WD rating scale reflecting the extent of neurological impairment was reported by Czlonkowska et al. in 2007 [17]. It was extended by hepatic and psychiatric subscales that were evaluated in total by Leinweber et al. in 2008 [18]. The GAS for WD, considerably shorter than the UWDRS, is comprised of two tiers scoring global disability (Tier 1) and neurological dysfunction (Tier 2) and was proposed by Aggarwal et al. in 2009 [19]. Potential difficulties that have arisen from both rating scales in daily practice are the relatively long duration of the complete clinical assessment and the formal requirement of two to three different medical specialists (i.e., neurology, gastroenterology, and psychiatry).

So far the UWDRS and the GAS for WD have not been directly compared, and it remains unclear which rating scale may be superior. Hence, the goal of the present study is to evaluate the UWDRS and the GAS for WD in routine clinical practice and to propose a less time consuming patient reported prescreening tool for use outside scientific trials, the "minimal UWDRS".

Methods

Patients

This prospective, monocentric, cross-sectional study was carried out between 2014 and 2015. The ethics committee at the University of Heidelberg (Heidelberg, Germany) approved the study. A total of 65 patients with treated WD were evaluated according to the UWDRS and the GAS for WD. Patients older than 14 years of age who had been diagnosed with WD according to the diagnostic and phenotypic classification of WD [2] by the Department of Gastroenterology at Heidelberg University Hospital were enrolled after giving written informed consent. For patients who were under 18 years of age, written informed consent was obtained from the parents or the legal guardians. Patient related information including gender, age at assessment, age at the time of diagnosis, initial mode of manifestation, treatment at assessment, and clinical parameters were collected.

Clinical evaluation of the UWDRS and the GAS for WD

The full UWDRS (maximum score 320 points) consists of three subscales representing three main features of clinical manifestation in WD: a neurological subscale (27 items, 208 points), a hepatic subscale (9 items, 36 points), and a psychiatric subscale (19 items, 76 points). Of the 55 items in total, the patient has to answer 26 questions, whereas 29 items need to be scored by the observer. Each item is scored on an ascending five point scale (0 points "no symptoms" and 4 points "worst characteristic possible") [17, 18].

The GAS for WD contains two parts. Tier 1 scores global disability in four areas: liver, cognition and behavior, motor, and osseomuscular (with an ascending six point scale (0–5); the scores of each item are not summed up). Tier 2 scores neurological dysfunction and consists of 14 items with an ascending five point scale (0–4). The items of Tier 2 are summed for a possible maximum of 56 points [19]. All clinical assessments were performed by a resident in internal medicine (H. M. Volpert) supervised by both an attending hepatologist (K. H. Weiss) and an attending neurologist (M. Weiler). Disagreements between the investigators were resolved by discussion.

The "minimal UWDRS"

The first nine items of the UWDRS neurological subscale were selected to develop a minimal neurological subscale, newly determined as the "minimal UWDRS." Since this reduced rating scale exclusively represented a questionnaire whose items are reported by the patient or their family (usually referring to the previous two to four weeks), the resulting score can be assessed before the consultation with the treating physician. The selected items are: item 1 "mobility", item 2 "falling", item 3 "salivation", item 4 "swallowing", item 5 "feeding", item 6 "dressing", item 7 "taking a bath or shower", item 8 "grooming", and item 9 "toilet use". Apart from items 3 and 4, all other questions assess the level of independence for ADL.

Statistical analysis

Comparison of the UWDRS with the GAS for WD

UWDRS and GAS for WD were compared by correlating the scores of the rating scales and subscales in scatter diagrams and by calculating the Pearson's correlation coefficient. Correlation coefficients were interpreted as weak ($r < 0.5$), moderate ($r = 0.5–0.79$), and strong ($r \geq 0.80$) [20]. To validate the UWDRS hepatic subscore and the GAS for WD Tier 1 "liver" domain, these items were each correlated with the Model for End

Stage Liver Disease (MELD) score and the Child-Pugh score [21, 22]. The frequencies of scoring 1, 2, 3, or 4 points were calculated as well as the percentage of scoring >0 points for each item. Internal consistencies were evaluated using Cronbach's alpha (values of ≥0.7 were interpreted as "good", and ≥0.9 were interpreted as "very good") [18]. Cronbach's alpha was used to compare our results with the results of previous studies that evaluated the two clinical rating scales [18, 19]. In addition, single item total score correlations were assessed.

Evaluation of the "minimal UWDRS"

The score of the newly developed "minimal UWDRS" was correlated with the scores of the UWDRS and the GAS for WD including their neurological subscores. A p value <0.05 was considered statistically significant. For statistical analysis, SPSS™ (version 20.0, IBM Germany, Ehningen) was used.

Results

Descriptive analysis

Table 1 gives an overview of the clinical characteristics of the 65 WD patients examined. Patients that presented with hepatic symptoms as the initial mode of manifestation totalled 70.8%. Table 2 shows the results of the UWDRS and the GAS for WD both in general and in dependence from the initial mode of manifestation (i.e., hepatic, neurological, combined hepatic/neurological, and asymptomatic). As indicated by the relatively low medians, patients with severe WD symptoms were rare throughout the entire study. When patients were assessed depending on their initial mode of manifestation, the UWDRS total score and the UWDRS neurological subscore differed significantly (p values 0.026 and 0.012, respectively), which reflected the neurological disease burden in this subgroup. Additional file 1: Table S1 shows significantly differing results of the UWDRS and the GAS for WD when comparing clinical subgroups with respect to gender, Kayser-Fleischer rings (KFR) at assessment, and liver cirrhosis at the time of diagnosis. The prevalence of subscores of each item including the respective single item total score correlations are listed in the supporting data (Additional file 1: Figure S1).

Correlations of the UWDRS, GAS for WD, and "minimal UWDRS"

The correlation of the UWDRS total score with the UWDRS neurological subscore is shown in Fig. 1a (correlation coefficient of $r = 0.96$; level of significance of r: $p < 0.001$). The UWDRS total score correlated with the UWDRS hepatic subscore to a lower extent (correlation coefficient of $r = 0.37$; level of significance of r: $p = 0.003$; Fig. 1b) than the UWDRS total score with the UWDRS psychiatric subscore (correlation coefficient of $r = 0.83$; level of significance of r: $p < 0.001$; Fig. 1c). Moreover, the UWDRS neurological subscore correlated with the GAS for WD Tier 2 score (correlation coefficient of $r = 0.80$; level of significance of r: $p < 0.001$; Fig. 1d).

Figure 2 depicts the correlations of the UWDRS hepatic subscore and the score of the GAS for WD Tier 1 "liver" domain, respectively, with each the MELD and the Child-Pugh score. The UWDRS hepatic subscore correlated weakly with both the MELD score (correlation coefficient of $r = 0.44$; level of significance of r: $p < 0.001$; Fig. 2a) and the Child-Pugh score (correlation coefficient of $r = 0.32$; level of significance of r: $p = 0.015$; Fig. 2b). For the score of the GAS for WD Tier 1 "liver" domain, results were similar: correlations with each the MELD score (correlation coefficient of $r = 0.28$; level of significance of r: $p = 0.027$; Fig. 2c) and the Child-Pugh score (correlation coefficient of $r = 0.12$; level of significance of r: $p = 0.376$; Fig. 2d) were weak.

The "minimal UWDRS" score significantly correlated with each the UWDRS total score ($r = 0.86$; Fig. 3a), the UWDRS neurological subscore ($r = 0.89$; Fig. 3b), and the GAS for WD Tier 2 score ($r = 0.86$; Fig. 3c).

Single item total score correlation and Cronbach's alpha

Single item total score correlations are listed in the supporting data (Additional file 1: Figure S1, right). Cronbach's alpha for the total UWDRS was 0.95, for the UWDRS neurological subscale it was 0.96, for the UWDRS hepatic subscale it was 0.65, and for the psychiatric subscale it was 0.83. No item could be deleted in order to improve Cronbach's alpha for the UWDRS neurological subscale. After omitting item 30 "fecal blood", Cronbach's alpha for the UWDRS hepatic subscale changed to 0.66. The three items 39a "sexual interest increased", 50 "voice/noise level", and 52b "mood depressed" were left out to improve the internal consistency of the UWDRS psychiatric subscale to 0.84. The internal consistency of the GAS for WD Tier 2 score (Cronbach's alpha of 0.82) was slightly lower than the one for the UWDRS neurological subscale. After omitting item 13 "KFR", Cronbach's alpha improved to 0.84.

Discussion

In the clinical management of WD, thorough clinical monitoring including early detection of potential medical side effects and therapy failure is crucial to improve the patient's motivation and adherence [23]. Therefore, liver function tests and the calculation of MELD and Child-Pugh scores on an every three months basis are recommended [6, 21, 24]. During the initial phase of treatment, the modified Nazer score is a reliable tool to identify patients at risk for hepatic treatment failure requiring liver transplantation [25, 26].

Table 1 Clinical characteristics of the 65 examined patients with WD

	N	Percentage	Median	Range
Gender				
Female	33	50.8		
Male	32	49.2		
Age at assessment (yr)				
All			35	15–62
Female			40	15–62
Male			29.5	16–62
Age at onset of symptoms (yr)			16	1–47
Age at time of diagnosis (yr)			17	3–54
Initial mode of manifestation				
Hepatic	46	70.8		
Hepatic + neurological	10	15.4		
Neurological	6	9.2		
Asymptomatic	3	4.6		
Liver cirrhosis at time of diagnosis	21	32.3		
By initial mode of manifestation				
Hepatic [*n* = 46]	15	32.6		
Hepatic + neurological [*n* = 10]	6	60.0		
Liver status at assessment				
MELD score [missing data *n* = 4]			7.3	6–17
Child-Pugh score [missing data *n* = 7]			5	5–11
KFR at time of diagnosis [missing data *n* = 8]	28	49.1		
KFR at assessment	19	29.2		
Treatment at assessment in all patients (*n* = 65)				
D-Penicillamine	38	58.5		
Trientine	16	24.6		
Zinc	7	10.8		
D-Penicillamine + zinc	2	3.1		
Trientine + zinc	2	3.1		
Treatment at assessment in neurologically symptomatic patients (*n* = 16)				
Chelating agents	13	81.2		
Zinc with or without chelating agent	3	18.8		
Duration of treatment (yr)			15	0.4–47

Abbreviations: KFR Kayser-Fleischer ring, *pts.* patients, *yr.* years

Additionally, ultrasound of the liver visualizes the status of cirrhotic reorganization. However, an adequate assessment of neurological impairment has long been neglected due to the lack of a suitable tool for evaluation. Standardized neurological assessment allows for both intra- and inter-individual comparison of symptoms, which improves follow up and adds the ability of quantifying the severity of neurological symptoms. Especially for clinical trials on effects and side effects of medical treatments in WD, neurological rating scales are invaluable [27, 28]. This study presents the first systematic comparison of two clinical rating scales previously developed for WD, the UWDRS and the GAS for WD, and evaluates their feasibility in routine clinical practice. Additionally, we introduce the patient reported part of the UWDRS neurological subscale, the "minimal UWDRS", as a handy and time saving prescreening tool for the assessment of WD patients in routine clinical practice outside scientific trials.

The significant differences in the UWDRS total score and the UWDRS neurological subscore observed in our study show that the results differ depending on the

Table 2 Overview of the UWDRS and GAS for WD Tier 2 (sub)scores

	Total score median (range)				*P* value
UWDRS total score	10 (0–97)				
UWDRS neurological subscore	5 (0–74)				
UWDRS hepatic subscore	2 (0–13)				
UWDRS psychiatric subscore	1 (0–26)				
GAS for WD Tier 2 score	3 (0–24)				
	Initial mode of manifestation				
	Hepatic	Hepatic + neurological	Neurological	Asymptomatic	
UWDRS total score	9 (0–55)	32.5 (2–97)	18.5 (5–76)	4 (3–5)	0.026*
UWDRS neurological subscore	6 (0–49)	21.5 (1–66)	14 (3–74)	4 (2–4)	0.012*
UWDRS hepatic subscore	2 (0–13)	2.5 (0–12)	1 (0–5)	1 (0–1)	0.546
UWDRS psychiatric subscore	1 (0–12)	1.5 (0–26)	2 (2–7)	0 (0–0)	0.081
GAS for WD Tier 2 score	2 (0–24)	5 (0–23)	4.5 (1–11)	2 (1–3)	0.099

*, *P* value statistically significant

initial mode of manifestation (Table 2). The strong correlation of the UWDRS total score with the UWDRS neurological subscore (Fig. 1a) demonstrates that the UWDRS neurological subscale represents the UWDRS total scale very well. As the UWDRS neurological subscore can total 208 points at maximum, or 65% of the total score, one reason for the strong correlation is that the UWDRS neurological subscore largely represents the UWDRS total score. In contrast, the correlation of the UWDRS total score with the UWDRS hepatic subscore is weak (Fig. 1b). Hence, the UWDRS hepatic scale does not reflect chronic compensated liver disease, which is common in WD [6]. The moderate correlation of the UWDRS total score with the UWDRS psychiatric score (Fig. 1c) reveals that patients with severe neurological or hepatic symptoms do not necessarily have pronounced concomitant psychiatric symptoms [14, 29]. More than 20% of the patients in the study were found to have failing memory (item 40), concentration difficulties (item 41), and reduced social contact (item 42), all being

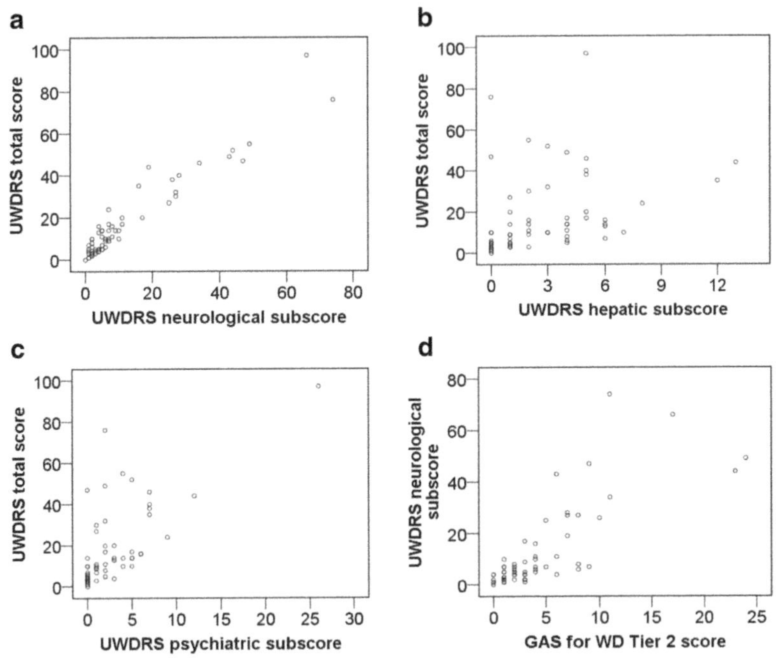

Fig. 1 **a** Correlation of the UWDRS total score with the UWDRS neurological subscore. **b** Correlation of the UWDRS total score with the UWDRS hepatic subscore. **c** Correlation of the UWDRS total score with the UWDRS psychiatric subscore. **d** Correlation of the UWDRS neurological subscore with the GAS for WD Tier 2 score

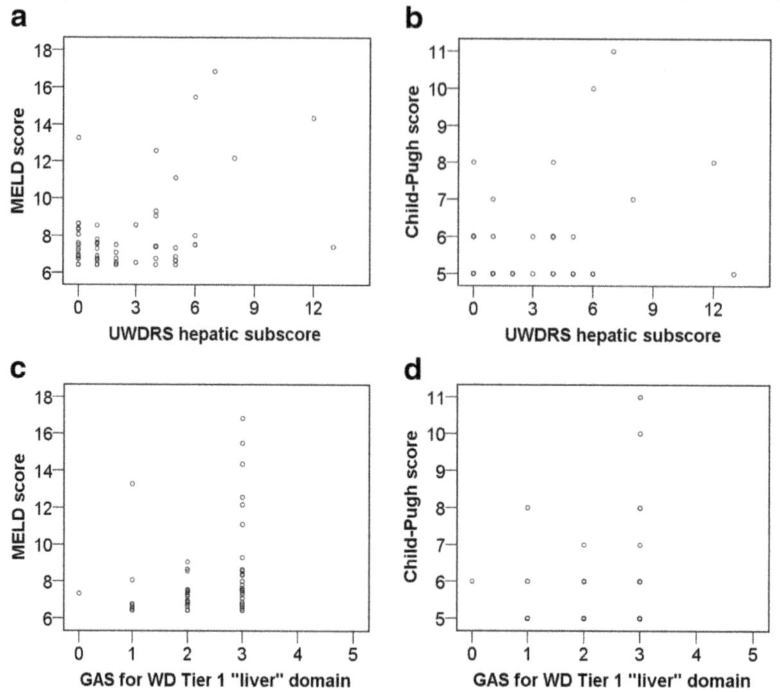

Fig. 2 **a** Correlation of the MELD score with the UWDRS hepatic subscore. **b** Correlation of the Child-Pugh score with the UWDRS hepatic subscore. **c** Correlation of the MELD score with the GAS for WD Tier 1 "liver" domain. **d** Correlation of the Child-Pugh score with the GAS for WD Tier 1 "liver" domain

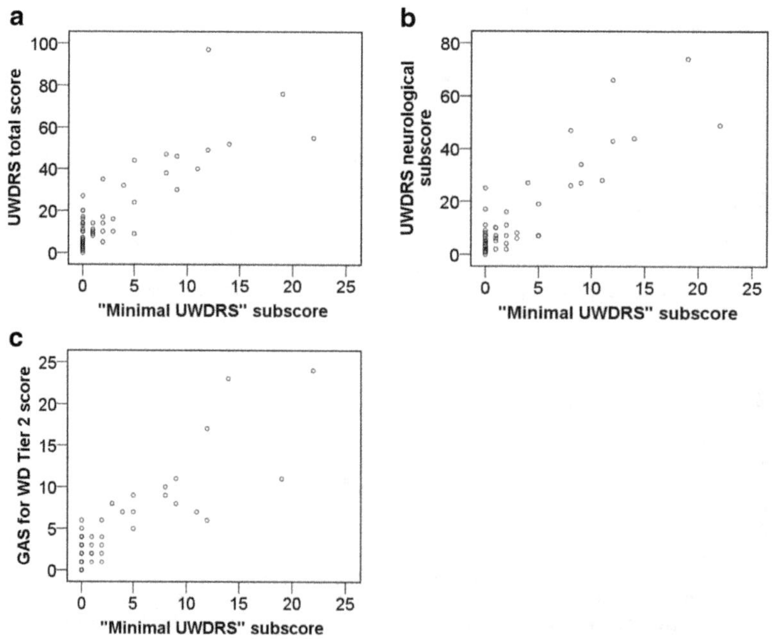

Fig. 3 **a** Correlation of the UWDRS total score with the UWDRS minimal neurological ("minimal UWDRS") subscore. **b** Correlation of the UWDRS neurological subscore with the UWDRS minimal neurological ("minimal UWDRS") subscore. **c** Correlation of the GAS for WD Tier 2 score with the UWDRS minimal neurological ("minimal UWDRS") subscore

psychiatric disabilities frequently seen in patients with WD [8, 30, 31]. A brief global psychiatric assessment as provided by the UWDRS psychiatric subscale is doubtlessly inappropriate to reflect such disorders. Nevertheless, it can be supportive in identifying patients with WD who would benefit from referral to a psychiatrist for further exploration.

The UWDRS neurological subscore correlates strongly with the GAS for WD Tier 2 score (Fig. 1d). Since the UWDRS scale includes a larger number of neurology and psychiatry related items than the GAS for WD scale, it documents these disabilities in greater detail (with the caveat that GAS for WD includes Kayser-Fleischer rings as a feature, while the UWDRS does not). However, this comes at some cost. In routine clinical practice, the larger number of items in the neurological and psychiatric subscales of the UWDRS requires significantly more time to assess than the Tier 2 score of the GAS for WD. However, this may not be a concern in clinical trials, particularly in those that assess therapeutic effects when detailed documentation of a change in a single neurological symptom is inevitable [32]. More significantly, many of the detailed neurological signs in the UWDRS scale are difficult to reliably discern in practice, as is reflected in the low interrater reliability (i.e., small values for intraclass correlation coefficients [ICC] for some of the individual items of the scale) [18]. In contrast, all the individual items of the GAS for WD have ICC values in the high range (i.e., can be assessed reliably) [19]. Whether a larger number of detailed items or a smaller number of reliably assessable items are of greater benefit will depend on the goal and the design of the individual clinical trial, as well as the consistency in raters. For instance, a trial interested in a specific neurological feature (e.g., autonomic disturbances) that is included only in the UWDRS is probably preferable. Likewise, the GAS for WD may be more suitable for a longitudinal trial with the goal of assessing a change in item scores in individual patients over a long period of time involving many different raters, as it reduces rater induced variance.

The weak correlation of the UWDRS hepatic subscore with the MELD score (Fig. 2a) and the Child-Pugh score (Fig. 2b) demonstrates that the UWDRS hepatic subscore does not mirror the current liver status very well. The correlation of the GAS for WD Tier 1 "liver" domain with the MELD score (Fig. 2c) and the Child-Pugh score (Fig. 2d) is also weak (i.e., this item does not represent the liver status very well either). Furthermore, we could not reproduce the correlation coefficient of $r = 0.65$ with respect to the Tier 1 "liver" domain and the Child-Pugh score published by Aggarwal et al. in 2009 (in our study: $r = 0.12$). However as the Child-Pugh score, as well as the MELD score to a lower extent, might have a limitation in detecting significant changes of the hepatic function in clinically stable or non-cirrhotic liver patients, the most meaningful mode of evaluation for the hepatic system in a WD specific rating scale has yet to be established.

The "minimal UWDRS" score correlates strongly with the UWDRS total score (Fig. 3a), the UWDRS neurological subscore (Fig. 3b), and the GAS for WD Tier 2 score (Fig. 3c). Outside clinical trials, the "minimal UWDRS" is a convenient and time saving prescreening tool to document neurological impairments in WD patients. The neurological questionnaire can be handed to the patient in the waiting area before the medical appointment without the requirement of a neurologist. Consequently, the questionnaire will help to better structure the consultation as the patient would have already deliberated his actual complaints and would be more prepared for the physician's questions. Besides, a short questionnaire, likely to be applied more frequently than an extensive neurological assessment, will support self reflection on disease symptoms and thus improve coping strategies as well as adherence to the treatment. Furthermore, the use of a questionnaire is more economical (after an initial detailed assessment), since it can be applied to figure out which impairments should be focused on and reevaluated at future follow up examinations. As seven out of nine items in the "minimal UWDRS" score the level of independence in the ADL, the physician will learn rapidly whether the neurological symptoms limit the patient's ADL. Constrictively, the questionnaire does not interrogate the exact reasons underlying potential impairments of the ADL. A further limitation is the "minimal UWDRS" may not adequately capture the full breadth of neurological disability in patients with WD. For instance, the "minimal UWDRS" may miss mild limb dystonia or new onset Kayser-Fleischer rings, which can be early signs of noncompliance or inadequate treatment. Thus, the time saving will come at some cost to patient care.

Altogether, our study collective suffered from relatively mild to moderate WD symptoms (Table 2, Additional file 1: Figure S1). Hence, we can not use a single item total score correlation to select single items for a minimal neurological scale. Otherwise, a minimal neurological scale will be inappropriate to be applied for patients with severe WD symptoms. Internal consistencies of the UWDRS total score and its subscales, as well as the internal consistency of the GAS for WD neurological assessment, are all very similar to those reported by Leinweber et al. 2008 and Aggarwal et al. 2009 [18, 19]. In our study, Cronbach's alpha for the UWDRS total score is 0.95 compared with 0.92 reported by Leinweber et al., the UWDRS neurological subscale is 0.95 compared with 0.94, the UWDRS hepatic subscale is 0.65 compared with 0.59, and the UWDRS psychiatric subscale is 0.83

compared with 0.76 [18]. Cronbach's alpha for the GAS for WD Tier 2 in our study (0.82) and in the first report (0.89) is also similar [19]. In summary, we largely confirm the internal consistencies for both the UWDRS and the GAS for WD as reported by the previous two articles.

The high prevalence of the hepatic initial mode of manifestation (70.8% in this study vs. an average of 45% in the literature) observed in our study collective may be due to selection bias caused by the fact that all patients were recruited in a WD outpatient clinic in a Department of Gastroenterology. The low median MELD (7.3) and Child-Pugh (5) scores show that most patients suffered from compensated liver cirrhosis. In general, our study collective is only mildly to moderately affected, which is probably due to the median duration of treatment at study inclusion being 15 years (Table 1). Despite the relatively long median time of pretreatment, patients still were clinically impaired. This finding underlines the importance of future studies focusing on improvement of the medication utilized to treat WD.

Conclusions

The main conclusions of our study are the following:

i) The UWDRS neurological and psychiatric subscales are valuable tools for a detailed assessment of neurological and psychiatric impairment in patients with WD.
ii) The GAS for WD Tier 2 can be considered as an alternative to gain an overview of the extent of neurological impairment.
iii) The UWDRS hepatic subscale, similar to the GAS for WD Tier 1, shows weak correlation to established hepatologic scores like MELD or Child-Pugh. This finding underlines the need for further assessment of liver specific rating scales in WD.
iv) We propose the patient reported "minimal UWDRS" (a nine item questionnaire) is a feasible, economical prescreening tool for the evaluation of the neurological status in WD patients with mild to moderate neurological symptoms.
v) Future studies are required to further evaluate the UWDRS, the GAS for WD, and the "minimal UWDRS" in WD patients with severe clinical symptoms.

Abbreviations

ADL: Activities of daily living; GAS for WD: Global assessment scale for wilson's disease; GeNeMove: German network of hereditary movement disorders; KFR: Kayser-fleischer rings; MELD score: Model of end stage liver disease score; UWDRS: Unified wilson's disease rating scale; WD: Wilson's disease

Acknowledgements

We thank the patients and their families for the support of this study. We are grateful to Dr. A. Aggarwal for thoroughly revising the manuscript and adding important aspects to the discussion. We acknowledge financial support by Deutsche Forschungsgemeinschaft and Ruprecht-Karls-Universität Heidelberg within the funding program Open Access Publishing.

Funding

This research received no specific funding.

Authors' contributions

HMV collected, analyzed, and interpreted the data. HMV also wrote the first draft of the manuscript. JP, JBG, WS, DNG and MS collected data and revised the manuscript critically for intellectual content. KHW and MW designed and supervised the study; collected, analyzed, and interpreted the data; and revised the manuscript critically for intellectual content. MW wrote the final manuscript. All authors read and approved the final manuscript.

Competing interests

KHW advises for Univar BV, Wilson Therapeutics, GMPO, BMS, and Bayer, and received grant support from Univar BV, Wilson Therapeutics, BMS, Novartis, Merck, and Bayer. KHW also received lecturer fees from Bayer, Orphan.

Author details

[1]Department of Internal Medicine IV, Heidelberg University Hospital, Im Neuenheimer Feld 410, Heidelberg, Germany. [2]Department of Neurology, Heidelberg University Hospital, Im Neuenheimer Feld 400, 69120 Heidelberg, Germany. [3]Department of Internal Medicine I, Heidelberg University Hospital, Im Neuenheimer Feld 410, Heidelberg, Germany.

References

1. Ferenci P. Pathophysiology and clinical features of Wilson disease. Metab Brain Dis. 2004;19:229–39.
2. Ferenci P, Caca K, Loudianos G, Mieli-Vergani G, Tanner S, Sternlieb I, Schilsky M, Cox D, Berr F. Diagnosis and phenotypic classification of Wilson disease. Liver Int. 2003;23:139–42.
3. Caca K, Ferenci P, Kuhn HJ, Polli C, Willgerodt H, Kunath B, Hermann W, Mossner J, Berr F. High prevalence of the H1069Q mutation in east German patients with Wilson disease: rapid detection of mutations by limited sequencing and phenotype-genotype analysis. J Hepatol. 2001;35:575–81.
4. Gromadzka G, Schmidt HH, Genschel J, Bochow B, Rodo M, Tarnacka B, Litwin T, Chabik G, Czlonkowska A. P.H1069Q mutation in ATP7B and biochemical parameters of copper metabolism and clinical manifestation of Wilson's disease. Mov Disord. 2006;21:245–8.
5. Shah AB, Chernov I, Zhang HT, Ross BM, Das K, Lutsenko S, Parano E, Pavone L, Evgrafov O, Ivanova-Smolenskaya IA, et al. Identification and analysis of mutations in the Wilson disease gene (ATP7B): population frequencies, genotype-phenotype correlation, and functional analyses. Am J Hum Genet. 1997;61:317–28.
6. Roberts EA, Schilsky ML. American Association for Study of liver D. Diagnosis and treatment of Wilson disease: an update. Hepatology. 2008;47:2089–111.
7. Svetel M, Kozic D, Stefanova E, Semnic R, Dragasevic N, Kostic VS. Dystonia in Wilson's disease. Mov Disord. 2001;16:719–23.
8. Oder W, Grimm G, Kollegger H, Ferenci P, Schneider B, Deecke L. Neurological and neuropsychiatric spectrum of Wilson's disease: a prospective study of 45 cases. J Neurol. 1991;238:281–7.
9. Starosta-Rubinstein S, Young AB, Kluin K, Hill G, Aisen AM, Gabrielsen T, Brewer GJ. Clinical assessment of 31 patients with Wilson's disease. Correlations with structural changes on magnetic resonance imaging. Arch Neurol. 1987;44:365–70.
10. Brewer GJ. Neurologically presenting Wilson's disease: epidemiology, pathophysiology and treatment. CNS Drugs. 2005;19:185–92.

11. Portala K, Levander S, Westermark K, Ekselius L, von Knorring L. Pattern of neuropsychological deficits in patients with treated Wilson's disease. Eur Arch Psychiatry Clin Neurosci. 2001;251:262–8.
12. Portala K, Westermark K, von Knorring L, Ekselius L. Psychopathology in treated Wilson's disease determined by means of CPRS expert and self-ratings. Acta Psychiatr Scand. 2000;101:104–9.
13. Walter G, Lyndon B. Depression in hepatolenticular degeneration (Wilson's disease). Aust N Z J Psychiatry. 1997;31:880–2.
14. Zimbrean PC, Schilsky ML. Psychiatric aspects of Wilson disease: a review. Gen Hosp Psychiatry. 2014;36:53–62.
15. Czlonkowska A, Tarnacka B, Litwin T, Gajda J, Rodo M. Wilson's disease—cause of mortality in 164 patients during 1992-2003 observation period. J Neurol. 2005;252:698–703.
16. Brewer GJ, Terry CA, Aisen AM, Hill GM. Worsening of neurologic syndrome in patients with Wilson's disease with initial penicillamine therapy. Arch Neurol. 1987;44:490–3.
17. Czlonkowska A, Tarnacka B, Moller JC, Leinweber B, Bandmann O, Woimant F, Oertel WH. Unified Wilson's disease rating scale – a proposal for the neurological scoring of Wilson's disease patients. Neurol Neurochir Pol. 2007;41:1–12.
18. Leinweber B, Moller JC, Scherag A, Reuner U, Gunther P, Lang CJ, Schmidt HH, Schrader C, Bandmann O, Czlonkowska A, et al. Evaluation of the unified Wilson's disease rating scale (UWDRS) in German patients with treated Wilson's disease. Mov Disord. 2008;23:54–62.
19. Aggarwal A, Aggarwal N, Nagral A, Jankharia G, Bhatt M. A novel global assessment scale for Wilson's disease (GAS for WD). Mov Disord. 2009;24:509–18.
20. Fahrmeir L. Statistik: der Weg zur Datenanalyse. 7th ed. Berlin, Heidelberg [u. a.]: Springer; 2010.
21. Kamath PS, Wiesner RH, Malinchoc M, Kremers W, Therneau TM, Kosberg CL, D'Amico G, Dickson ER, Kim WR. A model to predict survival in patients with end-stage liver disease. Hepatology. 2001;33:464–70.
22. Child CG, Turcotte JG. The liver and portal hypertension. In: Child CG, editor. Surgery and portal hypertension. Philadelphia: Saunders; 1964. p. 50–64.
23. Ala A, Walker AP, Ashkan K, Dooley JS, Schilsky ML. Wilson's disease. Lancet. 2007;369:397–408.
24. Benedeto-Stojanov D, Nagorni A, Bjelakovic G, Stojanov D, Mladenovic B, Djenic N. The model for the end-stage liver disease and child-Pugh score in predicting prognosis in patients with liver cirrhosis and esophageal variceal bleeding. Vojnosanit Pregl. 2009;66:724–8.
25. Nazer H, Ede RJ, Mowat AP, Williams R. Wilson's disease: clinical presentation and use of prognostic index. Gut. 1986;27:1377–81.
26. Weiss KH, Schafer M, Gotthardt DN, Angerer A, Mogler C, Schirmacher P, Schemmer P, Stremmel W, Sauer P. Outcome and development of symptoms after orthotopic liver transplantation for Wilson disease. Clin Transpl. 2013;27:914–22.
27. Weiss KH, Gotthardt DN, Klemm D, Merle U, Ferenci-Foerster D, Schaefer M, Ferenci P, Stremmel W. Zinc monotherapy is not as effective as chelating agents in treatment of Wilson disease. Gastroenterology. 2011;140:1189–98. e1181
28. Weiss KH, Stremmel W. Clinical considerations for an effective medical therapy in Wilson's disease. Ann N Y Acad Sci. 2014;1315:81–5.
29. Arguedas D, Stewart J, Hodgkinson S, Batchelor J. A neuropsychological comparison of siblings with neurological versus hepatic symptoms of Wilson's disease. Neurocase. 2015;21:154–61.
30. Iwanski S, Seniow J, Lesniak M, Litwin T, Czlonkowska A. Diverse attention deficits in patients with neurologically symptomatic and asymptomatic Wilson's disease. Neuropsychology. 2015;29:25–30.
31. Wenisch E, De Tassigny A, Trocello JM, Beretti J, Girardot-Tinant N, Woimant F. Cognitive profile in Wilson's disease: a case series of 31 patients. Rev Neurol (Paris). 2013;169:944–9.
32. Czlonkowska A, Gajda J, Rodo M. Effects of long-term treatment in Wilson's disease with D-penicillamine and zinc sulphate. J Neurol. 1996;243:269–73.

11

Relationship between serum uric acid level and mild cognitive impairment in Chinese community elderly

Miao Liu[1,2*†], Jianhua Wang[1,2†], Jing Zeng[1,2] and Yao He[1,2,3]

Abstract

Background: To evaluate the association between SUA levels within a normal to high range and the risk of mild cognitive impairment (MCI) among community elderly.

Methods: The present study was based on 2102 community elderly from a cross-sectional study conducted in a representative urban area of Beijing between 2009 and 2010. The mean age were 71.2 ± 6.6 years old, 59.7% were female. Mini-Mental State Examination (MMSE) was used to assess cognitive function by trained neurology doctors.

Results: The prevalence of hyperuricemia and MCI was 16.7% and 15.9% respectively. With the increase of SUA levels, the prevalence of MCI showed a strong decreasing linear trend. Multiple logistic regression analysis showed ORs for MCI were 1.01(95% CI: 0.69–1.48), 1.50(95% CI: 0.85–2.64), 1.65(95% CI: 1.12–2.43) and 1.53(95% CI: 1.00–2.33), 1.84(95% CI: 1.27–2.90), 1.92(95% CI: 1.02–3.35) for the second, third and highest quarters among men and women respectively (with the lowest quartile as the reference).

Conclusions: Higher SUA levels, when in the normal range, were positively associated with cognitive function among Chinese community elderly, but this association was not robust among participants with hyperuricemia.

Keywords: Chinese, Elderly, Epidemiology, Mild cognitive impairment, Uric acid

Background

With the acceleration in the population aging, dementia has become one of the most important health problems over the world [1]. Studies have estimated that the total number of population affected by dementia is about 46.8 million globally, and the number keeps increasing [2, 3]. According to WHO' report, the patients affected by dementia will double every 20 years, and most of them live in developing countries [4]. In China, dementia is also a serious problem along with the large elder population. It was estimated people with dementia in China increased from 3.68 million in 1990 to 9.19 million in 2010 [5]. On the other hand, the disease burden of dementia is huge. It will not only cause disability, reduce life quality of patients, and also causes burdens to caregivers and take up health and social care resources [6–8]. Hence, it's of critical importance to carry out early prevention and control of dementia.

Several studies have focused on serum uric acid (SUA) level and cognitive function [9–15]. Like the old saying, gout unlike any other disease, kills more wise men than simple, which means that gout patients have higher SUA levels and also higher intelligence quotient (including cognitive function) [16].Although a number of studies have revealed the relationship, the conclusion remains controversial. Some studies found that higher SUA level was beneficial to cognitive function and prevent cognitive impairment [12, 13]. But other studies also came to the opposite conclusion; SUA was a risk factor for cognitive function, like for cardiovascular disease [10]. Also, most studies only included the normal SUA levels, but missed the very high SUA level [17–19]. Thus, SUA levels within a normal range have not been fully studied with cognitive function. Therefore, we examined the association of SUA level in the normal range and also in

* Correspondence: liumiaolmbxb@163.com
†Equal contributors
1Institute of Geriatrics, Chinese PLA General Hospital, 28 Fuxing Road, Beijing 100853, China
2Beijing Key Laboratory of Aging and Geriatrics, Beijing, China
Full list of author information is available at the end of the article

the hyperuricemia range for related risk of MCI in an urban community elderly population of Beijing, China.

Methods

Study population

The sampling methods were reported in our previous study [20]. In brief, this was a population-based cross-sectional survey conducted in a metropolitan area representative of urban community in Beijing, China. A two-stage stratified clustering sampling method was used. First, 9 residents were randomly selected from the total 94 residents in Wanshoulu district. Second, all the individuals aged ≥60 years that had lived in the selected residence for more than 1 year were recruited. A total of 2162 residents aged 60–95 years were selected and invited for screening. Besides the 60 elderly with incomplete data, the left 2102 residents (848 men, 1254 women) completed the survey, and the participants accounted for about 10% of total elderly in Wanshoulu community.

All the nurses and doctors who took part in the field survey had strict training. Face-face interview was carried out, all the detail health condition of the participants were asked using a standardized questionnaire, including demographic factors, medical history, family history, and lifestyles. Physical examinations was carried out by specially trained nurses, including height, weight, waist circumstance (WC). We also calculated body mass index (BMI). Two blood pressures were measured using sphygmomanometer in a sitting position after 30 min' rest. Fasting blood specimens of all participants were obtained for standard tests of glucose, blood lipids and SUA level.

Definitions

Hyperuricemia was defined positive if SUA level was ≥7.0 mg/dL (417 μmol/L) in men or ≥6.0 mg/dL (357 μmol/L) in women, or positively diagnosed [21]. SUA levels of participants with and without hyperuricemia were categorized into 4 levels using the quartiles (P_{25}, P_{50} and P_{75}) as cut-off values by gender.

We used the Mini-Mental State Examination (MMSE) to assess cognitive function by trained neurology doctors. The MMSE scale was proved to be feasible among Chinese for dementia screening [22]. MCI was defined according the guideline, which is as follows: (1) for illiteracy participants, MMSE score less than a score of 17; (2) for participants with 1–6 education years, MMSE score less than a score of 20; (3) for participants with more than 7 education years, MMSE score less than a score of 24 [23, 24].

Prevalence of cerebral vascular disease and kidney disease was defined according to previous medical diagnosis by hospitals of second level and above. Current smoking was defined as those who currently smoked at least one cigarette daily; current alcohol drinking was defined as drinking alcohol at least once weekly for the past year. Physical activity was divided into two categories: ≥0.5 h/day or <0.5 h/day.

Statistical analysis

For the basic characteristics, $\bar{x} \pm s$ were used for continuous variables like age, WC, BMI, blood pressure, blood lipid, glycaemia and SUA level. *n* (%) were used for categorical variables like gender(male or female), education level (less than 6 years, or more than6 years), marriage status (married or unmarried), current smoking (yes or no), current drinking(yes or no), physical activity ≥ 0.5 h/day (yes or no), family history (yes or no). T test and Chi-square test were used to examine differences in continuous and categorical variables. Linear multiple regression and logistic multivariable regression was used to estimate the βand odds ratio (OR) of gender-specific SUA level with cognitive function. All analyses were conducted using SPSS (19.0, No. of Serial: 5,076,595).

Results

Clinical features of participants with and without hyperuricemia

The mean SUA level was 5.3 ± 1.4 mg/dL (range, 1.4–11.3 mg/dL), men had a higher SUA level than women (5.8 ± 1.3 vs 5.2 ± 1.4, $p < 0.001$). The general characteristics according to gender and hyperuricemia were shown in Table 1. The mean age were 71.2 ± 6.6 years old, 59.7% were female. The education level was high, 72.4% of all the participants had at least gone to junior middle school. Participants with hyperuricemia had older age, greater WC, higher BMI, higher TG, level and lower HDL-C levels. However, there were no significant differences in blood pressure and FPG. In women, besides these differences, we also observed higher levels of 2hPG in participants with hyperuricemia than those without. The percentage of participants who were married, better educated, current smoking and drinking did not differ with hyperuricemia. For MMSE score, participants with hyperuricemia had higher MMSE score in men (27.7 ± 2.6 vs 27.0 ± 3.8, $p = 0.014$) but not in women (27.0 ± 3.5 vs 26.7 ± 3.8, $p = 0.057$).

Age and gender-specific prevalence of hyperuricemia and MCI of the study participants

The prevalence of hyperuricemia and MCI in this community elderly was 16.7% and 15.9% respectively. Prevalence of both two diseases increased linearly with increasing age group ($p < 0.001$). Women have a statistically higher prevalence of MCI than men (18.0% vs. 12.9%, $P = 0.001$). For hyperuricemia, men had a relatively higher prevalence in the elderly aged less than 70 yrs., but women had increased at a faster rate than men, however, the difference was not statistically significance ($p > 0.05$). The results were listed in Table 2.

Table 1 General characteristics of the participants by hyperuricemia

Characteristic	Male (*n* = 848)				Female (*n* = 1254)				Total (*n* = 2102)
	hyperuricemia (*n* = 148)	No hyperuricemia (*n* = 700)	*P*	subtotal	hyperuricemia (*n* = 204)	No hyperuricemia (*n* = 1050)	*P*	subtotal	
$\bar{x} \pm s$									
Age (yrs)	73.5 ± 6.9	72.1 ± 6.8	0.028	72.3 ± 6.9	71.8 ± 6.0	70.1 ± 6.3	0.001	70.4 ± 6.2	71.2 ± 6.6
WC(cm)	94.0 ± 8.4	90.6 ± 8.4	<0.001	91.2 ± 8.5	90.3 ± 9.5	85.6 ± 8.6	<0.001	86.4 ± 8.9	88.3 ± 9.1
BMI(kg/m2)	25.7 ± 3.0	24.8 ± 3.1	0.002	24.9 ± 3.1	26.4 ± 3.8	24.8 ± 3.5	<0.001	25.0 ± 3.6	25.0 ± 3.4
SBP(mm Hg)	136.8 ± 17.5	136.6 ± 18.0	0.927	136.7 ± 17.9	141.9 ± 20.4	140.2 ± 20.9	0.285	140.5 ± 20.8	139.0 ± 19.8
DBP(mmHg)	77.4 ± 9.4	78.6 ± 9.7	0.191	78.4 ± 9.7	75.9 ± 10.4	76.8 ± 9.9	0.273	76.6 ± 10.0	77.3 ± 9.9
TC(mmol/L)	5.0 ± 1.1	4.9 ± 0.9	0.131	4.9 ± 0.9	5.5 ± 1.0	5.5 ± 1.0	0.550	5.5 ± 1.0	5.3 ± 1.0
TG(mmol/L)	1.8 ± 1.0	1.5 ± 0.8	0.001	1.5 ± 0.9	2.1 ± 1.0	1.7 ± 0.9	<0.001	1.8 ± 0.9	1.7 ± 0.9
HDL-C(mmol/L)	1.2 ± 0.3	1.3 ± 0.4	0.016	1.3 ± 0.4	1.4 ± 0.4	1.5 ± 0.4	<0.001	1.5 ± 0.4	1.4 ± 0.4
LDL-C(mmol/L)	3.1 ± 0.9	3.0 ± 0.8	0.338	3.1 ± 0.8	3.4 ± 0.8	3.4 ± 0.9	0.506	3.4 ± 0.9	3.3 ± 0.8
FPG(mmol/L)	6.0 ± 1.3	6.1 ± 1.6	0.428	6.1 ± 1.5	6.1 ± 1.3	6.1 ± 1.8	0.704	6.1 ± 1.8	6.1 ± 1.7
2hPG(mmol/L)	8.1 ± 2.6	8.2 ± 3.0	0.707	8.2 ± 3.0	9.2 ± 3.3	8.2 ± 3.3	<0.001	8.4 ± 3.3	8.3 ± 3.2
MMSE score	27.7 ± 2.6	27.0 ± 3.8	0.014	27.1 ± 3.6	27.0 ± 3.5	26.7 ± 3.8	0.057	26.8 ± 3.7	26.9 ± 3.7
n (%)									
Education ≥ 7 yrs	124(83.8)	576(82.3)	0.663	700(82.5)	142(69.6)	680(64.8)	0.183	822(65.6)	1522(72.4)
Married	131(88.5)	650(92.9)	0.075	781(92.1)	157(77.0)	836(79.6)	0.392	993(79.2)	1774(84.4)
Current smoking	27(18.2)	153(21.9)	0.329	180(21.2)	7(3.4)	44(4.2)	0.615	51(4.1)	231(11.1)
Current alcohol drinking	58(39.2)	267(38.1)	0.812	325(38.3)	14(6.9)	86(8.2)	0.522	100(8.0)	425(20.2)
Physical activity (≥0.5 h/day)	88(59.5)	422(60.3)	0.852	510(60.1)	121(59.3)	603(57.4)	0.618	724(57.7)	1234(58.7)
Family history of dementia	10(6.8)	32(4.6)	0.266	42(5.1)	10(4.9)	50(4.8)	0.932	60(4.8)	102(4.9)
Cerebral vascular disease	28(18.9)	90(12.9)	0.053	118(13.9)	25(12.3)	124(11.8)	0.857	149(11.9)	267(12.7)
Kidney disease	31(20.9)	52(7.4)	<0.001	83(9.8)	5(2.5)	17(1.6)	0.408	22(1.8)	105(5.0)

Data are mean ± SD for continuous values or n (%) for category values
TC total cholesterol, *TG* triglyceride, *LDL-C* low density lipoprotein cholesterol

Mean MMSE score and prevalence of MCI for participants with and without hyperuricemia

The mean MMSE score showed an increasing trend along with quarters of SUA levels among those without hyperuricemia in both genders (p for trend <0.05). The prevalence of MCI also showed the same trend, which decreased from 20.9% to 13.7% (p = 0.030). Among those participants who had hyperuricemia, the mean score of MMSE and the prevalence of MCI did not show statistically significant changing trend with SUA levels. The results were listed in Table 3. Also, we can see from Table 3, the mean score kept increasing for the first two quarters among

Table 2 Prevalence of hyperuricemia and MCI by gender and age group

	Prevalence of hyperuricemia (%)				Prevalence of MCI (%)			
	Men	Female	*p*	Subtotal	Men	Female	*p*	Subtotal
Age group								
60–69 yrs	14.8	12.3	0.300	13.2	7.4	9.9	0.048	9.0
70–79 yrs	17.8	18.7	0.704	18.3	12.9	22.4	<0.001	18.5
≥ 80 yrs	22.6	24.1	0.815	23.2	26.1	38.0	0.039	30.9
P_{trend}	0.036	0.002		<0.001	<0.001	<0.001		<0.001
subtotal	17.5	16.3	0.475	16.7	12.9	18.0	0.001	15.9

Table 3 MMSE score and MCI Prevalence According to SUA quartiles by gender and hyperuricemia

	SUA quartiles by gender and hyperuricemia					
	Q_1	Q_2	Q_3	Q_4	P_{trend}	total
Participants without hyperuricemia						
MMSE score						
Male	26.9 ± 3.9	27.0 ± 4.0	27.1 ± 3.4	27.2 ± 3.7	0.038	27.0 ± 3.8
Female	26.3 ± 3.8	26.5 ± 4.1	27.0 ± 3.9	27.1 ± 3.2	0.048	26.7 ± 3.8
Subtotal	26.6 ± 3.9	26.8 ± 4.1	27.0 ± 3.7	27.1 ± 3.4	0.031	26.8 ± 3.8
Prevalence of MCI						
Male	28(15.7)	23(13.7)	24(13.6)	21(11.9)	0.039	96(13.7)
Female	68(25.8)	52(20.1)	39(14.8)	36(13.6)	0.008	195(18.6)
Subtotal	96(20.9)	75(16.7)	63(15.2)	57(13.7)	0.030	291(16.6)
Participants with hyperuricemia						
MMSE score						
Male	27.8 ± 3.2	27.7 ± 2.5	27.7 ± 2.8	27.5 ± 2.2	0.965	27.7 ± 2.6
Female	26.7 ± 3.6	27.4 ± 2.7	27.2 ± 4.1	26.5 ± 3.4	0.549	27.0 ± 3.5
Subtotal	27.2 ± 3.4	27.5 ± 2.5	27.3 ± 3.6	27.0 ± 3.1	0.772	27.2 ± 3.1
Prevalence of MCI						
Male	5(13.5)	3(8.1)	4(10.8)	1(2.7)	0.155	13(8.8)
Female	9(18.8)	7(13.0)	4(7.8)	11(21.6)	0.854	31(15.2)
Subtotal	14(16.5)	10(11.0)	8(9.1)	12(13.6)	0.526	44(12.5)

those with hyperuricemia, and got decreased for the highest two quarters of SUA levels. The prevalence also decreased from 16.5% to 9.1% for the first three quarters, and changed to 13.6% for the highest quarter of SUA level.

Multivariate associations of SUA level with MMSE score and MCI prevalence

Table 4 showed the multivariate associations between SUA and with MMSE score and MCI prevalence. This table showed that after adjusted age, gender, education, marital status, current smoking, current alcohol drinking, BMI, physical activity ≥ 0.5 h/day, family history of dementia, hypertension, cerebral vascular disease and diabetes, participants with higher SUA levels were at significantly elevated risk for MCI prevalence among those without hyperuricemia. For MMSE score, the β (95% CI) of SUA were 0.14(95% CI: 0.04–0.42) and 0.28(95% CI: 0.02–0.53) for men and women respectively. For MCI prevalence, the OR (95% CI) of quarters of SUA showed an increasing trend. The ORs were

Table 4 Multiple linear and logistic regression of SUA level for MMSE score and MCI prevalence

	SUA level (continuous)		SUA level (quartiles by gender)				
MMSE score	β(95% CI)	*P*	Q1	Q2 β(95% CI)	Q3 β(95% CI)	Q4 β(95% CI)	P_{trend}
Participants with hyperuricemia							
Male	−0.03(−0.56–0.39)	0.721	1.00(Ref)	0.97(0.66–1.43)	0.92(0.58–1.26)	0.99(0.87–1.13)	0.544
Female	−0.01(−0.43–0.37)	0.882	1.00(Ref)	1.07(0.80–1.27)	1.05(0.78–1.31)	1.00(0.92–1.18)	0.922
Participants without hyperuricemia							
Male	0.14(0.04–0.42)	0.048	1.00(Ref)	1.01(0.69–1.48)	1.50(0.85–2.64)	1.65(1.12–2.43)	0.027
Female	0.28(0.02–0.53)	0.037	1.00(Ref)	1.53(1.00–2.33)	1.84(1.27–2.90)	1.92(1.02–3.35)	0.017
Prevalence of MCI	OR (95% CI)	*P*	Q1	Q2 OR (95% CI)	Q3 OR (95% CI)	Q4 OR (95% CI)	P_{trend}
Participants with hyperuricemia							
Male	1.06(0.47–1.64)	0.126	1.00(Ref)	0.48(0.10–2.33)	0.54(0.12–2.40)	0.10(0.01–0.97)	0.256
Female	1.02(0.67–1.56)	0.915	1.00(Ref)	0.59(0.18–1.90)	0.32(0.08–1.23)	1.08(0.36–3.20)	0.246
Participants without hyperuricemia							
Male	0.82(0.68–0.99)	0.047	1.00(Ref)	0.95(0.50–1.78)	0.91(0.49–1.70)	0.72(0.38–1.36)	0.025
Female	0.80(0.65–0.97)	0.034	1.00(Ref)	0.87(0.45–1.70)	0.72(0.44–1.77)	0.64(0.39–1.06)	0.008

Adjusted for age, education, marital status, BMI, current smoking, current drinking, physical activity ≥ 0.5 h/day, family history of dementia, hypertension, cerebral vascular disease and diabetes

1.01(95% CI: 0.69–1.48), 1.50(95% CI: 0.85–2.64), 1.65(95% CI: 1.12–2.43) and 1.53(95% CI: 1.00–2.33), 1.84(95% CI: 1.27–2.90), 1.92(95% CI: 1.02–3.35) for the second, third and highest quarters among men and women respectively (with the lowest quartile as the reference). Among the participants with hyperuricemia, the β (95% CI) for MMSE score were −0.03(95% CI: -0.56-0.39) and −0.01(95% CI: -0.43-0.37) for men and women. In the model of MCI prevalence, the ORs were also not statistically significant among participants with hyperuricemia.

We also ascertained the association of SUA level with MMSE score and MCI prevalence in the sensitivity analysis and the results were similar (Additional file 1: Appendix Table S1 and S2). When participants with cerebral vascular disease (n = 267, 12.7%) and kidney disease (n = 105, 5.0%) were excluded, the βs and ORs were similar with that in the Table 4. Higher SUA level was related with better cognitive function when SUA was in the normal range. There was also still no significant association among participants with hyperuricemia.

Discussion

In this representative community elderly based study; we evaluated the association of SUA level and cognitive function. The results that higher SUA level within normal range were positively associated with a decreased prevalence of MCI even after adjusting for demographic and other potential confounders. However, this association was not significant among participants with hyperuricemia.

Different from the high risk and harm of SUA level and cardiovascular diseases [25], a number of studies have provided evidence that SUA had protective effect on cognitive function and is beneficial to reduce dementia [14–16]. In this representative sample of Chinese urban elderly, we also found a graded positive association between hyperuricemia and cognitive function. When in the normal range, higher SUA level was associated with higher MMSE score and lower risk of MCI prevalence. And cognitive function was found to rise along with the increase of quarters of SUA levels. This is in accordance with previous studies. Molshatzki found that after 10 years follow-up, low uric acid levels in patients with preexisting cardiovascular disease are associated with poorer cognitive function [14]. Méndez-Hernández revealed that higher levels of uric acid are associated with a decreased risk of dementia using a case-control study in a Mexican population [13]. Yili Wu found that among Chinese aged 50–74 years, prevalence of cognitive disorder declined across UA tertiles [9]. The mechanism between higher SUA level and better cognitive function was not clear; one possible explanation was oxidative stress. SUA is a water-soluble antioxidant, which accounts for more than half of the free radical scavenging activity [17]. SUA could exert neuro-protective effects against Alzheimer's disease via its antioxidant capacities [16].

The present study also provides evidence that elevated SUA level was not associated with MCI among those participants with hyperuricemia. When SUA level was higher than the normal range, there was no statistically significant positive correlation with cognitive function. This result confirmed previous studies. A study about elderly women from U.S. showed higher baseline SUA levels was associated with poorer cognitive performance (p = 0.048). Another study from Italy showed that participants who had the highest SUA tertile had higher risk (OR = 3.32, 95%CI: 1.06–10.42) to suffer from dementia based on 1016 community-dwellings. On the other hand, there were several studies revealed that higher SUA levels were related to higher prevalence of gout and cardiovascular diseases [26, 27]. So the key question is what is the appreciate cut point for SUA levels. There is urgent need for long-time follow-up cohort studies to verify the optimal diagnostic boundary value, which would maximize the benefits, not only for gout and cardiovascular diseases, but also for MCI and dementia.

The study had several potential limitations. First, the SUA level was measured once, and may not reflect the true value, and did not consider the fluctuation. Second, the limitations of cross-sectional study lowered strength of evidence for causal inference. Long time follow up study are needed to confirm the results. Third, results among hyperuricemia individuals are based on very few cases of MCI patients, thus results might not be reliable. Fourth, there were several possible confounding factors we didn't consider ApoE genotype and drug treatment status. On the other hand, the study also some advantages. We used strict training process and quality assurance programs during the whole study. The selected community was representative metropolitan area of the geographic and economic characteristics in Beijing, and the response rate was high. So this population-based study with large sample and high response rate would have a good chance to better analysis the association between SUA level and cognitive function. Second, the SUA level in this study was carefully analyzed using the normal range and higher SUA level in hyperuricemia, which is different from most previous studies. The results also showed that it's not the simple "the higher the better" or "no correlation" or "the lower the better". The association results were different with SUA levels.

Conclusion

In summary, the present study showed higher SUA level are related to lower prevalence of MCI and better cognitive function, only when SUA level was in the normal range among Chinese community elderly population. This indicated that further studies should focus on the appropriate SUA level, which is helpful to reduce both dementia and cardiovascular diseases.

Acknowledgements
We thank Nurse Kang, Head Nurse Wang from PLA general hospital for research assistance and all the participants in flied works.

Funding
This study is supported by research grants from Beijing Natural Science Foundation (7174350), Beijing Municipal Science and Technology Commission (Z161100005016021), National key research and development program (2016YFC1303603) and State Key Development Program of Basic Research of China (973 programs, 2013CB530800). The funding body had no involvement in any stage of the study.

Authors' contributions
ML and YH contributed to the design of the study. All authors were involved in the analysis and interpretation of the data. JHW, and JZ conducted the statistical analysis. ML and YH worked on the drafting of the manuscript. All authors read and approved the final manuscript.

Competing interests
The author (s) declared no conflicts of interest with respect to the research, authorship, funding, and/or publication of this article.

Author details
[1]Institute of Geriatrics, Chinese PLA General Hospital, 28 Fuxing Road, Beijing 100853, China. [2]Beijing Key Laboratory of Aging and Geriatrics, Beijing, China. [3]State Key Laboratory of Kidney Disease, Chinese PLA General Hospital, 28 Fuxing Road, Beijing 100853, China.

References

1. Lambert MA, Bickel H, Prince M, Fratiglioni L, Von Strauss E, Frydecka D, et al. Estimating the burden of early onset dementia; systematic review of disease prevalence. Eur J Neurol. 2014;21:563–9.
2. Prince M, Bryce R, Albanese E, Wimo A, Ribeiro W, Ferri CP. The global prevalence of dementia: a systematic review and metaanalysis. Alzheimers Dement. 2013;9:63–75.
3. Wortmann M. Dementia: a global health priority - highlights from an ADI and World Health Organization report. Alzheimers Res Ther. 2012;4:40.
4. Alzheimer's Association. 2014 Alzheimer's disease facts and figures. Alzheimers Dement. 2014;10(2):e47–92.
5. Chan KY, Wang W, Wu JJ, Liu L, Theodoratou E, Car J, et al. Epidemiology of Alzheimer's disease and other forms of dementia in China, 1990-2010: a systematic review and analysis. Lancet. 2013;381:2016–23.
6. Yu R, Chau PH, McGhee SM, Cheung WL, Chan KC, Cheung SH, et al. Trends in prevalence and mortality of dementia in elderly Hong Kong population: projections, disease burden, and implications for long-term care. Int J Alzheimers Dis. 2012;2012:406852.
7. Prince M, Acosta D, Ferri CP, Guerra M, Huang Y, Jacob KS, et al. The association between common physical impairments and dementia in low and middle income countries, and, among people with dementia, their association with cognitive function and disability. A 10/66 dementia research group population-based study. Int J Geriatr Psychiatry. 2011;26:511–9.
8. Li N, Zhang L, Du W, Pang L, Guo C, Chen G, et al. Prevalence of dementia-associated disability among Chinese older adults: results from a national sample survey. Am J Geriatr Psychiatry. 2015;23:320–5.
9. Wu Y, Zhang D, Pang Z, Jiang W, Wang S, Tan Q. Association of serum uric acid level with muscle strength and cognitive function among Chinese aged 50-74 years. Geriatr Gerontol Int. 2013;13:672–7.
10. Vannorsdall TD, Kueider AM, Carlson MC, Schretlen DJ. Higher baseline serum uric acid is associated with poorer cognition but not rates of cognitive decline in women. Exp Gerontol. 2014;60:136–9.
11. Gonzalez-Aramburu I, Sanchez-Juan P, Sierra M, Fernandez-Juan E, Sanchez-Quintana C, Berciano J, et al. Serum uric acid and risk of dementia in Parkinson's disease. Parkinsonism Relat Disord. 2014;20:637–9.
12. Cicero AF, Desideri G, Grossi G, Urso R, Rosticci M, D'Addato S, et al. Serum uric acid and impaired cognitive function in a cohort of healthy young elderly: data from the Brisighella study. Intern Emerg Med. 2015;10:25–31.
13. Mendez-Hernandez E, Salas-Pacheco J, Ruano-Calderon L, Tellez-Valencia A, Cisneros-Martinez J, Barraza-Salas M, et al. Lower uric acid linked with cognitive dysfunction in the elderly. CNS Neurol Disord Drug Targets. 2015;14:564–6.
14. Molshatzki N, Weinstein G, Streifler JY, Goldbourt U, Tanne D. Serum uric acid and subsequent cognitive performance in patients with pre-existing cardiovascular disease. PLoS One. 2015;10:e120862.
15. Tuven B, Soysal P, Unutmaz G, Kaya D, Isik AT. Uric acid may be protective against cognitive impairment in older adults, but only in those without cardiovascular risk factors. Exp Gerontol. 2017;89:15–9.
16. De Giorgi A, Fabbian F, Pala M, Tiseo R, Parisi C, Misurati E, et al. Uric acid: friend or foe? Uric acid and cognitive function "gout kills more wise men than simple". Eur Rev Med Pharmacol Sci. 2015;19:640–6.
17. Euser SM, Hofman A, Westendorp RG, Breteler MM. Serum uric acid and cognitive function and dementia. Brain. 2009;132:377–82.
18. Ruggiero C, Cherubini A, Lauretani F, Bandinelli S, Maggio M, Di Iorio A, et al. Uric acid and dementia in community-dwelling older persons. Dement Geriatr Cogn Disord. 2009;27:382–9.
19. Li J, Dong BR, Lin P, Zhang J, Liu GJ. Association of cognitive function with serum uric acid level among Chinese nonagenarians and centenarians. Exp Gerontol. 2010;45:331–5.
20. Liu M, He Y, Jiang B, Wu L, Yang S, Wang Y, et al. Association between serum uric acid level and metabolic syndrome and its sex difference in a Chinese community elderly population. Int J Endocrinol. 2014;2014:754678.
21. B L, T W, Hn Z, Ww Y, Hp Y, Cx L, et al. The prevalence of hyperuricemia in China: a meta-analysis. BMC Public Health. 2011;11:832.
22. Xu G, Meyer JS, Huang Y, Du F, Chowdhury M, Quach M. Adapting mini-mental state examination for dementia screening among illiterate or minimally educated elderly Chinese. Int J Geriatr Psychiatry. 2003;18:609–16.
23. Peng D, Xu X, Liu J, Jiao Y, Zhuang H, Meng X, et al. Discussion on application of MMSE for senile dementia patients. *Chinese Journal of Neuroimmunology and Neurology*2005. 12:187–90.
24. Liu M, He Y, Jiang B, Wu L, Wang J, Yang S, et al. Association between metabolic syndrome and mild cognitive impairment and its age difference in a Chinese community elderly population. Clin Endocrinol. 2015;82:844–53.
25. Braga F, Pasqualetti S, Ferraro S, Panteghini M. Hyperuricemia as risk factor for coronary heart disease incidence and mortality in the general population: a systematic review and meta-analysis. Clin Chem Lab Med. 2016;54:7–15.
26. Galassi FM, Borghi C. A brief history of uric acid: from gout to cardiovascular risk factor. Eur J Intern Med. 2015;26:373.
27. Abeles AM. Hyperuricemia, gout, and cardiovascular disease: an update. Curr Rheumatol Rep. 2015;17:13.

12

Evoked potentials after painful cutaneous electrical stimulation depict pain relief during a conditioned pain modulation

Oliver Höffken[1*], Özüm S. Özgül[1], Elena K. Enax-Krumova[1], Martin Tegenthoff[1] and Christoph Maier[2]

Abstract

Background: Conditioned pain modulation (CPM) evaluates the pain modulating effect of a noxious conditioning stimulus (CS) on another noxious test stimulus (TS), mostly based solely on subjective pain ratings. We used painful cutaneous electrical stimulation (PCES) to induce TS in a novel CPM-model. Additionally, to evaluate a more objective parameter, we recorded the corresponding changes of cortical evoked potentials (PCES-EP).

Methods: We examined the CPM-effect in 17 healthy subjects in a randomized controlled cross-over design during immersion of the non-dominant hand into 10 °C or 24 °C cold water (CS). Using three custom-built concentric surface electrodes, electrical stimuli were applied on the dominant hand, inducing pain of 40–60 on NRS 0–100 (TS). At baseline, during and after CS we assessed the electrically induced pain intensity and electrically evoked potentials recorded over the central electrode (Cz).

Results: Only in the 10 °C-condition, both pain (52.6 ± 4.4 (baseline) vs. 30.3 ± 12.5 (during CS)) and amplitudes of PCES-EP (42.1 ± 13.4 μV (baseline) vs. 28.7 ± 10.5 μV (during CS)) attenuated during CS and recovered there after (all $p < 0.001$). In the 10 °C-condition changes of subjective pain ratings during electrical stimulation and amplitudes of PCES-EP correlated significantly with each other ($r = 0.5$) and with CS pain intensity ($r = 0.5$).

Conclusions: PCES-EPs are a quantitative measure of pain relief, as changes in the electrophysiological response are paralleled by a consistent decrease in subjective pain ratings. This novel CPM paradigm is a feasible method, which could help to evaluate the function of the endogenous pain modulation processes.

Keywords: CPM, Electrically evoked potentials, Cold pressor test, Pain relief

Background

Conditioned pain modulation (CPM) describes the analgesic effect of a noxious conditioning stimulus (CS) on a noxious test stimulus (TS), based on the diffuse noxious inhibitory control [1–3]. Impaired endogenous pain inhibition has been demonstrated in several chronic pain states [4]. Furthermore, ineffective endogenous analgesia seems to represent a risk for developing chronic postoperative pain and opioid-induced hyperalgesia [5–8]. Remarkably, patients with painful diabetic neuropathy and insufficient endogenous analgesia respond better to duloxetine, a serotonin-noradrenalin-reuptake-inhibitor supposed to enhance the function of the descending inhibitory pathways [5].

Different fMRI studies focused on the neural mechanism of CPM. For example, using heat as TS and intramuscular injection of hypertonic saline as CS, the signal intensity increases during each TS in the presence of the CS were reduced in three brainstem regions: the caudalis subdivision of the spinal trigeminal nucleus, i.e., the primary synapse, the region of the subnucleus reticularis dorsalis and in the dorsolateral pons near the parabrachial nucleus [9]. These changes also correlated with the

* Correspondence: oliver.hoeffken@rub.de
[1]Department of Neurology, Berufsgenossenschaftliches Universitätsklinikum Bergmannsheil GmbH, Ruhr-University Bochum, Bürkle-de-la-Camp-Platz 1, 44789 Bochum, Germany
Full list of author information is available at the end of the article

magnitude of analgesia. A further study using phasic heat as TS and heterotopic ice-cold as CS reported the psychophysical effect to be directly proportional to the cold-induced modulation of the laser-induced BOLD response in left posterior insula/SII, correlating also with changes in the anterior cingulate, orbitofrontal and lateral prefrontal cortices [10]. Obermann et al. combined functional magnetic resonance imaging and electrically evoked pain- related potentials (PREP) in healthy subjects showing that increasing stimulus intensity results in a similar increase of pain ratings, PREP, and BOLD responses within the pACC (posterior part of the anterior cingulate cortex), PCC (posterior cingulate cortex), insula, and somatosensory cortex (SII) [11].

Hitherto, there is no commonly accepted protocol for CPM-assessment [12]. Numerous paradigms with different TS and CS (pressure, heat, cold, ischemia, electricity, laser) have been introduced, with high variability in the magnitude of the CPM-effect across subjects and studies [13]. Several studies have evaluated the CPM-effect using electrophysiological findings to objectively quantify the CPM effect, based on the spinal nociceptive flexion reflex (changes of amplitude [14] or threshold [15]), the R2-response of the blink reflex [16], as well as on sensory evoked potentials (SEP) after CO_2-laser stimulation [17–19], electrical tooth stimulation [20, 21], contact-heat stimulation [2] and chemonasal CO_2-stimulation [22]. All of them showed significant effects across the study populations, however, they report of variable effects on individual subject level, and not all studies reported the number of subjects in whom the CPM-effect was detectable [23]. This is an important issue, because under optimal circumstances one needs a CPM protocol using reliable test and conditioning stimuli, which, as a control condition, is also able to elicit a CPM-effect in healthy subjects. Otherwise, in case that during CPM assessment a patient has no CPM-effect, one would not be able to differentiate whether this is due to methodological reasons or whether it is an abnormal finding due to the underlying disease.

Until now, and despite their clinical relevance in the assessment of small fiber function based on the pain-related evoked potentials [24–27], and the early scientific interest in electrically induced cortical potentials [28], the CPM-effect has not been investigated using painful cutaneous electrical stimulation (PCES) induced by K^2 stimulation electrodes generating evoked potentials (PCES-EP) as TS. PCES-EP are recorded after activation of intraepidermal nociceptive fibers using custom-built concentric surface electrodes with small anode-cathode distance (K^2 stimulation electrodes) [29], inducing a pinprick-like sensation. Although estimated mean conduction velocity was reported to be 11.61 ± 5.12 m/s, which is close to conduction velocity of A-delta fibers [29], this type of stimulation cannot exclude the possibility of low-threshold mechanoreceptors being involved. Interestingly, the individual pain ratings during PCES and amplitudes of PCES-EP have been shown to correlate significantly [29, 30]. Therefore, PCES-EP induced by using K^2 stimulation electrodes has a potential to provide a link between subjective pain estimation and objective electrophysiological measures. Furthermore, it has been shown that both the amplitude of the PCES-EP as well as the induced pain intensity has a high test-retest reliability [31].

The aim of the study was to investigate the capability of PCES-EP to objectively evaluate the CPM-effect electrophysiologically. Therefore, we applied PCES as TS and recorded both the subjective pain ratings induced by PCES-EP, and the amplitude of PCES-EP at baseline, during and after CS. As CS we chose the immersion of the hand into cold water as it is commonly used and elicits stronger CPM-effects compared to other CS [32] and has been also shown to be a reliable stimulus in terms of the induced pain intensity [33].

Methods

Participants

After approval by the local ethics committee (Reg. Nr. 15-5300; 06–16-2015) 18 healthy subjects (age > 18 years) were recruited after informed consent, using recently recommended inclusion and exclusion criteria [34]. The study was conducted in the department of Neurology, University Hospital Bergmannsheil Bochum, Germany between June and August 2015. Exclusion criteria included current pain, neuropathy, nerve lesions, topical drug treatment, history of neurological, psychiatric or severe cardiovascular diseases. A sample size calculation was performed using data on changes of the N2-P2-amplitudes of contact heat evoked potentials (CHEP) from a study examining the conditioned pain modulation with CHEP as a test stimulus and painful heat as conditioning stimulus [2] and revealed for a power of 80%, type I error of 0.05 and an estimated drop-out rate of 5% a sample size of at least 14 subjects per study arm in a crossover design.

Before stimulation we determined handedness by the German version of the Edinburgh Handedness Inventory [35].

PCES-EP

We denoted the pain perceived during painful cutaneous electrical stimulation of the intraepidermal nociceptive fibers for PCES-EP-recording as '*PCES pain*'. '*PCES-EP -amplitude*' was the corresponding peak-to-peak amplitude N1-P1 recorded over central electrode Cz according to the international 10–20-System.

For PCES, we placed three custom-built concentric surface electrodes (K^2 electrodes used to induces pain-related evoked potentials (PREP) in previous studies) [36] on the dominant hand in a triangular formation (distance of 1.5–2 cm at the dorsum of the hand, supply area of the superficial radial nerve). The stimulation electrodes are connected in parallel to a stimulator (Digitimer DS7A). We fixed the electrodes as such that all of the stimuli were applied at the same location. One electrical stimulus applied simultaneously by all three stimulation electrodes consisted of a train of three monopolar squares waves of 200 μs duration with 5 ms interval in between (see Fig. 1). We applied 20 triple trains in 5 blocks with a variable intertrain interval of 4–6 s in a pseudorandomized manner, with a fixed interblock interval of 12 s. Thus, each of the 5 blocks consisted of 4 triple trains à 10.6 ms and lasted 15.04 s, thus the whole procedure with application of 20 triple trains lasted about 96.17 s.

After every 4 triple trains subjects reported the current PCES-pain intensity to the examiner as a rating on the 101-point numerical rating scale (NRS, 0 = no pain and 100 = strongest pain imaginable) after they have been instructed and familiarized with the NRS prior to the experiment, thus resulting in a total of 5 ratings per PCES-EP-session. As the 5 values within the baseline period were stable (data not shown), the PCES pain intensity was defined as the mean of the 5 ratings for further statistics.

According to the international 10–20-System, the recording electrode was at Cz, referred to linked earlobes (A1 and A2). Impedances were kept below 5 kΩ. PCES-EPs were recorded and stored for offline analysis with a 32-channel-amplifier (Brain Amp, Brain Products, Germany; bandwidth: 1 Hz-1 kHz, sampling rate: 5 kHz). PCES-EPs were analyzed in sweeps from 200 ms before and 800 ms after onset of the triple pulses, and averaged. We determined the latency of N1-peak and N1-P1 peak-to-peak amplitude. In accordance to previous studies [11, 29, 30], we rejected the first sweep to avoid contamination by startle response. Prior to averaging, one experienced investigator evaluated all records individually to exclude technical or blink artifacts.

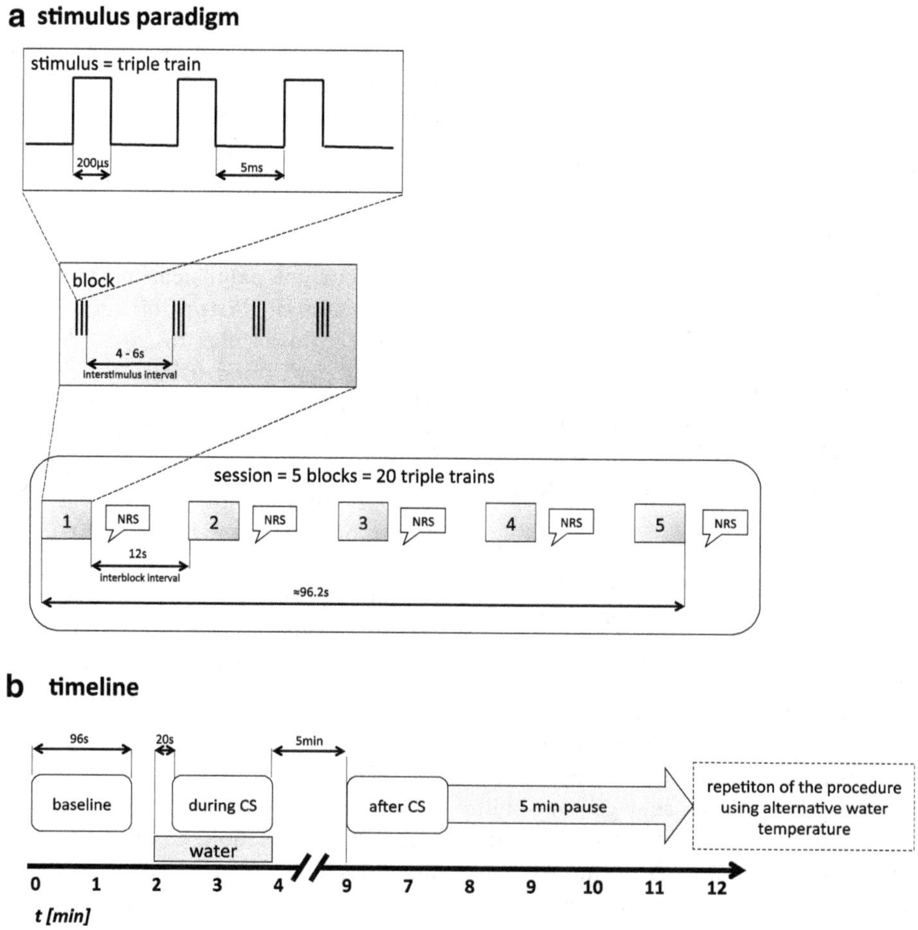

Fig. 1 Stimulation paradigm (**a**) and timeline of experimental procedure (**b**)

Experimental procedure

The study was designed as a randomized placebo-controlled crossover study.

During the experiment subjects sat in a comfortable chair in an air-conditioned room.

The conditioned pain modulation was assessed using the PCES as TS. As CS we used immersion of the non-dominant hand into a container filled with cold water at a temperature of 10 ± 2 °C (cold and intended to be painful), or – as a control condition – water of 24 ± 2 °C (cold, but intended to be non-painful), in a crossover design. Participants were randomized via a paper-pencil-based lot to sequence A (first 24 °C cold water; then 10 °C) or to sequence B (vice versa). During the whole experiment, an infrared thermometer measured the skin temperature next to the used K^2-stimulation electrodes before and after every PCES-EP-session.

The CPM-assessment consisted of three blocks denoted as 'baseline, 'during CS and 'after CS. At first, subjects were familiarized with the stimulus characteristic by applying current intensities inducing subthreshold (i.e. painless tingling) and suprathreshold (i.e. pinprick-like pain) sensations. Then, the 'baseline'-block started with a PCES-EP -session to receive stable PCES-EP and stable PCES-pain corresponding to NRS 40–60, estimating the pain intensity after every 4 electrical stimuli. Therefore, stimulus intensity of presented triple pulses was adjusted until subjects perceived a stable electrically-induced pain level of 5 successive stimuli. We defined the pain intensity as stable, if the value of four successive pain ratings did not change more than 5 points on the NRS (0–100). In the 'during CS'-block subjects immersed their non-dominant hand into 24 °C or 10 °C cold water, depending on the randomization. An investigator (OH) not involved in the documentation of pain and analysis of PCES-EP prepared the conditioning stimulus (temperature of cold-water) and generated the random allocation sequence. The second examiner (ÖÖ) was blinded to the intervention. Additionally, the subjects were blinded for the aim of the experiments.

Immediately after hand immersion into the water, subjects estimated the pain intensity induced by the coldness on the NRS (0–100). After 20 s, the PCES-EP recordings were repeated during CS, and after every 4 stimuli the subjects estimated the pain intensity both induced by electrical stimulation and cold water. Finally, after about 2 min, subjects took their hand out of the water. Five min later, the PCES-EP-session 'after CS' was performed. After additional 5 min, the procedure was repeated using the alternative water temperature, thus the interval between the end of the conditioning stimulus of the first test session and the begin of the testing stimulus of the second test session was 10 min, as previously recommended [12].

Definition of the CPM-effect

The CPM-effect_{PAIN} was calculated as difference between the mean of the 5 pain ratings during CS and the mean of the 5 pain ratings at baseline (each after electrical stimulus No. 4, 8, 12, 16 and 20) [5, 37].

CPM-effect$_{PAIN}$ *= Mean of 5 pain ratings (during) – Mean of 5 pain ratings (baseline).*

Additionally, we calculated the $\text{CPM-effect}_{AMPLITUDE}$ as difference between the mean of the 19 PCES-EP-amplitudes during CS and the mean of the 19 PCES-EP-amplitudes at baseline:

CPM-effect$_{AMPLITUDE}$ *= Mean of 19 PCES-EP-amplitudes (during) – Mean of 19 PCES-EP-amplitudes (baseline).*

According to Granot, Yarnitsky et al., every difference < 0 was suggested to represent an efficient pain inhibition [5, 37], both for CPM-effect_{PAIN} and $\text{CPM-effect}_{AMPLITUDE}$. However, others have suggested that some allowance should be made for measurement error, though using another CPM-protocol, based on pressure pain thresholds as test stimulus [38]. Yet, the current recommendations for CPM-practice stated no cut-off value for definition of a sufficient CPM-effect [12].

Statistical analysis

All analyses were conducted using SPSS version 19 (IBM, New York, NY), with statistical significance at $p < 0.05$.

Descriptive statistics are presented as means and standard deviations. Nominal parameters were analyzed using χ2-tests.

ANOVA for repeated measures was performed for the dependent variables PCES-EP-amplitude, PCES-pain, and PCES-EP-N1-latency with between-subjects factors group of subjects (sequence A and B), levels of "temperature levels" (24 °C and 10 °C water temperature), and within-subjects factor "time period" (baseline, during and after cold water stimulation).

Differences in the CPM-effect based on PCES-pain and PCES-EP-amplitude between both temperature conditions (10 °C-water and 24 °C-water as CS) were evaluated using two-tailed paired t-tests. Pearson correlation analysis was performed between PCES-EP-amplitude and PCES-pain, between their changes during CPM-assessment (based on the difference, i.e. CPM-effect_{PAIN} as well as $\text{CPM-effect}_{AMPLITUDE}$, and based on the ratios for pain intensity and amplitude of the evoked potentials, i.e. "during CS" divided by "baseline"). Further on, the changes during CPM-assessment were correlated to the cold water pain intensity. Additionally, linear regression analysis was performed with 'changes of PCES-EP-amplitude' as dependent variable, and 'changes of PCES-pain' and 'pain induced by the cold water' as independent variables.

Results

Participants

One subject failed to perceive pain with a reproducible intensity of 40–60 on the NRS during TS application, and was therefore excluded. Hence, 17 participants (age: 28.1 ± 2.1 years (mean ± SEM), range 19–45 years; 9 female) were included from further analysis. Eight subjects were allocated to sequence A (firstly exposed to 24 °C cold water; then to 10 °C) and 9 to sequence B (firstly exposed to 10 °C cold water; then to 24 °C). There were no unintended side effects during the experiments.

Stimulation intensity

The mean stimulus intensity to induce a pain of NRS 50–60 was 7.3 ± 5.4 mA (range 1.6 – 20 mA). Please note that in our stimulation setting all 3 electrodes were connected in parallel to a single stimulator. Hence, the given current intensities are proportionally distributed over all electrodes. The stimulation was well tolerated without evoking any muscle twitches, and no one quit study participation due to intolerably painful stimuli.

CPM-effect

N1-P1-amplitude, N1- and P1-latency of PCES-EP were normally distributed according to the Kolmogorov–Smirnov test and visual inspection of data histograms. Both for PCES-pain and PCES-EP-amplitude, ANOVA yielded a significant effect of the factor "time period" (PCES-pain: $F_{2;60} = 35.212$, $p < 0.001$; PCES-EP-amplitude: $F_{2;60} = 42.423$, $p < 0.001$) and a significant effect of "temperature level" (PCES-pain: $F_{2;60} = 12.686$, $p < 0.001$; PCES-EP-amplitude: $F_{2;60} = 21.404$, $p < 0.001$), while there was no interaction between "time period" and "temperature level" (PCES-pain: $F_{2;60} = 0.319$, $p = 0.728$; PCES-EP-amplitude: $F_{2;60} = 0.529$, $p = 0.592$). We found a significant effect of "sequence" on the PCES-EP-amplitude ($F = 11.843$, $p < 0.005$), probably due to differences in the amplitudes between both subject populations, at the aimed pain intensity of NRS 60 on the 101-point rating scale (see Fig. 2b). However, there was no significant effect of "sequence" on the pain intensity ($F_{2;60} = 1.561$, $p = 0.221$), and more importantly, there was no significant interaction of "time period" and "sequence" (PCES-pain: $F_{2;60} = 1.297$, $p = 0.281$; PCES-EP-amplitude: $F_{2;60} = 0.870$, $p = 0.424$, Fig. 2). Thus, the CPM-conditions were analyzed independently from the sequence.

For N1-latency, ANOVA yielded a significant effect of the factor "time period" ($F_{2;60} = 3.568$, $p = 0.034$), but there was no effect of "sequence", "temperature level" and interaction of "time period" and "sequence". Independent of factor "sequence" and "temperature" level N1-latency increased significantly from "baseline" (131.5 ± 11.2 ms) to "during CS" (133.7 ± 12.2 ms; $P = 0.025$), while there was no change from "during CS" to "after CS" (133.9 ± 12.1 ms; $P = 0.823$).

Skin temperature

ANOVA for repeated measurements yielded neither significant skin temperature changes during the experiment (factor "time period": $F_{2;64} = 0.142$, $p = 0.868$), nor significant differences between the 10 °C- and 24 °C-conditions (factor "temperature level": $F_{1;32} = 0.037$, $p = 0.849$), and no significant interaction between both factors ($F_{2;64} = 0.457$, $p = 0.635$).

Cold water pain, PCES-pain, and PCES-EP-*amplitude during CPM-assessment*

In the 10 °C-condition the average rating of the cold water pain was significantly higher (58.9 ± 25.4, range: 0–90.8 NRS), compared to the 24 °C-condition (6.9 ± 1.8, range: 0–41.7 NRS, $p < 0.001$).

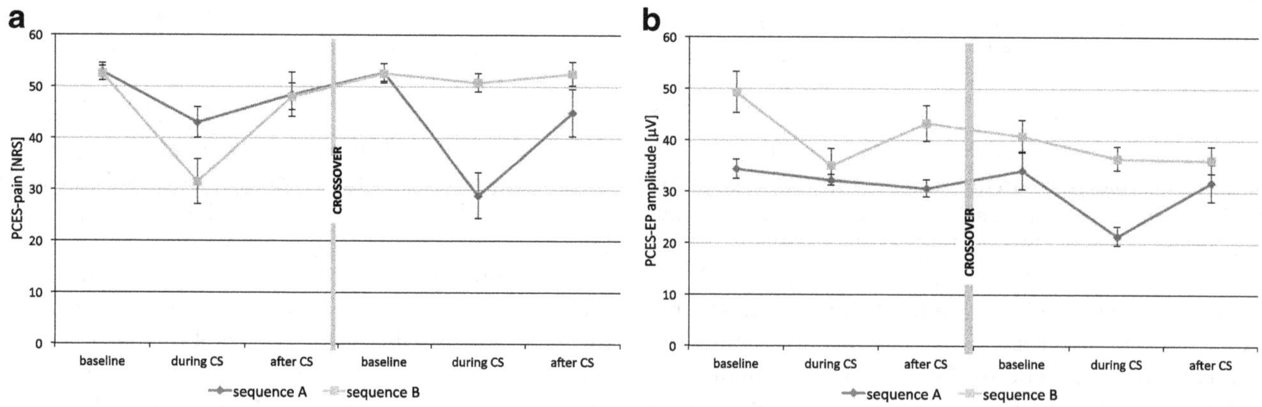

Fig. 2 Time course of PCES-pain (**a**) and PCES-EP-amplitude (**b**) in sequence A (firstly 24 °C cold water; then 10 °C cold water as conditioning stimulus) and B (firstly 10 °C cold water; then 24 °C cold water as conditioning stimulus)

In the 10 °C-condition, both PCES-EP-amplitude (p = 0.003) and PCES-pain (p < 0.001) decreased between the 'baseline' and 'during CS' session (Table 1). After CS-termination, both PCES-pain (p < 0.001) and PCES-EP-amplitude (p = 0.022) increased. In the 24 °C-condition only PCES-pain decreased significantly 'during CS' compared to 'baseline' (p = 0.019), but not PCES-EP-amplitude (p = 0.194) (see Fig. 3). After CS-termination we found no changes of both parameters (PCES-EP-amplitude p = 0.678; PCES-pain p = 0.256).

Regarding the PCES-pain ratings, 16 subjects (94%) had a CPM-effect$_{PAIN}$ < 0 in the 10 °C-condition versus 12 subjects (71%) in the 24 °C-condition (p = 0.072). Regarding the PCES-EP-amplitudes, all subjects had a CPM-effect$_{PCES}$ < 0 in the 10 °C-condition versus 13 subjects (76%) in the 24 °C-condition (p = 0.003). However, both CPM-effect$_{PAIN}$ and CPM-effect$_{AMPLITUDE}$ were significantly higher in the 10 °C-condition than in the control condition (both p < 0.00001, Table 1).

CPM-assessment based on the PCES-EP-amplitude (N1-P1) and PCES-EP-latency (N1), as well as the PCES-pain; CPM-effects are shown for absolute (abs.) and relative (rel.) changes from baseline to during CS; data was accumulated disregarding the randomization sequence (sequence A or B), as there was no evidence for a sequence-effect on the results.

Relation between cold water pain, PCES-pain and PCES-EP-amplitude during CPM-assessment

In the 10 °C-condition, we assessed the interaction between cold water pain, changes of PCES-EP-amplitudes and changes of PCES-pain. Analyzing the changes of PCES-pain and PCES-EP-amplitude as ratios ('during CS'/'baseline'), the ratios for PCES-pain and PCES-EP-amplitude correlated significantly (r = 0.50, p < 0.05, Fig. 4).

The cold water pain intensity correlated with the PCES-EP-amplitude ratios (r = −0.5, p < 0.05) and with the PCES-pain ratios (r = −0.6, p < 0.01). PCES-EP-latency correlated with PCES-pain (r = −0.65; p < 0.01), but not with cold pain (r = 0.05; p = 0.429) or PCES-EP-amplitude (r = −0.2; p = 429).

Discussion

Applying PCES using K^2 stimulation electrodes as TS, we could induce endogenous pain inhibition by hand immersion in 10 °C cold water, and assessed the CPM-effect both subjectively based on pain ratings, and objectively using electrophysiological measures. On a group level, during the 10 °C-condition, the PCES-induced pain and the PCES amplitude was reduced on average by 42% and 32%, respectively (vs. 10% and 7%, respectively, during the control condition). On single-subject level, the PCES-EP-amplitude decreased in all subjects and the PCES-pain intensity decreased in 94% of the cases, in contrast to other published protocols, which were not able to induce a CPM-effect in all subjects, e.g. [23, 38]. More important, the reported changes in subjective pain intensity and the objectively measured changes in PCES-EP-amplitude correlated significantly. On a group level, the changes in both subjective pain ratings and objective electrophysiological measures were significant only in the painful water condition, but not in the control condition where the PCES-EP-amplitude did not change significantly.

PCES as TS

The magnitudes of this CPM-effect based on subjective pain ratings during PCES in our study (42 ± 24%) is comparable to previous studies using painful cold as CS, where the CPM-effect based on subjective pain ratings varied between 10% and 60% from the baseline [13, 39, 40].

We investigated the feasibility of PCES-pain to assess the CPM-effect as this technique provides several advantages over other TS. The very confined stimulation zone of K^2 stimulation electrodes (3 × 19.6 mm^2 = 58.8 mm^2) enables stimulation of small skin areas, whereas heat as most often used TS is usually being applied via thermodes with a contact area of 900mm^2. Another advantage of PCES using K^2 stimulation electrodes is the brief, distinct and well-tolerable pinprick-like pain. The electrical stimuli are safe and can be repeated without relevant risk of tissue damage. While using repeated heat pain as TS is limited due to habituation of both pain ratings and contact heat evoked potentials (CHEP) [41, 42], in our study the PCES-pain intensity showed no habituation and remained stable over 20 stimuli with

Table 1 Parameters of the Conditioned Pain Modulation (CPM)

	10° condition			24° condition		
	PCES-induced pain (NRS 0–100)	PCES- amplitude (μV)	PCES-latency (ms)	PCES-induced pain (NRS 0–100)	PCES-amplitude (μV)	PCES-latency (ms)
baseline	52.6 ± 4.4	42.1 ± 13.4	130.7 ± 10.5	52.7 ± 5.0	37.8 ± 8.3	132.2 ± 12.1
during CS	30.3 ± 12.5	28.7 ± 10.5	133.5 ± 11.9	47.1 ± 7.8	34.5 ± 5.8	133.9 ± 12.8
after CS	46.6 ± 10.4	37.9 ± 11.7	133.3 ± 12.8	50.6 ± 9.6	33.6 ± 7.1	134.5 ± 11.8
CPM-effect (abs.)	−22.4 ± 13.6	−13.5 ± 6.4	2.8 ± 6.2	−5.6 ± 6.5	−3.3 ± 4.7	1.6 ± 4.8
CPM-effect (rel.)	42.0 ± 24.3%	32.0 ± 10.7%	−2.1 ± 5.1%	10.5 ± 12.6%	7.2 ± 11.0%	−1.3 ± 3.7

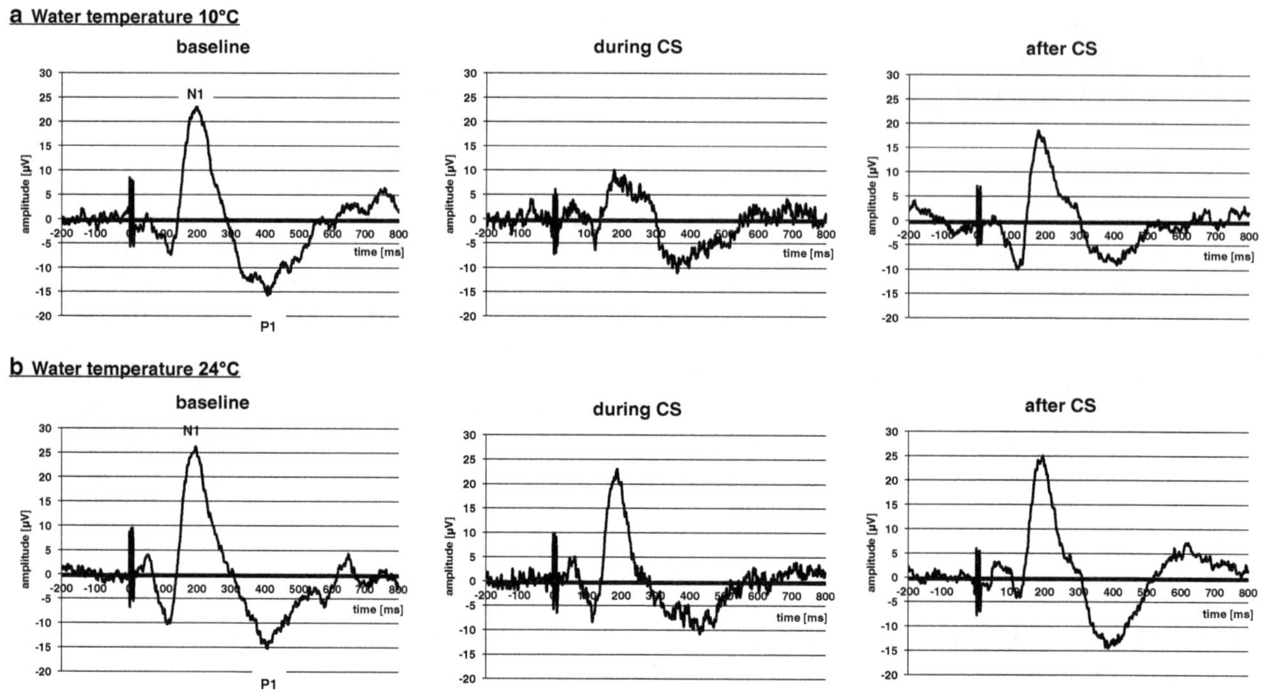

Fig. 3 PCES-EPs of one participant shown at baseline, during CS, and after CS in both conditions: **a**) water temperature 10 °C, and **b**) water temperature 24 °C

pseudorandomized intertrain intervals of 4–12 s (data not shown). Thus, CPM-paradigms using heat pain as TS need longer interstimulus intervals to prevent habituation and longer latencies to raise thermode temperature from neutral skin temperature (~32 °C) to painful heat (~43°-47 °C). In contrast, using concentric electrodes to elicit PCES-EP enable a reliable judgment of pain intensity and a quick adjustment to target pain intensity by modifying current intensity [31].

CPM-effect on the PCES-EP-amplitude and PCES-EP-N1-latency

In our CPM-paradigm, the PCES-EP-amplitude significantly decreased during CS by 32 ± 11%, which was much more pronounced than CHEP-amplitudes [2] or SEP-amplitudes after chemonasal CO_2-stimulation [22] as TS. Furthermore, the PCES-EP-amplitude is comparable to studies assessing SEP-amplitudes after CO_2 laser stimulation [17], and after electrical tooth stimulation [20, 21].

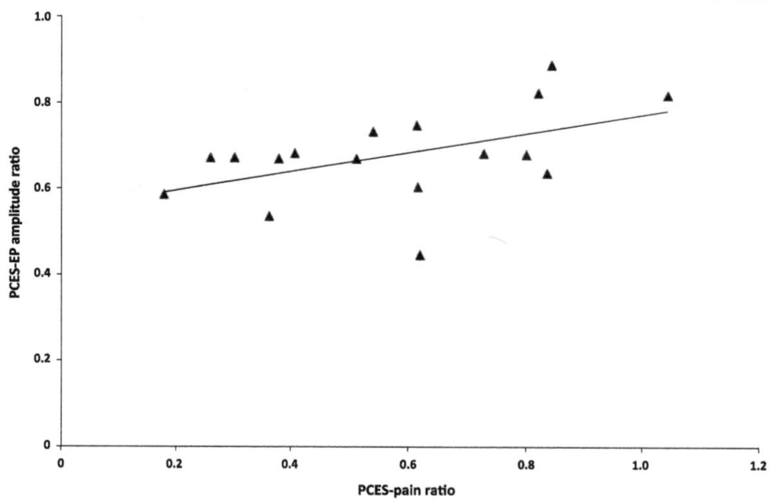

Fig. 4 Changes of PCES-EP amplitude and changes of PCES-pain in subjects in the 10° cold water condition, expressed as ratios (during CS/ baseline)

There was a significant, yet moderate correlation between the changes in PCES-EP-amplitudes and PCES-pain intensity. A correlation between the decrease of EP amplitudes and the pain intensity has been also reported, albeit lower, for CPM-models using CHEP as TS and hot water pain as CS [2], and SEP after CO_2-laser stimulation as TS and heat as CS (no detailed data presented) [18]. CHEP reflect C-fiber transmission, whereas pinprick-like pain during cortically recorded so-called pain-related evoked potentials (PREP) is assumed to represent mainly A-delta-fiber function [25, 29], though the latter type of stimulation cannot exclude the possibility of also low-threshold mechanoreceptors being involved. Thus, the interpretation of differences in the effects of both techniques needs to be done with care. A study recording SEP after electrical tooth stimulation as TS and CO_2-laser stimulation as CS have also found a significant CPM-effect for both pain intensity and EP-amplitudes, without presenting any data on their correlation [17].

Another study investigated CPM using chemo-somatosensory evoked potentials (CSSEPs) elicited by CO_2-gas as TS and tonic heat pain as CS, and found significantly reduced CSSEP-amplitudes and prolonged latencies during CS [22]. The authors postulated that earlier CSSEP-components reflect the sensory input, while later components reflect the cerebral signal processing, and based on their findings they concluded the analgesic effects of CPM at a cerebral level. Although the local origin of PCES-EP-components was not investigated, previous PREP-studies indicated that the investigated N1-component reflects an early cortical processing [29, 30]. Therefore, the CPM-induced reduction of PCES-EP-amplitudes in our study mainly refers to modulation of the sensory input. In contrast to our results, CPM-induced changes of CSSEP were not reflected by the subjects' pain ratings [22].

Based on previous studies, PCES-EP induced by K^2 stimulation electrodes are recorded after activation of intraepidermal nociceptive fibers [27, 29, 30]. The concentric design and small anode–cathode distance of K^2 stimulation electrodes produce high current density at low current intensities, resulting predominantly in stimulation of nociceptive Aδ-fibers [11, 36]. Furthermore, the well-localized, sharp, pin-prick like sensation and the conduction velocity measured corresponds to Aδ-fiber activation [43].

Results of functional magnetic resonance imaging studies demonstrate that PCES induces activation within the pACC (posterior part of the anterior cingulate cortex), PCC (posterior cingulate cortex), insula, and somatosensory cortex (SII) [11].

Here, an increase of PCES stimulus intensity resulted in increasing pain ratings, increasing PCES-EPs and increasing BOLD response within these brain regions [11]. Although PCES-EP showed a high test-retest-reliability concerning the commonly used parameters N1-latency and N1P1-amplitude [31], the present study demonstrates that PCES-induced pain and PCES-EPs can be modulated by CPM.

To this point, it remains open which targets in the sensory pathway are mainly involved. Using a different kind of electrical skin stimulus, Bromm et al. demonstrated that the opioid agonist tilidin is able to reduce pain ratings and evoked potentials [44].

Based on the concept of the diffuse noxious inhibitory controls (DNIC), an activation of the spino-bulbo-spinal mechanism or descending pathways are of major importance to modulate pain perception by inhibition or facilitation of noxious information [2, 45]. Further studies are required to identify the exact link between the amplitudes of PCES-EPs and pain perception. Here, a combination of CPM paradigms including PCES-EPs recorded at a cortical level and nociceptive flexion reflex responses evaluating mainly the spinal modulation may be beneficial to explore more detailed the exact mechanisms of the endogenous analgesia.

Furthermore, we analyzed the changes of N1-latency of cortical PCES-EP during CPM. We found a significant increase of N1-latency only from 'baseline' to 'during CS' application. This is in accordance to previous studies using chemo-somatosensory evoked potentials as test stimulus and tonic heat pain as conditioning stimulus to induce CPM [22]. Interestingly, in both conditions of 10° and 24°cold water as CS, the N1-latency increased. However, some subjects perceived the 24 °C cold water which was intended to be a non-painful control CS, also as a painful, similarly to another study using a conditioning stimulus of 25 °C, which was also rated as painful on an NRS on average by 2.3 ± 0.4 [46]. Hence, this may explain the missing difference between both conditions.

It should be noted that a CPM-effect was in fact elicited in 71–76% (depending on the outcome measure) of participants in the control condition, though it was to a lesser extent than in the 10 °C condition. Similarly to Treister et ale46], examining a CPM model with conditioning stimulus of 25 °C, where a mean CPM-effect amounted to 22% (in our study 10.5 ± 12.6%). Such non-noxious inhibitory control-like effects have already been previously discussed as potentially representing the amount of habituation or psychological effects, like anxiety-related increased pain at the beginning of a series of experimental trials [46].

Relation between cold water pain and CPM-magnitude

The cold water pain intensity induced significantly changes of both PCES-pain and PCES-EP-amplitudes.

The more painful the subjects rated the cold water (as conditioning stimulus), the less painful they rated the PCES-pain during CS and the smaller were the PCES-EP-amplitudes during CS. This is in contrast to previous results, where the magnitude of the CPM-effect, using hot water hand immersion as CS and contact heat pain as TS, depended only from the CS-temperature, but not from the perceived CS-pain intensity [47]. However, our results are consistent with another study showing that pain inhibition under CPM seems to depend on the perceived level of the CS pain rather than solely its physical intensity [48]. Interestingly, the cold water pain intensity showed no effect on PCES-EP latency, suggesting that the CPM-effect based on the electrophysiological response reflects different central processing compared to the CPM-effect based on subjective pain ratings. Further studies are needed to explore this issue.

Limitations

Some limitations must be considered when interpreting the findings of the present study. Despite randomization of participants there was a difference of the initial N1-P1 amplitudes of PCES-EP between group A and B. This might result from the interindividual variation of PCES-EP-amplitudes, as our study was powered to detect differences between the PCES-EP-amplitudes before and after application of a conditioning stimulus. Considering this, we analyzed changes of amplitudes and pain ratings during the CPM by calculating ratios in addition to the calculated differences (representing the CPM-effect as per definition recommended) to avoid an impact of the individual variation of the amplitude on the results.

Another possible limitation is the fact that, retrospectively, subjects perceived the difference in temperature between both immersions of the hand. However, they were blinded for the aim of the study. Also, we found no carry over effect, suggesting that the limitation on blinding the water temperature to the subjects is not relevant for the study. As discussed above, during the non-painful control condition about 50% of the subjects reported painful perception after immersion in painful 24 °C cold water, here, about 20% estimated pain levels above 10 of NRS. Using a higher temperature as a neutral control condition could have reduced pain perception and, hence, a comparison of distinct painful and non-painful conditions may have result in even greater differences between the CPM-effect induced by both different CS. Taken this into account, we assessed the interaction between cold water pain, changes of PCES-EP-amplitudes and changes of PCES-pain independently from the CPM-condition (see above). Though, it should be mentioned that calculating a Pearson correlation based on 24 datasets where the CS was rated as painful (see results section), represents a statistical limitation.

In a previous study the CPM-effect based on pain intensity after electrical stimulation, induced by cold pressor test showed acceptable reliability [1]. However, results regarding the re-test reliability of different CPM testing protocols vary widely between studies, and seem to depend on the used CS and TS as well as the time interval (for discussion see Gehling et al. 2016 [33]), therefore the reliability of the introduced CPM model here should be further investigated. Nevertheless, the used TS and CS were shown to be reliable, in terms of the induced pain intensity (for TS and CS) and evoked potentials [31, 33].

Also, some limitations regarding the selective activation of nociceptive fibers during electrical stimulation of the used concentric electrodes must be admitted. Recent studies have questioned whether such electrical stimulation through specially designed electrodes selectively activates nociceptive A-delta fibers [49]. Furthermore, different stimulation intensities and electrode designs (resulting in different spreading of current due to different resistances during intracutan or surface stimulation) make a direct comparison impossible. Further studies are needed to clarify this issue and to examine the underlying mechanisms of reduction of the PCES-EP-amplitude and N1-latency during painful CS application.

There is inconsistent data about the influence of menstrual cycle on CPM [50–53]. In the present study, we did not control for the stage of menstrual cycle of female participants. This might be seen as a limitation of the study, however, detecting such differences was not in the scope of the present study and as both CPM assessments were performed on the same day, differences in the results between both conditions due to menstrual cycle can be excluded.

Conclusions

In summary, we present a novel CPM-paradigm being able to induce a significant decrease of the subjective pain intensity in healthy subjects by hand immersion in painful cold water. More importantly, and to our knowledge for the first time, we were able to demonstrate a concomitant decrease of the PCES-EP-amplitude during CPM and the perceived intensity of the PCES induced pinprick-like pain, which both correlated with the pain intensity of the conditioning stimulus. Thus, this CPM model is a feasible and cost-effective novel method to objectify and evaluate interventions related to the function of endogenous pain modulation.

Abbreviations

CHEP: Contact heat evoked potential; CPM: Conditioned pain modulation; CS: Conditioning stimulus; CSSEP: Chemo-somatosensory evoked potential; DNIC: Diffuse noxious inhibitory controls; NRS: Numerical rating scale; pACC: Posterior part of the anterior cingulate cortex; PCC: Posterior cingulate cortex; PCES: Painful cutaneous electrical stimulation; PCES-EP: PCES-evoked potential; PREP: Pain-related evoked potential; SEP: Sensory evoked potential; SII: Secondary somatosensory cortex; TS: Test stimulus

Acknowledgements
We are indebted to the subjects who participated in the study for their consent and cooperation.

Funding
This work was supported by SFB 874, TP A1. The funding body had no role in the design of the study and collection, analysis, and interpretation of data and in writing the manuscript.

Authors' contributions
OH, ÖÖ, EKE-K, MT and CM contributed to the conception and design of the study, collaborated on the statistical analysis of the data, discussed the results, participated in writing the manuscript and approved the final version. ÖÖ and OH conducted all study experiments. All authors read and approved the final manuscript.

Competing interests
The authors declare that they have no competing interests.

Author details
[1]Department of Neurology, Berufsgenossenschaftliches Universitätsklinikum Bergmannsheil GmbH, Ruhr-University Bochum, Bürkle-de-la-Camp-Platz 1, 44789 Bochum, Germany. [2]Department of Pain Medicine, Berufsgenossenschaftliches Universitätsklinikum Bergmannsheil GmbH, Ruhr-University Bochum, Bürkle-de-la-Camp-Platz 1, 44789 Bochum, Germany.

References
1. Biurrun Manresa JA, Fritsche R, Vuilleumier PH, Oehler C, Morch CD, Arendt-Nielsen L, Andersen OK, Curatolo M. Is the conditioned pain modulation paradigm reliable? A test-retest assessment using the nociceptive withdrawal reflex. PLoS One. 2014;9(6):e100241.
2. Moont R, Crispel Y, Lev R, Pud D, Yarnitsky D. Temporal changes in cortical activation during conditioned pain modulation (CPM), a LORETA study. Pain. 2011;152(7):1469–77.
3. Nahman-Averbruch H, Yarnitzky D, Granovsky Y, Gerber E, Dagul P, Granot M. The role of stimulation parameters on the conditioned pain modulation response. Scand J Pain. 2013;4:10–4.
4. Lewis GN, Rice DA, McNair PJ. Conditioned pain modulation in populations with chronic pain: a systematic review and meta-analysis. J Pain. 2012; 13(10):936–44.
5. Yarnitsky D, Granot M, Nahman-Averbuch H, Khamaisi M, Granovsky Y. Conditioned pain modulation predicts duloxetine efficacy in painful diabetic neuropathy. Pain. 2012;153(6):1193–8.
6. Grosen K, Vase L, Pilegaard HK, Pfeiffer-Jensen M, Drewes AM. Conditioned pain modulation and situational pain catastrophizing as preoperative predictors of pain following chest wall surgery: a prospective observational cohort study. PLoS One. 2014;9(2):e90185.
7. Ram KC, Eisenberg E, Haddad M, Pud D. Oral opioid use alters DNIC but not cold pain perception in patients with chronic pain - new perspective of opioid-induced hyperalgesia. Pain. 2008;139(2):431–8.
8. Petersen KK, Graven-Nielsen T, Simonsen O, Laursen MB, Arendt-Nielsen L. Preoperative pain mechanisms assessed by cuff algometry are associated with chronic postoperative pain relief after total knee replacement. Pain. 2016;157(7):1400–6.
9. Youssef AM, Macefield VG, Henderson LA. Pain inhibits pain; human brainstem mechanisms. NeuroImage. 2016;124(Pt A):54–62.
10. Bogdanov VB, Vigano A, Noirhomme Q, Bogdanova OV, Guy N, Laureys S, Renshaw PF, Dallel R, Phillips C, Schoenen J. Cerebral responses and role of the prefrontal cortex in conditioned pain modulation: an fMRI study in healthy subjects. Behav Brain Res. 2015;281:187–98.
11. Obermann M, Pleger B, de Greiff A, Stude P, Kaube H, Diener HC, Katsarava Z. Temporal summation of trigeminal pain in human anterior cingulate cortex. NeuroImage. 2009;46(1):193–200.
12. Yarnitsky D, Bouhassira D, Drewes AM, Fillingim RB, Granot M, Hansson P, Landau R, Marchand S, Matre D, Nilsen KB, et al. Recommendations on practice of conditioned pain modulation (CPM) testing. Eur J Pain. 2015;19(6):805–6.
13. Pud D, Granovsky Y, Yarnitsky D. The methodology of experimentally induced diffuse noxious inhibitory control (DNIC)-like effect in humans. Pain. 2009;144(1–2):16–9.
14. Piche M, Arsenault M, Rainville P. Cerebral and cerebrospinal processes underlying counterirritation analgesia. J Neurosci. 2009;29(45):14236–46.
15. Sandrini G, Ruiz L, Capararo M, Danilov A, Beretta A, Nappi G. Effects of dothiepin on nociceptive flexion reflex and diffuse noxious inhibitory controls in humans. Eur J Pharmacol. 1993;243(1):99–102.
16. Drummond PD. The effect of trigeminal nociceptive stimulation on blink reflexes and pain evoked by stimulation of the supraorbital nerve. Cephalalgia. 2003;23(7):534–40.
17. Fujii-Abe K, Oono Y, Motohashi K, Fukayama H, Umino M. Heterotopic CO2 laser stimulation inhibits tooth-related somatosensory evoked potentials. Pain Med. 2010;11(6):825–33.
18. Kakigi R. Diffuse noxious inhibitory control. Reappraisal by pain-related somatosensory evoked potentials following CO2 laser stimulation. J Neurol Sci. 1994;125(2):198–205.
19. Watanabe S, Kakigi R, Hoshiyama M, Kitamura Y, Koyama S, Shimojo M. Effects of noxious cooling of the skin on pain perception in man. J Neurol Sci. 1996;135(1):68–73.
20. Motohashi K, Umino M. Heterotopic painful stimulation decreases the late component of somatosensory evoked potentials induced by electrical tooth stimulation. Brain Res Cogn Brain Res. 2001;11(1):39–46.
21. Motohashi K, Umino M, Fujii Y. An experimental system for a heterotopic pain stimulation study in humans. Brain Res Brain Res Protoc. 2002;10(1):31–40.
22. Kunz M, Mohammadian P, Renner B, Roscher S, Kobal G, Lautenbacher S. Chemo-somatosensory evoked potentials: a sensitive tool to assess conditioned pain modulation? Somatosens Mot Res. 2014;31(2):100–10.
23. Kennedy DL, Kemp HI, Ridout D, Yarnitsky D, Rice AS. Reliability of conditioned pain modulation: a systematic review. Pain. 2016;157(11):2410–9.
24. Mueller D, Obermann M, Koeppen S, Kavuk I, Yoon MS, Sack F, Diener HC, Kaube H, Katsarava Z. Electrically evoked nociceptive potentials for early detection of diabetic small-fiber neuropathy. Eur J Neurol. 2010;17(6):834–41.
25. Obermann M, Katsarava Z, Esser S, Sommer C, He L, Selter L, Yoon MS, Kaube H, Diener HC, Maschke M. Correlation of epidermal nerve fiber density with pain-related evoked potentials in HIV neuropathy. Pain. 2008;138(1):79–86.
26. Uceyler N, Kahn AK, Kramer D, Zeller D, Casanova-Molla J, Wanner C, Weidemann F, Katsarava Z, Sommer C. Impaired small fiber conduction in patients with Fabry disease: a neurophysiological case-control study. BMC Neurol. 2013;13:47.
27. Uceyler N, Zeller D, Kahn AK, Kewenig S, Kittel-Schneider S, Schmid A, Casanova-Molla J, Reiners K, Sommer C. Small fibre pathology in patients with fibromyalgia syndrome. Brain. 2013;136(Pt 6):1857–67.
28. Bromm B, Meier W. The intracutaneous stimulus: a new pain model for algesimetric studies. Methods Find Exp Clin Pharmacol. 1984;6(7):405–10.
29. Katsarava Z, Ayzenberg I, Sack F, Limmroth V, Diener HC, Kaube H. A novel method of eliciting pain-related potentials by transcutaneous electrical stimulation. Headache. 2006;46(10):1511–7.
30. Oh KJ, Kim SH, Lee YH, Kim JH, Jung HS, Park TJ, Park J, Shinn JM. Pain-related evoked potential in healthy adults. Ann Rehabil Med. 2015;39(1):108–15.
31. Ozgul OS, Maier C, Enax-Krumova EK, Vollert J, Fischer M, Tegenthoff M, Hoffken O. High test-retest-reliability of pain-related evoked potentials (PREP) in healthy subjects. Neurosci Lett. 2017;647:110–6.
32. Oono Y, Nie H, Matos LM, Wang K, Arendt-Nielsen L. The inter- and intra-individual variance in descending pain modulation evoked by different conditioning stimuli in healthy men. Scand J Pain. 2011;2:162–9.
33. Gehling J, Mainka T, Vollert J, Pogatzki-Zahn EM, Maier C, Enax-Krumova EK. Short-term test-retest-reliability of conditioned pain modulation using the cold-heat-pain method in healthy subjects and its correlation to parameters of standardized quantitative sensory testing. BMC Neurol. 2016;16:125.
34. Gierthmuhlen J, Enax-Krumova EK, Attal N, Bouhassira D, Cruccu G, Finnerup NB, Haanpaa M, Hansson P, Jensen TS, Freynhagen R, et al. Who is healthy? Aspects to consider when including healthy volunteers in QST-based studies- a consensus statement by the EUROPAIN and NEUROPAIN consortia. Pain. 2015;156(11):2203–11.

35. Oldfield RC. The assessment and analysis of handedness: the Edinburgh inventory. Neuropsychologia. 1971;9(1):97–113.
36. Kaube H, Katsarava Z, Kaufer T, Diener H, Ellrich J. A new method to increase nociception specificity of the human blink reflex. Clin Neurophysiol. 2000;111(3):413–6.
37. Granot M, Weissman-Fogel I, Crispel Y, Pud D, Granovsky Y, Sprecher E, Yarnitsky D. Determinants of endogenous analgesia magnitude in a diffuse noxious inhibitory control (DNIC) paradigm: do conditioning stimulus painfulness, gender and personality variables matter? Pain. 2008;136(1–2):142–9.
38. Locke D, Gibson W, Moss P, Munyard K, Mamotte C, Wright A. Analysis of meaningful conditioned pain modulation effect in a pain-free adult population. J Pain. 2014;15(11):1190–8.
39. Edwards RR, Ness TJ, Weigent DA, Fillingim RB. Individual differences in diffuse noxious inhibitory controls (DNIC): association with clinical variables. Pain. 2003;106(3):427–37.
40. Baad-Hansen L, Poulsen HF, Jensen HM, Svensson P. Lack of sex differences in modulation of experimental intraoral pain by diffuse noxious inhibitory controls (DNIC). Pain. 2005;116(3):359–65.
41. Agostinho CM, Scherens A, Richter H, Schaub C, Rolke R, Treede RD, Maier C. Habituation and short-term repeatability of thermal testing in healthy human subjects and patients with chronic non-neuropathic pain. Eur J Pain. 2009;13(8):779–85.
42. Greffrath W, Baumgartner U, Treede RD. Peripheral and central components of habituation of heat pain perception and evoked potentials in humans. Pain. 2007;132(3):301–11.
43. Katsarava Z, Yaldizli O, Voulkoudis C, Diener HC, Kaube H, Maschke M. Pain related potentials by electrical stimulation of skin for detection of small-fiber neuropathy in HIV. J Neurol. 2006;253(12):1581–4.
44. Bromm B, Seide K. The influence of tilidine and prazepam on withdrawal reflex, skin resistance reaction and pain rating in man. Pain. 1982;12(3):247–58.
45. Sprenger C, Bingel U, Buchel C. Treating pain with pain: supraspinal mechanisms of endogenous analgesia elicited by heterotopic noxious conditioning stimulation. Pain. 2011;152(2):428–39.
46. Treister R, Eisenberg E, Gershon E, Haddad M, Pud D. Factors affecting - and relationships between-different modes of endogenous pain modulation in healthy volunteers. Eur J Pain. 2010;14(6):608–14.
47. Nir RR, Granovsky Y, Yarnitsky D, Sprecher E, Granot M. A psychophysical study of endogenous analgesia: the role of the conditioning pain in the induction and magnitude of conditioned pain modulation. Eur J Pain. 2011;15(5):491–7.
48. Nir RR, Yarnitsky D, Honigman L, Granot M. Cognitive manipulation targeted at decreasing the conditioning pain perception reduces the efficacy of conditioned pain modulation. Pain. 2012;153(1):170–6.
49. Perchet C, Frot M, Charmarty A, Flores C, Mazza S, Magnin M, Garcia-Larrea L. Do we activate specifically somatosensory thin fibres with the concentric planar electrode? A scalp and intracranial EEG study. Pain. 2012;153(6):1244–52.
50. Wilson H, Carvalho B, Granot M, Landau R. Temporal stability of conditioned pain modulation in healthy women over four menstrual cycles at the follicular and luteal phases. Pain. 2013;154(12):2633–8.
51. Tousignant-Laflamme Y, Marchand S. Excitatory and inhibitory pain mechanisms during the menstrual cycle in healthy women. Pain. 2009;146(1–2):47–55.
52. Rezaii T, Hirschberg AL, Carlstrom K, Ernberg M. The influence of menstrual phases on pain modulation in healthy women. J Pain. 2012;13(7):646–55.
53. Palit S, Bartley EJ, Kuhn BL, Kerr KL, DelVentura JL, Terry EL, Rhudy JL. Endogenous inhibition of pain and spinal nociception in women with premenstrual dysphoric disorder. J Pain Res. 2016;9:57–66.

13

The usefulness of chief complaints to predict severity, ventilator dependence, treatment option, and short-term outcome of patients with Guillain-Barré syndrome

Ying Wang[1*], Pei Shang[1], Meiying Xin[1], Jing Bai[1], Chunkui Zhou[1*] and Hong-Liang Zhang[1,2*]

Abstract

Background: It remains an urgent need for early recognition of disease severity, treatment option and outcome of Guillain-Barré syndrome (GBS). The chief complaint may be quickly obtained in clinic and is one of the candidates for early predictors. However, studies on the chief complaint are still lacking in GBS. The aim of the study is to describe the components of chief complaints of GBS patients, and to explore association between chief complaints and disease severity/treatment option/outcome of GBS, so as to aid the early prediction of the disease course and to assist the clinicians to prescribe an optimal early treatment.

Methods: A total of 523 GBS patients admitted to the First Hospital of Jilin University from 2003 to 2013 were enrolled for retrospective analysis. The data of chief complaints, clinical manifestations, and treatment options, etc. were collected. The clinical severity was evaluated by the Medical Research Council sum score and the Hughes Functional Grading Scale. The prognosis at 6 month after discharge was described by modified Erasmus GBS outcome score. The clinic GBS severity evaluation scale (CGSES), a newly established model in our study, was used to explore the role of chief complaints to predict intravenous immunoglobulin (IVIg).

Results: The major components of the chief complaints of GBS patients were weakness, numbness, pain, cranial nerve involvement, dyspnea, ataxia and autonomic dysfunction. Chief complaint of weakness was a predictor of severe disease course and poor short-term outcome, while chief complaint of numbness and cranial nerve involvement were promising predictors. Cranial nerve involvement was the predictor of ventilator dependence. The percentages of 366 GBS patients, who need IVIg treatment at nadir with CGSES ranging from 1 to 4, were 50.00, 67.34, 80.61, and 90.67%, respectively.

Conclusions: Chief complaints are clinic predictors of disease severity, ventilator dependence and short-term outcome. IVIg treatment during hospitalisation could be predicted in clinic using CGSES score.

Keywords: Guillain-Barré syndrome, Chief complaint, Retrospective study, Clinical manifestations, Disease severity

* Correspondence: yingwangki@outlook.com; zhouchunkui@163.com; drzhl@hotmail.com
[1]Neuroscience Centre, Department of Neurology, the First Hospital of Jilin University, Xinmin Street 71#, Changchun 130021, China
Full list of author information is available at the end of the article

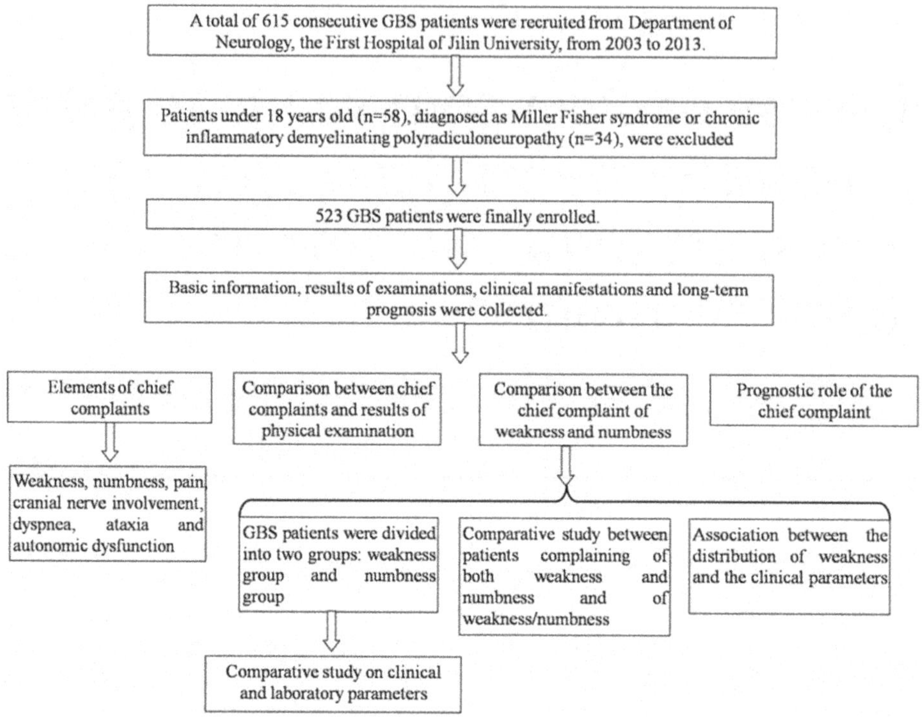

Fig. 1 Flow chart of subject enrollment. This investigation was on the base of the clinical information of 615 consecutive Guillain-Barré syndrome (GBS) patients. Patients with younger age, Miller Fisher syndrome or chronic inflammatory demyelinating polyradiculoneuropathy were excluded. The association between the chief complaint and the severity as well as prognosis was explored. The elements of the chief complaint were depicted, and the differences between GBS patients with distinct chief complaints were studied

Background

Most of the studies on the clinical features of Guillain-Barré syndrome (GBS) are based on objective parameters including medical history, physical examinations, laboratory examinations and electrophysiological examinations, etc. [1]. However, chief complaints, the most significantly subjective experience on the disease that drive patients to doctors have not received equal focus of attention [1, 2]. The importance of the chief complaint is emphasised in some of diseases [3]. For example, subjective cognitive impairment is the definition given to the subjects whose results on neuropsychological tests are normal but with complaints of memory impairment; a growing body of evidence indicates that subjective cognitive impairment could be a pre-clinical phase of Alzheimer's disease [3]. The association between the chief complaint of patients with GBS and the severity/prognosis of disease remains unknown. A systematic study of the chief complaint of GBS is warranted for the following reasons. Firstly, chief complaints, the most significant symptoms reported by patients are not always in parallel with the results of physical examinations [4, 5]. Empirically, for most of the time chief complaints reflect the most significant part of the clinical manifestations, and for some time, chief complaints contain symptoms that could not be found by physical examinations. For example, an 82-year-old woman complained of back pain and glove-and-stocking paraesthesia for 5 days, but her neurological examination could be unremarkable [5]. Secondly, the chief complaint is potentially an early predictor of the severity, treatment option and prognosis of GBS. GBS is a devastating disease mainly characterised by progressively symmetrical flaccid paralysis [1, 2]. In severe cases, patients may develop respiratory muscle paralysis and need intensive care [1, 2]. Thus, early prediction of the disease course could assist clinicians to provide an optimal management to the patients at admission. For example, if a patient has a high risk to develop respiratory muscle paralysis at nadir, a respiratory monitor could be used at admission. Currently, the chief complaint is not on the list of predictors for GBS. The prognostic factors for death in GBS patients are age, the severity of disease and the speed of progression [6]. For the survivors, various predictors of prognosis have been addressed, such as an older age, severe disability at admission, cranial nerve involvement, ventilator dependence, autonomic dysfunction, neck flexor weakness and acute motor axonal neuropathy, and so forth [7–9]. Moreover, a clinical prognostic scoring model has been established to depict the outcome of GBS [10]. Age, antecedent diarrhea, and Hughes Functional Grading Scale (HFGS) score at 2 weeks after entry have been identified as predictors for the outcome of GBS 6 month after discharge [10].

Table 1 Demographics, clinical manifestations and laboratory findings of patients with Guillain-Barré syndrome (GBS)

Basic information	
Male/female ratio	311/212
Age (years), median (IQR)	36 (26–45)
Duration in hospital (days), median (IQR)	15 (10–20)
Symptoms of antecedent infection ($n = 523$)	
Interval between infection and onset (days), median (IQR)	5 (2–9)
Diarrhea, No. (%)	137 (26.20)
Upper respiratory tract infection, No. (%)	153 (29.25)
Severity of disease ($n = 523$)	
MRC sum score at admission, median (IQR)	48 (42–56)
HFGS at admission, median (IQR)	3 (2–4)
MRC sum score at nadir, median(IQR)	48 (36–54)
HFGS at nadir, median (IQR)	3 (2–4)
Interval between onset and nadir (days), median (IQR)	8 (6–12)
MRC sum score at discharge, median (IQR)	56 (49–60)
HFGS at discharge, median(IQR)	2 (1–3)
Clinical manifestations ($n = 523$)	
Cranial nerve involvement, No. (%)	236 (45.12)
Hyporeflexia/areflexia, No. (%)	484 (92.54)
Superficial sensation deficits, No. (%)	223 (43.05)
Autonomic deficits, No. (%)	289 (55.26)
Dyspnea, No. (%)	134 (25.62)
Ventilator dependence, No. (%)	64 (12.24)
Blood routine examination at admission ($n = 523$)	
White blood cell, mean (SD), 10^9/L	9.00 (3.61)
Neutrophil, mean (SD), %	68.75 (3.63)
Lymphocyte, mean (SD), %	23.36 (0.10)
Lumbar puncture ($n = 287$)	
Protein concentration, mean (SD), g/L	1.05 (0.88)
White blood cell, mean (SD), 10^6/L	3 (2–7)
Albumin-cytologic dissociations, No. (%)	192 (66.90)
IgG concentration, mean (SD), mg/L	189.24 (205.63)
Nerve conduction studies ($n = 165$)	
Demyelinating group, No. (%)	89 (53.94)
Axonal group, No. (%)	46 (27.88)
Overlap group, No. (%)	30 (18.18)

The chief complaint is the first information that physicians obtain from patients, and it may assist clinicians to make an early recognition of the severity and prognosis of the disease. However, chief complaints are rarely taken into account when the predictors for severity/prognosis of GBS are explored [6–10]. Herein, we retrospectively investigate the components of chief complains so as to further explore their role in predicting disease severity, treatment option and prognosis.

Methods

The aim of the study is to explore the important role of the chief complaint in GBS, and the study design is showed in Fig. 1.

Study subjects

A total of 615 consecutive GBS patients were enrolled from Department of Neurology, the First Hospital of Jilin University, during the time interval between 2003 and 2013 (Fig. 1). Thirty-four patients, with the diagnosis of Miller Fisher syndrome or later identified chronic inflammatory demyelinating polyradiculoneuropathy, were excluded. Fifty-eight subjects with the age under 18 years old were also ruled out due to their different clinical characteristics from adult patients [11]. Finally, a cohort of 523 GBS patients fulfilling the inclusion criteria [12] and contradictive to the exclusion criteria were included for data analysis. For these patients, data of demographics, chief complaints, antecedent infection, history of past illness, clinical manifestations, results of blood and cerebrospinal fuild examinations, results of electrophysiological study and ventilation dependence were subsequently collected. The short-term prognosis was described by HFGS at discharge, and by the modified Erasmus GBS outcome score (mEGOS), ranging from 0 to 9, at 6 months after discharge [10].

Measurement of disability

The clinical severity and functional impairment of GBS patients were assessed by two widely used scales, i.e. the Medical Research Council (MRC) sum score and HFGS score. The MRC sum score, ranging from 0 (tetraplegic) to 60 (normal strength), described the strength of six pairs of symmetrical muscles in both upper and lower extremities [13]. The definition of the HFGS score was that, 0: healthy state; 1: minor symptoms and capable of running; 2: able to walk 5 m or more without assistance but unable to run; 3: able to walk 5 m across an open space with help; 4: bedridden or chair-bound; 5: requiring assisted ventilation for at least part of the day; 6: dead [14]. The nadir of the disease course was identified as the day during hospitalisation when the lowest MRC sum score was observed.

The clinic GBS severity evaluation scale (CGSES)

A model, namely CGSES, for predicting the disease severity and guiding the treatment option during hospitalisation was established based on the information that could be easily obtained in clinic after a quick inquiry. Finally, four of the clinical parameters, which could predict the progress of GBS during hospitalisation, were quantified to build

CGSES, including duration between onset to admission, chief complaints of weakness, numbness and cranial nerve involvement. The data of 373 GBS patients recruited from 2003 to 2011 were employed to establish the CGSES, and the data of the other 150 patients admitted from 2012 to 2013 were utilised to validate the model. The severe GBS patients, among whom the immunotherapy was needed, were defined as the patients with an HFGS score equal to or more than 3 at nadir. The proportions of severe GBS patients with continuous CGSES scores ranging from 1 to 4 were analysed.

Statistics

The Statistical Program for Social Science (SPSS, IBM, West Grove, PA, USA) version 18.0 was employed to accomplish the statistical analysis of all the data. For categorical variables, differences of proportion were analysed by Chi-square or Fisher exact test while qualitative variables by Mann-Whitney U test. The Student-t test was used to compare the values of normal continuous variables between two groups. Correlation between the values of two groups of normal continuous variable was tested by Pearson rank correlation coefficient (r) while between categorical variable and non-categorical variable by Spearman rank correlation coefficient (rs). The ordinal logistic regression was utilised to analyse the prognostic role of chief complaints, and the odds ratio (OR) was used to express the strength of prognostic effects. All tests were two-tailed, and the p value < 0.05 was set as the level of significance.

Results

Chief complaints are composed of seven elements

The clinical parameters of enrolled patient are presented in Table 1. Seven basic elements including weakness, numbness, pain, cranial nerve involvement, dyspnea, ataxia and autonomic dysfunction were found to compose the chief complaints of GBS patients. The details are provided in Table 2. In addition, 125 (23.90%) out of 523 patients reported these distinct kinds of symptoms with combinations thereof. Seventy patients complained of weakness and paraesthesia (including numbness and pain), 19 of weakness and cranial nerve involvement, 2 of weakness and autonomic disturbance, 12 of paraesthesia and autonomic dysfunction, 8 of paraesthesia and cranial nerve deficits as well as 1 of autonomic disorder and cranial nerve damage. The chief complaints of 13 GBS patients comprised at least 3 different kinds of elements, among whom 1 patient complained of four kinds.

Doctors find more than patients report

A comparative study was conducted between the results of neurological examinations and the chief complaints (Fig. 2). Neurologists tended to find more symptoms

Table 2 Chief complaints in Guillain-Barré syndrome (GBS) patients

Chief complaint	Number of patients	Details, No. (%)
Weakness	384	Four limbs 294 (76.56), lower extremities 47 (12.24), upper extremities 20 (5.21), hands and feet 2 (0.52), hands 4 (1.04), asymmetric weakness 17 (4.43)
Numbness	161	Four limbs 100 (62.11), lower extremities 12 (7.45), upper extremities 6 (3.73), hands and feet 14 (8.70), hands 6 (3.73), feet 2 (1.24), fingers 4 (2.48), toes 1 (0.62), fingers and toes 1 (0.62), face 1 (0.62), whole body 1 (0.62), tongue 1 (0.62), tongue and face 1 (0.62), asymmetric numbness 1 (0.62)
Pain	19	Details were missing.
Cranial nerve involvement	73	Oculomotor and/or abducent nerve 25 (34), facial nerve 17 (23), glossopharyngeal and vagus nerve 35 (48), trigeminal nerve 2 (3)
Dyspnea	10	
Ataxia	2	
Autonomic dysfunction (including pain)	23	Pain 19 (83), palpitation 1 (4), urinary retention 1 (4), sweating 1 (4), swelling on hands 1 (4).

after performing a careful physical examination than GBS patients initially demonstrated. For all the symptoms investigated including weakness, paraesthesia, cranial nerve involvement and autonomic dysfunction, significant differences were observed (Fig. 2). Weakness was not only the most frequent clinical manifestation, but also the most recognisable symptom by GBS patients. About 383 (73.42%) of 523 patients noticed weakness in their limbs, but neurologists observed that weakness occurred in 461 (88.15%) of all patients. Thus, only 383 (83.29%) of 461 patients could recognise the weakness that disturbed their daily lives and drove them to the doctors. In contrast, autonomic dysfunction was the most ignorable presentation; only 23 (4.40%) out of 523 patients complained of it, while neurologists actually identified it in 289 (55.26%) of these patients.

Chief complaints aid prediction of disease severity and clinical manifestations

The prognostic role of weakness, numbness and cranial nerve involvement, which were among the most frequent chief complaints of GBS patients, was explored. The severity of GBS was related to the chief complaints of patients. Weakness is the most common symptoms among GBS patients [1], and MRC sum score and HFGS are designed to evaluated the disease severity based on strength deficits

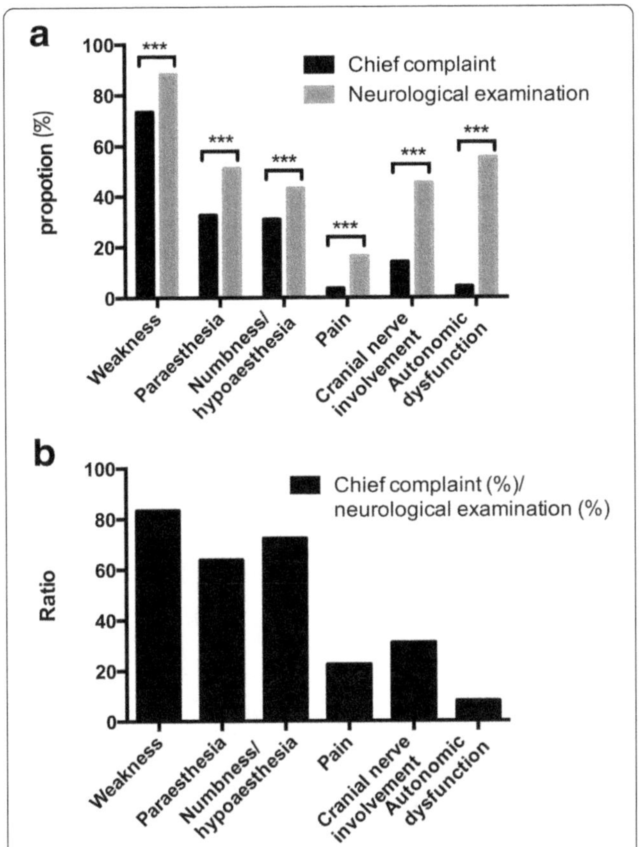

Fig. 2 Neurological examinations and chief complaints. **a** Weakness, paraesthesia (including numbness/hypoaesthesia and pain), numbness/hypoaesthesia, pain, cranial nerve involvement, and autonomic dysfunction (including pain) were reported by 384 (73.42%), 170 (32.50%), 161 (30.78%), 19 (3.63%), 73 (13.96%) and 23 (4.40%) of 523 Guillain-Barré syndrome (GBS) patients. After neurological examination, doctors demonstrated that the symptoms mentioned above occurred in 461 (88.15%), 267 (51.05%), 223 (43.05%), 85 (16.25%), 236 (45.12%), and 289 (55.26%) of 523 GBS patients. Significant differences were observed for all the symptoms ($p < .001$). **b** The proportion was calculated by chief complaint (%)/neurological examination (%). It revealed that 83.29%, 63.67%, 72.19%, 22.34%, 30.93% and 7.96% of the GBS patients presented with weakness, paraesthesia, numbness/hypoaesthesia, pain, cranial nerve involvement, ataxia and autonomic dysfunction recognised these symptoms and contained them in their chief complaints. $*p < 0.05$, $**p < 0.01$, $***p < 0.001$

[13, 14]. It was not surprising that the patients with the chief complaint of weakness had significantly lower MRC sum scale score and higher HFGS at admission and nadir, while those with the chief complaint of numbness had significantly higher MRC sum scale score and lower HFGS at admission and nadir (Table 3).

Furthermore, chief complaints were related to the clinical features of GBS patients. A significantly large proportion of GBS patients complaining weakness had younger age, antecedent infection of diarrhea, decreased reflexes, but had less possibility to develop cranial nerve involvement and autonomic deficits during the hospitalisation than patients without this chief complaint (Table 3). Patients reporting numbness were more likely to have antecedent infection of upper respiratory tract infection and were more easily to develop cranial nerve involvement, hyporeflexia and sensory deficits (Table 2). Other negative results are also showed in Table 3.

Among 73 patients who were complaining of symptoms associated with cranial nerve involvement in clinic, such as dysphagia, ptosis and diplopia, cranial nerve involvement, dyspnea and ventilator dependence were more frequently observed than in 450 patients without the chief complaint of cranial nerve involvement [69 (93.85%) vs 172 (38.21%), $p < .001$; 28 (38.46%) vs 91 (20.31%), $p = .001$; 15 (20.00%) vs 44 (9.83%), $p = .014$]. GBS patients with the chief complaint of cranial nerve involvement also had significantly higher MRC sum scores/ lower HFGS at admission, nadir and discharge [MRC sum score, median (IQR): 54 (44–60), 48 (34.5–60), 58 (48–60) vs 44 (36–51), 40 (25–48), 50 (41.5–56), $p < .001$, $< .001$, $< .001$; HFGS: 3 (1–4), 3 (1–4), 1 (1–3) vs 3 (3–4), 4 (3–4), 3 (1–4), $p < .001$, .027, $< .001$].

Chief complaints are predictors for prognosis

The short-term outcome of GBS was analysed at discharge and 6 months after discharge, respectively. The disease severity at discharge described by the MRC sum score and HFGS could be predicted by chief complaints. Patients with the chief complaint of weakness had significantly lower MRC sum scale score and higher HFGS at discharge, while with the chief complaint of numbness had significantly higher MRC sum scale score and lower HFGS at discharge (Table 3).

In addition, the prognosis 6 months after discharge was evaluated by mEGOS. The median of mEGOS of all enrolled patients was 2, with IQR of 1 to 4. GBS patients with weakness as the chief complaint had a significantly higher mEGOS, while numbness and cranial nerve involvement a lower one (Fig. 3a). After preforming ordinal logistic regression, none of chief complaints of weakness, numbness or cranial nerve involvement lost the prognostic role ($p = 0.016$, 0.006 and 0.005), and the OR were 1.61, 0.60, and 0.49, respectively.

Establishment of CGSES

Except for chief complaints of weakness, numbness and cranial nerve involvement, the duration between onset and admission was also included as a variable in the model due to its correlation to HFGS at nadir. The median of the duration between onset and admission for all GBS patients was 5 days with IQR of 3 to 8, and the duration was negatively correlated to the HFGS at nadir ($p < .001$, $rs = -0.264$). The CGSES was presented in Table 4A. Among 373 GBS patients, 7 patients were ruled out because of the missing of data. The

Table 3 Relation between chief complaints and clinical features

	Complaint with/without weakness			Complaint with/without numbness		
	with	Without	*P* value	with	without	*P* value
Basic information						
Number of patient	384	139		161	362	
Male/female ratio	234/150	77/62	.23	90/71	222/140	.23
Age, median (IQR)	39 (29–48)	47 (34.25–58.75)	.042	41 (31–56)	40 (29.5–50)	.30
Antecedent infection						
Diarrhea, No. (%)	111 (28.80)	27 (19.59)	.031	36 (22.64)	100 (27.75)	.21
Upper respiratory tract infection, No. (%)	103 (26.93)	49 (35.14)	.063	64 (39.62)	90 (24.73)	.001
Clinical manifestations						
Cranial nerve involvement, No. (%)	152 (39.49)	79 (56.72)	< .001	82 (50.76)	157 (43.26)	< .001
Hyporeflexia, No. (%)	361 (94.03)	119 (85.96)	.002	99 (61.24)	134 (37.02)	< .001
Sensory deficits, No. (%)	160 (41.67)	65 (46.58)	.34	94 (58.22)	132 (36.39)	< .001
Autonomic deficits, No. (%)	200 (52.00)	88 (63.51)	.017	97 (60.38)	192 (53.02)	.14
Dyspnea, No. (%)	101 (26.40)	33 (23.65)	.16	32 (20.13)	101 (28.02)	.053
Ventilator dependence, No. (%)	46 (12.00)	18 (12.84)	.79	14 (8.81)	46 (12.74)	.11
Severity of disease						
MRC sum score at admission, median (IQR)	45 (32.75–52)	47 (37.5–56)	< .001	48 (42–56)	42.5 (31.25–51.5)	< .001
HFGS at admission, median (IQR)	4 (2.75–4)	3 (1.75–4)	< .001	3 (2–4)	4 (2–4)	< .001
MRC sum score at nadir, median (IQR)	42 (28–48.25)	42 (34–54.5)	< .001	46 (36–54)	36 (21–48)	< .001
HFGS at nadir, median (IQR)	4 (3–4)	3.5 (2–4)	.001	3 (3–4)	4 (3–4)	< .001
MRC sum score at discharge, median (IQR)	54 (44–57.25)	54 (42–60)	.002	55 (48–60)	48.5 (36.5–58)	< .001
HFGS as discharge, median (IQR)	2 (2–4)	1 (0–1.25)	.002	2 (1–3.75)	3 (1–4)	.009

percentages of severe GBS patients with the sum of the score ranging from −1 to 4, were 10 (50.00%), 20 (66.67%), 46 (67.65%), 79 (80.61%), 90 (89.11%) and 46 (93.88%), respectively. The patients scored −2 were not available. As the percentages of severe patients with the score of 0 and 1, 3 and 4 were close to each other, a converted score, which was defined as CGSES, was set in Table 4B. The percentages of severe patients with CGSES score ranging from 1 to 4 were presented in Fig. 3b. The median of the CGSES of 366 patients was 3 with the IQR of 2 to 4, and the CGSES score was positively correlated to the HFGS at nadir ($p < .001$, rs = 0.283).

To validate our model, the data of the residual 150 patients were used. Seven patients with missing data were excluded. The percentages of severe GBS patients with CGSES scores ranging from 1 to 4 were 13 (53.85%), 45 (68.89%), 38 (78.95%) and 47 (91.49%), respectively. All of the values were within the 95% confidence intervals of the established model.

Discussion

We explored the role of the chief complaint to predict the severity and outcome of GBS, as well as how the chief complaint may guide treatment options. Although various components are available in the chief complaints of GBS patients, weakness, numbness and cranial nerve involvement were the most popular. The chief complaint only covers a part of the clinical manifestations, and some existing symptoms are not chief complaints. Chief complaints are associated with clinical parameters, and are predictors for disease severity, clinical manifestations and prognosis. CGSES score, which is able to be evaluated after a quick inquiry in clinic, has a potential role to predict the disease severity at nadir and to guide the treatment option.

Results of physical examination were widely used to depict the feature of GBS and to evaluate the efficiency of treatment [1, 9, 15]. However, the chief complaint, has not drawn enough attention in most of the studies on the clinical features of GBS [1, 2]. According to the results of our study, some new concerns of GBS have arisen. Firstly, our study has listed chief complaint as the candidate for the predictors for GBS disease course. A number of studies have focused on the predictors for the disease course of GBS [6–10]. However, the chief complaint of GBS only appears in some case reports to provide information of special individuals [16, 17], and retrospective studies to unravel the prognostic role of the chief complaint are missing. Our results

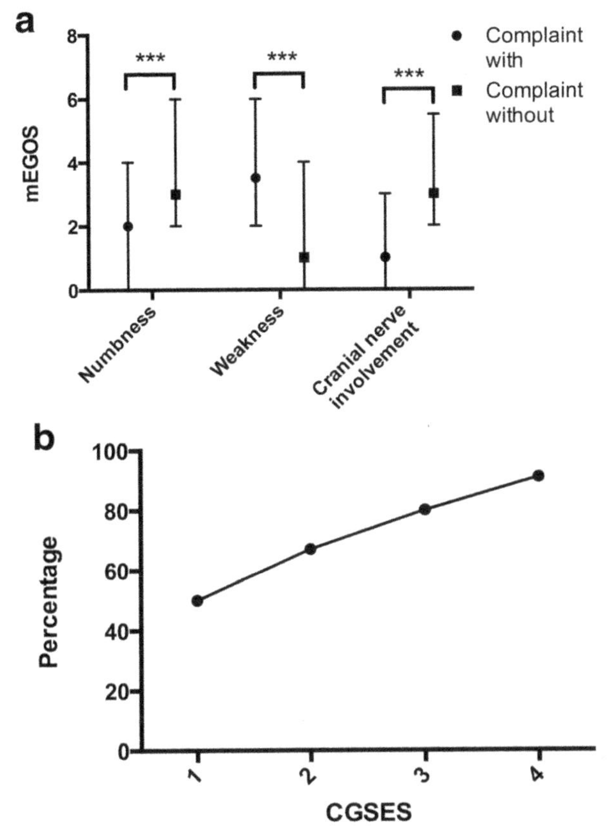

Fig. 3 The predictive role of chief complaints. **a** The Guillain-Barré syndrome (GBS) patients complaining of weakness had poor outcomes 6 months after discharge (modified Erasmus GBS outcome scores (mEGOS): 3.5 with IQR of 2–6 vs 1 with IQR of 0–4, $p < .001$). However, the patients with the chief complaints of numbness and cranial nerve involvement were observed to have better prognosis (mEGOS: 2 with IQR of 0–4 vs 3 with IQR of 2–6, $p < .001$; 1 with IQR of 0–3 vs 3 with IQR of 2–5.5, $p < .001$). **b** The numbers (percentage) of severe GBS patients, with clinic GBS severity evaluation scale (CGSES) scores ranging from 1 to 4, were 10 (50%) ($n = 20$), 66 (67%) ($n = 98$), 79 (80%) ($n = 98$), and 136 (91%) ($n = 150$), respectively

Table 4 Clinic Guillain-Barré syndrome severity evaluation scale (CGSES)

Predictors	Score
A.	
Chief complain of weakness	
with	1
without	0
Chief complain of numbness	
with	−1
without	0
Chief complain associated with cranial nerve involvement	
with	−1
without	0
Duration between onset and admission (days)	
0–2	3
3–5	2
6–10	1
> 10	0
sum of score	−2 to 4

B.

sum of score	−2	−1	0	1	2	3	4
CGSES	1	1	2	2	3	4	4

demonstrated that weakness, numbness and cranial nerve involvement were associated the severity and prognosis of GBS. Thus, chief complaint could assist clinicians to predict the disease course and the outcome of GBS at admission. As the MRC sum score and HFGS were designed based on the strength deficits among GBS patients, the chief complaint of weakness could be an important indicator for a severe disease course. When compared to the results of neurological examination, chief complaint is an easier and earlier obtained index to predict clinical severity and treatment options. A detailed neurological examination will be performed when the patients is hospitalised, and the results of the physical examination could imply the disease course. As a detailed examination is hardly available in clinic, chief complaint will be a more convenient parameter for clinicians to judge the severity of disease, especially to early recognise the risk of developing dyspnea.

Secondly, the results of our study imply that a type of "latent GBS" may exist without notation. The results of our study demonstrate that some patients may not recognise all their symptoms, and they tended to report only symptoms that obviously disturbed their life. Thus, a latent form of GBS presenting as a period time of mild weakness may be out of the view of the neurologists. Patients may not go to hospital or not report it to doctors because of the mildness of disease, so the missed diagnosis occurs at outpatient clinic. With this consideration, clinicians should proactively ask about weakness when the patients report paraesthesia or report symptoms indicating cranial nerve or autonomic nerve involvement to avoid a missed diagnosis at outpatient clinic [2]. It is thus necessary to perform the paresis test on patients with a suspect of GBS. Last but not the least, CGSES had a potential role to guide the treatment option. The treatment of GBS is a combination of supportive care and immunotherapy. The immunotherapy is recommended when the HGFS score is equal to or more than 3 [18]. Over 80% of the GBS patients with CGSES score of 3 or 4 had an HGFS score equal to or more than 3 at nadir. Thus, we recommend that the immunotherapy may be used at admission on patients with a CGSES score of 3 or 4, especially 4, aiming at improving the prognosis.

Our study has limitations. Retrospective studies could be less reliable than prospective studies since validation of retrospectively collected data is complicated. However, in the current study, 523 GBS patients have been enrolled, and such a large sample volume could kind of guarantee the validation of the conclusions. A few patients with acute-onset chronic inflammatory demyelinating polyradiculoneuropathy might be enrolled in the study [19]. Due to the inadequate follow-up data and electrophysiological data, the associations between chief complaints and long-term outcome/subtypes of GBS were not well explored. The features of GBS patients reporting ataxia, dyspnea and autonomic dysfunction were not investigated due to the small sample volume.

With these concerns, more attention and studies are warranted to disclose the incidence and features of mild form of GBS, as the characteristics for mildly and severely affected GBS patients are dissimilar, regarding age, sex and antecedent infection [14]. The role of the chief complaints of ataxia, dyspnea and autonomic dysfunction should be further explored. Studies are also warranted to explore whether distinct chief complaints indicate different immune response of GBS patients. CGSES score need to be further confirmed in prospective studies as well.

Conclusions

Weakness and numbness are the most common chief complaints among GBS patients. Chief complaints are predictors of disease severity, ventilator dependence and short-term outcome. Immunotherapy may be used at admission on patients with a CGSES score of 3 or 4.

Abbreviations

CGSES: Clinic GBS severity evaluation scale; GBS: Guillain-Barré syndrome; HFGS: Hughes functional grading scale; IVIg: Intravenous immunoglobulin; mEGOS: Modified erasmus GBS outcome score; MRC: Medical research council; OR: Odds ratio

Acknowledgements

Not applicable

Funding

The work was supported by grants from the Elite PHD Program of Bethune Health Science Centre, Jilin University (No. 470110000421) and Graduate Innovation Fund of Jilin University (No. 2016106). These two grants supported the analysis of the data and the writing of the manuscript.

Authors' contributions

YW contributed to study design, acquisition of data, analysis and interpretation of data and manuscript draft. PS and MYX contributed to the acquisition of data. JB contributed to the revision of manuscript. CKZ contributed to study design, analysis of data and revision of manuscript. HLZ contributed to study design, supervision of study process, revision of manuscript, and gave final approval of the version to be published. All authors read and approved the final manuscript.

Competing interests

The authors declare that they have no competing interests.

Author details

[1]Neuroscience Centre, Department of Neurology, the First Hospital of Jilin University, Xinmin Street 71#, Changchun 130021, China. [2]Current address: Department of Life Sciences, the National Natural Science Foundation of China, Beijing, China.

References

1. Fokke C, van den Berg B, Drenthen J, Walgaard C, van Doorn PA, Jacobs BC. Diagnosis of Guillain-Barré syndrome and validation of Brighton criteria. Brain. 2014;137:33–43.
2. Willison HJ, Jacobs BC, van Doorn PA. Guillain-Barré syndrome. Lancet. 2016;388:717–27.
3. Stewart R. Subjective cognitive impairment. Curr Opin Psychiatry. 2012;25:445–50.
4. Mishra A, Dave N, Mehta M. Fulminant Guillain-Barré syndrome with myocarditis. J Family Med Prim Care. 2014;3:84–5.
5. Parmentier C, Vandermeeren Y, Laloux P, Mormont E. Asymptomatic posterior reversible encephalopathy revealed by brain MRI in a case of axonal Guillain-Barré syndrome. Clin Neurol Neurosurg. 2012;144:1006–9.
6. van den Berg B, Bunschoten C, van Doorn PA, Jacobs BC. Mortality in Guillain-Barre syndrome. Neurology. 2013;80:1650–4.
7. Kalita J, Misra UK, Goyal G, Das M. Guillain-Barré syndrome: subtypes and predictors of outcome from India. J Peripher Nerv Syst. 2014;19:36–43.
8. Verma R, Chaudhari TS, Raut TP, Garg RK. Clinico-electrophysiological profile and predictors of functional outcome in Guillain-Barre syndrome (GBS). J Neurol Sci. 2013;335:105–11.
9. González-Suárez I, Sanz-Gallego I, Rodríguez de Rivera FJ, Arpa J. Guillain-Barré syndrome: natural history and prognostic factors: a retrospective review of 106 cases. BMC Neurol. 2013;13:95.
10. Walgaard C, Lingsma HF, Ruts L, van Doorn PA, Steyerberg EW, Jacobs BC. Early recognition of poor prognosis in Guillain-Barre syndrome. Neurology. 2011;76:968–75.
11. Roodbol J, de Wit MC, Walgaard C, de Hoog M, Catsman-Berrevoets CE, Jacobs BC. Recognizing Guillain-Barré syndrome in preschool children. Neurology. 2011;76:807–10.
12. Asbury AK, Cornblath DR. Assessment of current diagnostic criteria for Guillain-Barré syndrome. Ann Neurol. 1990;27(Suppl):s21–4.
13. Hughes RA, Newsom-Davis JM, Perkin GD, Pierce JM. Controlled trial prednisolone in acute polyneuropathy. Lancet. 1978;2:750–3.
14. Van Koningsveld R, Van Doorn PA, Schmitz PI, Ang CW, Van der Meché FG. Mild form of Guillain-Barré syndrome in an epidemiologic survey in The Netherlands. Neurology. 2000;54:620–5.
15. Bril V, Ilse WK, Pearce R, Dhanani A, Sutton D, Kong K. Pilot trial of immunoglobulin versus plasma exchange in patients with Guillain-Barré syndrome. Neurology. 1996;46:100–3.
16. Kim DJ, Lee J, Lee J, Kim MR, Ha IH. Guillain-Barré syndrome mistaken for a common spinal disorder: a case report. Altern Ther Health Med. 2015;21:64–7.
17. Aminzadeh V, Hassanzadeh RA. A report of guillain-Barré syndrome with myalgia and mild weakness. Iran J Child Neurol. 2014;8:70–2.
18. van Doom PA, Ruts L, Jacobs BC. Clinical features, pathogenesis, and treatment of Guillain-Barré syndrome. Lancet Neurol. 2008;7:939–50.
19. Sung JY, Tani J, Park SB, Kiernan MC, Lin CS. Early identification of 'acute-onset' chronic inflammatory demyelinating polyneuropathy. Brain. 2014;137:2155–63.

14

MR imaging features of benign retroperitoneal paragangliomas and schwannomas

Yanguang Shen[1†], Yan Zhong[1†], Haiyi Wang[1], Lu Ma[1], Yingwei Wang[1], Kun Zhang[2], Zhonghua Sun[3] and Huiyi Ye[1*]

Abstract

Background: To determine whether MRI feature analysis can differentiate benign retroperitoneal extra-adrenal paragangliomas and schwannomas.

Methods: The MRI features of 50 patients with confirmed benign retroperitoneal extra-adrenal paragangliomas and schwannomas were retrospectively reviewed by two radiologists blinded to the histopathologic diagnosis. These features were compared between two types of tumours by use of the Mann-Whitney test and binary logistic regression. The patients' clinical characteristics were reviewed.

Results: Analysis of MRI images from 50 patients revealed no significant differences in the quantitative MRI features of lesion size, ratio of diameter and apparent diffusion coefficient. There were significant differences in the qualitative MRI features of location, necrosis, cysts and degree of tumour enhancement for two readers, with no significant differences in the other qualitative MRI features between these tumours. The combination of necrosis with degree of tumour enhancement during the arterial phase increased the probability that a retroperitoneal mass would represent retroperitoneal extra-adrenal paraganglioma as opposed to schwannoma.

Conclusion: We have presented the largest series of MRI features of both benign retroperitoneal extra-adrenal paragangliomas and schwannomas. Some MRI features assist in the differentiation between these tumours, with imaging features consisting of necrosis and avid enhancement during the arterial phase, suggestive of retroperitoneal extra-adrenal paragangliomas.

Keywords: Paraganglioma, Schwannoma, Retroperitoneal space, Magnetic resonance imaging

Background

Primary neurogenic tumours, which constitute 10% to 20% of primary retroperitoneal tumours, occur in a younger age group and are usually benign [1]. These tumours can be classified as ganglion cell origin, paraganglionic system origin (pheochromocytomas and paragangliomas), or nerve sheath origin (neurilemmomas, neurofibromas, neurofibromatosis, and malignant nerve sheath tumours). Schwannomas and extra-adrenal pheochromocytomas are the most common benign soft-tissue tumours occurring in the retroperitoneum [2, 3]; extra-adrenal pheochromocytomas account for 1–3%, and schwannomas account for 4% of retroperitoneal tumours [4, 5]. Retroperitoneal paragangliomas can be divided into functional and non-functional paragangliomas, and functional tumours are often associated with hypertension, tachycardia, headache and diaphoresis [6]. However, non-functional paragangliomas can be completely clinically silent (they are referred to as "incidentalomas"). Since retroperitoneal benign schwannomas are usually asymptomatic, diagnostic difficulties are often encountered for differentiating retroperitoneal paragangliomas from schwannomas due to their nonspecific clinical and imaging features. However, any physical contact with these silent paragangliomas can precipitate cardiac arrhythmias and malignant hypertension [7]. Now,

* Correspondence: 13701100368@163.com
†Equal contributors
[1]Department of Radiology, Chinese PLA General Hospital, Fuxing Road 28, Box, Beijing 100853, China
Full list of author information is available at the end of the article

more than ever, urologists and radiologists should understand the imaging appearances of paragangliomas, as differential diagnosis between them is clinically essential in decision making on a therapeutic strategy.

To the best of our knowledge, description of the MRI features of retroperitoneal extra-adrenal paragangliomas and schwannomas has been reported on small sample sizes in the literature, and no joint assessment has been performed for the imaging appearances of these two similar entities, which may be expected to have overlapping imaging findings in view of their common pathologic characteristics. Therefore, the purpose of our study was to retrospectively analyse the MRI imaging differences of benign retroperitoneal extra-adrenal paragangliomas and schwannomas, particularly for those with non-functional paragangliomas.

Methods

Patients

This retrospective study was approved by our institutional review board with waiver of informed consent due to the retrospective nature. Between July 2008 and February 2016, retroperitoneal extra-adrenal paragangliomas and schwannomas were identified within the radiology databases and were confirmed by surgical resection and pathological findings in 50 patients who had undergone preoperative MRI. Of these 50 patients, 20 had undergone preoperative CT (13 paraganglioma and 7 schwannoma patients). All patients' medical histories were reviewed. In all, 50 patients (30 men and 20 women, mean age: 44.3 ± 12.1 years, age range: 17–79 years old) had a total of 50 tumours: 24 benign retroperitoneal extra-adrenal paragangliomas and 26 benign retroperitoneal schwannomas.

Magnetic resonance imaging protocol

MRI examinations were performed with a 1.5-T system ($n = 5$, Signa HDXT, GE Healthcare), 3.0-T system ($n = 28$, Signa EXCITE; GE Healthcare, Milwaukee, WI, USA) and a 3.0-T system ($n = 17$, Discovery 750, GE Healthcare, Milwaukee, WI, USA). A surface phased-array coil was used, with all patients in the supine position. Respiratory-triggered transverse and coronal T2-weighted fast spin-echo sequences were initially performed, followed by transverse T1-weighted dual-echo in-phase and out-of-phase sequences and three-dimensional fat-saturated T1-weighted dynamic contrast-enhanced sequences performed during suspended respiration. Transverse breath-hold diffusion-weighted imaging (DWI) was obtained using a single-shot, spin-echo echo-planar sequence prior to the administration of contrast material with tri-directional gradients and two sets of b values: 0 and 800 s/mm^2. A 15-mL bolus of contrast medium (Gadobenate dimeglumine, MultiHance; Bracco Sine, Shanghai, China) was injected intravenously at a flow rate of 2 mL/s using a power injector (Spectris; MedRad, Warrendale, PA, USA), followed by a 20-mL saline flush. Dynamic contrast-enhanced MRI (DCE-MRI) was performed in the transverse plane at baseline (precontrast) and during the arterial, venous and delayed phases.

The MR imaging parameters for T2-w FSE images were as follows: infinite/90–105 ms (repetition time ms/echo time ms); field of view (FOV), 36–44 cm; section thickness, 5 mm; intersection gap, 1 mm; and matrix, 320 × 224. The imaging parameters for T1-w dual-echo images were as follows: 260/(2.2–2.5; 5.5–5.8) ms; FOV, 36–44 cm; section thickness, 5 mm; intersection gap, 1 mm; and matrix, 256 × 192. The scanning protocol of DWI was as follows: 5400/50–60 ms; FOV, 36–40 cm; flip angle, 90°; matrix, 128 × 128; section thickness, 5 mm; intersection gap, 1 mm; all directions; one signal acquired, b values of 0, 800 s/mm^2. The parameters for three-dimensional (3D) DCE-MRI sequences were as follows: 3.0–3.9/1.2–1.6 ms; FOV, 34–40 cm; section thickness, 5 mm; interpolated section thickness, 2.5 mm; and matrix, 288 × 224.

Imaging features analysis

Two radiologists who had 10 and 5 years of experience in the interpretation of abdominal MR images independently reviewed all images. Readers who were blinded to the histologic diagnoses of the lesions evaluated and recorded each lesion for the presence of each of the following features [8, 9].

Quantitative MR image feature analysis (A) Tumour maximum size: the maximum size of each lesion was measured at its single largest diameter in three planes. (B) Ratio of diameter: two readers independently measured the maximum transverse diameter (TD) and longitudinal diameter (LD) of the mass in the coronal section. The means of maximum TD and LD of the tumour in the coronal section were recorded. Each measurement was conducted three times, with the mean value used as the final value to avoid intra- and inter-observer disagreements. Ratios of diameter were determined by the following equations: Ratio of diameter = Mean TD/ Mean LD. (C) Apparent diffusion coefficient (ADC) values: ADC maps were auto-generated. The region of interest (ROI) was placed corresponding to the most obvious enhancing region of the retroperitoneal tumours in the arterial phase according to visual assessment, with the aim of avoiding necrosis, haemorrhage and cystic changes (which are defined as those parts of the lesions showing no enhancement on DCE-MR images) and was performed using an Advantage Workstation (Advantage Workstation, version 4.6, GE Healthcare, Bue, France). In each patient and for each tumour, three ROIs, each measuring 30–60 mm^2, were drawn on three target anatomical structures. The mean ADC values in ROIs on three targets were calculated for each patient.

Qualitative MR image feature analysis (1) Position and peripheral location: The lesion was assessed according to whether it was located in the right paravertebral region or the left paravertebral region (near the spinal column and psoas muscle, adrenal region or kidney); anterior to the vertebrae (close to the abdominal aorta and the inferior vena cava, the origin of the inferior mesenteric artery or peripancreatic location); or in the pelvic cavity. (2) Shape: Tumours were round or oval/irregular. (3) Margin: Tumours were well-defined or partly poorly defined. (4) Microscopic lipid: There was an area of signal loss in the lesion on out-of-phase T1-weighted images. (5) Subacute haemorrhage: There were areas of increased T1 signal intensity on unenhanced fat suppressed T1-weighted images. (6) Cystic degeneration: Represented by areas with signal intensities (SIs) equal to that of cerebrospinal fluid on T2-weighted images; low SI on T1-weighted images; lack of enhancement; and lobulated morphology. (7) Necrosis: Represented by high SI on T2-weighted images, although not as high as the signal of cerebrospinal fluid; low SI on T1-weighted images; lack of enhancement; and central location within the tumour. (8) Degree of tumour enhancement: Subjective assessments of the MR imaging degree of mass enhancement compared with that of the renal cortex (avid enhancement, moderate enhancement or slight enhancement) were performed on Gd-enhanced MR images acquired during the arterial phase. (9) Other MR imaging features: Calcification, smooth expansion of a sacral nerve root exit foramen, fluid-fluid level, and subjective assessment of the MR imaging degree and pattern of mass enhancement during the venous and delayed phases.

Pathologic diagnosis

All specimens were retrospectively examined by two uropathologists who were unaware of the MRI findings (10 years of experience in uropathology) in consensus.

Statistical analysis

Continuous variables are expressed as the means ± SD and were analysed by independent t-tests for normally distributed data or Mann-Whitney tests for non-normally distributed data. For the qualitative variables, the Chi square test was used to compare the sample proportions of the two groups. Generalized estimating equations based on a binary logistic regression model were used to determine whether lesion type (retroperitoneal extra-adrenal paragangliomas or schwannomas) was associated with any of the individual binary factors. In this context, stepwise variable selection was performed to determine whether the combination of two or more of the aforementioned imaging features represented a significant independent predictor of schwannoma or paraganglioma. These tests were performed separately for each reader. Kappa coefficients were not used for this determination because the very high prevalence rates of certain imaging features for many of the binary factors was expected to produce misleadingly low values [8, 10]. All reported p values are two-sided and considered statistically significant when less than 0.05. SPSS version 19.0 software (IBM Corporation, Armonk, NY, USA) was used for all computations.

Results

Demographic data and clinical characteristics

In this study, a total of 50 lesions in 50 patients were identified for inclusion in the analysis, consisting of 24 retroperitoneal extra-adrenal paragangliomas (Fig. 1) and 26 retroperitoneal schwannomas (Fig. 2). All presenting clinical characteristics of these patients are summarized in Table 1. A total of 30 tumours were incidentally found in 50 patients. The 24-h urinary vanilmandelic acid and urinary catecholamine concentrations were measured for 22 of the patients, of which 9 were positive. No patient had a medical history of neurofibromatosis. The tumours were fully excised in all cases, with clear resection margins. The final histologic diagnosis was obtained by laparoscopic surgery (15 lesions), robot-assisted laparoscopy (11 lesions), and laparotomy (24 lesions).

Findings of the quantitative MR imaging features

The presenting quantitative MR imaging characteristics of mean maximum lesion size, ratio of diameter and ADC values of the 24 retroperitoneal extra-adrenal paragangliomas and 26 schwannomas are summarized in Table 2, with no significant differences in the assessments by two reviewers. Of the 50 lesions, the maximum diameter was greater than 5 cm in 34 cases (17 retroperitoneal extra-adrenal paragangliomas and 17 schwannomas), while in the remaining 16 cases, the maximum diameter was less than 5 cm (7 paragangliomas and 9 schwannomas).

Findings of the qualitative MR imaging features

(1) There were statistically significant differences in terms of lesion location, necrosis, cystic degeneration and degree of tumour enhancement for both readers ($p = 0.000–0.011$, 0.000–0.019 for readers 1 and 2, respectively), while there were no statistically significant differences between retroperitoneal extra-adrenal paragangliomas and schwannomas in terms of shape, boundaries, microscopic fat, and subacute haemorrhage findings for both readers ($p = 0.164–0.589$, 0.271–1.0 for readers 1 and 2, respectively) (Table 3).

(2) Concordance of the two readers for each of the assessed binary features was good to excellent, ranging from 52% to 98% for all features (Table 4).

(3) Only two features remained statistically significant in the stepwise multivariate logistic regression model: necrosis and degree of tumour enhancement. The combination of necrosis with degree of tumour enhancement during the arterial phase increased the probability that a

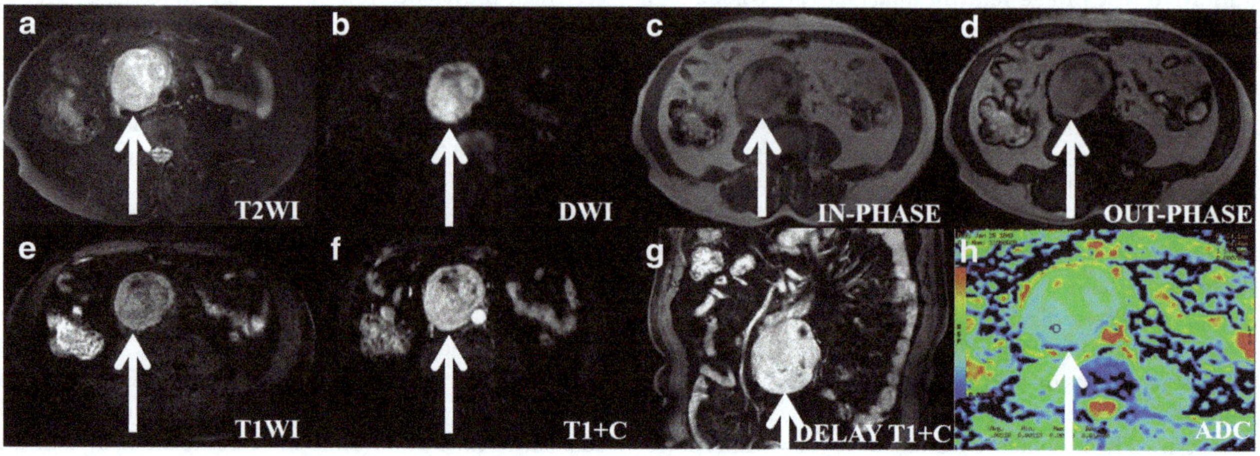

Fig. 1 A patient (age: 60–69) with hypertension and a histologically proven benign retroperitoneal paraganglioma in the right prevertebral region (between the inferior vena cava and aorta). The transverse and longitudinal diameters of the tumour are 8 cm and 9.25 cm, respectively. **a** On axial T2WI, the tumour appears with high signal intensity compared with the gluteal muscles. The intratumoural cystic areas are higher in signal intensity. **b** On axial DWI, the tumour appears circular and nodular, with high signal intensity. **c**, (**d**) and (**e**) In T1WI (in-phase, out-of-phase and pre-scanned imaging), part of the tumour signal is slightly lower than that of the gluteal muscle, and most of it is slightly higher than that of the gluteal muscle. **f** On contrast T1WI during the aerial phase, the tumour exhibits obvious and inhomogeneous enhancement. **g** On coronal T1WI during the delay phase, the tumour exhibits obvious and inhomogeneousenhancement. **h** On ADC imaging, the mean ADC value of the ROI of the tumour is 0.00119 mm^2/s

retroperitoneal mass would represent extra-adrenal paraganglioma versus schwannoma, with diagnostic accuracies (c statistic or area under the curve-AUC) of 0.893 (reader 1) and 0.853 (reader 2)and with 95% confidence intervals (CIs) of 0.807–0.978 for reader 1 and 0.748–0.9579 for reader 2 (Table 5).

(4) No retroperitoneal extra-adrenal paragangliomas were identified in the pelvis, though 4 schwannomas were identified in the pelvis, with 1 case located in the medial iliac arterial bifurcation, 2 cases in the wall of the basin, and another in the anterior sacral space. Approximately 54.17% of the paragangliomas were located in the prevertebral region, which is close to the aorta and the inferior vena cava. However, 50% of schwannomas were in the right paravertebral region (2 cases in the renal portal area, 10 cases in lumbar major muscles, and 1 case in the adrenal region).

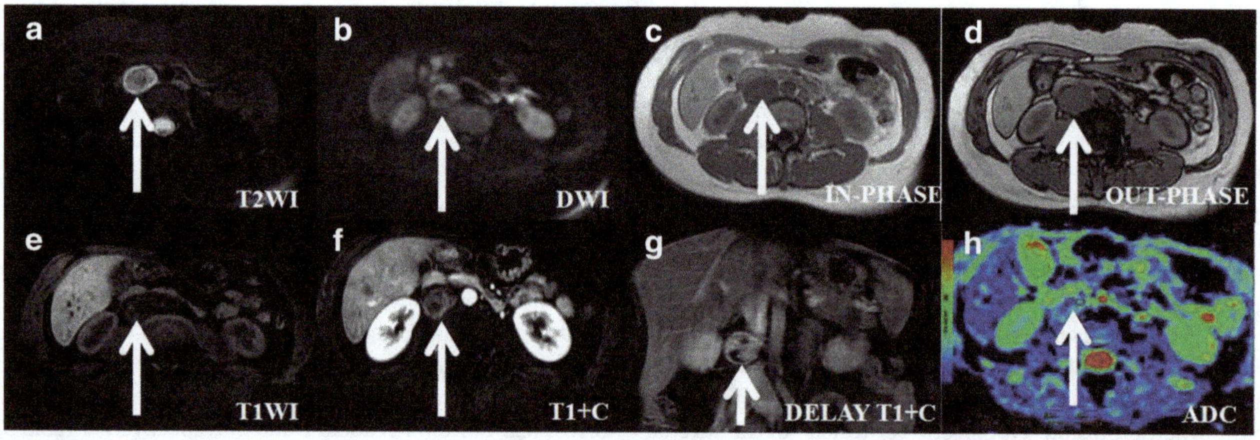

Fig. 2 An asymptomaticpatient (age: 30–39) with a histologically proven benign retroperitoneal schwannoma. The transverse and longitudinal diameters of the tumour are 2.19 cm and 3.51 cm, respectively. **a** On axial T2-weighted imaging, the tumour presents with heterogeneous signal intensity compared with the gluteal muscles. **b** On axial DWI, the tumour appears circular, with high signal intensity. **c**, (**d**) On T1-weighted imaging (in-phase, out-of-phase imaging), the tumour's signal is slightly lower and isointense compared with that of the gluteal muscle. The intratumoural microscopic fat areas are slightly lower in signal intensity on out-of-phase imaging. **e** On T1-weighted imaging (pre-scanned imaging), the tumour's signal is slightly lower, with isointense and hyperintense spots compared with that of gluteal muscle. The intratumoural subacute haemorrhage areas present as hyperintense spots in signal intensity on pre-scanned imaging. **f** On contrast T1-weighted imaging during the aerial phase, the tumour presents as slightly enhanced and inhomogeneous. **g** On coronal T1-weighted imaging during the delay phase, the tumour presents as moderately enhanced and inhomogeneous. **h** On ADC imaging, the mean ADC value of the ROI of the tumour is 0.00171 mm^2/s

Table 1 Patient demographics and clinical characteristics

Characteristic	Paragangliomas group ($n = 24$)	Schwannoma group ($n = 26$)	P-value
No. of patients (female)	24 (12)	26 (8)	–
[a]Age (years)	48.04 ± 9.70	40.88 ± 13.29	0.036
Hypertension (n)	11	1	0.001
CA-related symptoms (n)	3	0	0.001
Symptomless(n)	10	20	0.001
VMA/24 h (Positive)	22 (9)	0	0.001
CA/24 h (Positive)	22 (9)	0	0.001
^{131}I–MIBG positive	9	0	0.001
other symptoms			
Abdominal mass (n)	2	4	–
Lumbago (n)	3	2	–
dysuria (n)	0	1	–
Resection of tumor			
Laparoscopic surgery (n)	9	6	–
Robot-assisted laparoscopic (n)	10	1	–
Laparotomy (n)	5	19	–

[a]Values are mean values ± standard deviations. P values were calculated by using t test
Other data are numbers of patients (n). P values were calculated by using x^2 test.
CA-related symptoms catecholamine-related symptoms, *VMA* Vanilmandelic acid, *CA* Catecholamine, *MIBG* Metaiodobenzylguanidine scintigraphy

Findings of other MR imaging features

First, only small sub-centimetre flecks of calcification were seen in 2 schwannomas and 1 paraganglioma. Second, only two schwannomas were shown to demonstrate smooth expansion of a sacral nerve root exit foramen without including bony destruction of the sacrum. Third, all tumours showed inhomogeneous enhancement following gadolinium administration, with a non-enhancing component showing a fluid signal or necrotic component and peripheral enhancement of the solid elements. Only one paraganglioma had a fluid-fluid level inside the lesion. The degrees of enhancement of 21 paragangliomas and 26 schwannomas showed continuous signal increases in mass in the venous and delayed phases (the persistent pattern), and only 3 paragangliomas showed "washout" of signal intensity.

Discussion

Retroperitoneal extra-adrenal paragangliomas and schwannomas confined to the retroperitoneum are frequently encountered in clinical practice, and diagnostic difficulties are often encountered [11]. To the best of our knowledge, this study represents the largest series to date to describe the MRI features of both tumours, with the aim of differentiating them due to overlapping clinical, MR imaging and histologic features.

Paragangliomas are usually described on MRI as masses having characteristic high-signal intensity or a light bulb bright signal on T2WI with the use of fat suppression [12], which is used to differentiate them from other tumours, but further studies have proposed that this feature is neither specific nor sensitive and have indicated that the use of this sign leads to the misdiagnosis of paragangliomas in up to 35% of cases [13, 14]. The MRI characteristics of benign retroperitoneal schwannomas include hypointensity on T1WI and hyperintensity on T2WI [15, 16], and neither is specific. However, in our results, the MRI features consisting of tumour location, necrosis and tumour enhancement showed significant differences between these two retroperitoneal tumours.

More than 50% of paragangliomas were situated in the prevertebral region close to the inferior vena cava and aorta following the aorto-sympathetic chain, results that were consistent with other reports [17]. However, schwannomas were usually located in the paravertebral region and, less commonly, adjacent to the kidney, pre-sacral space, and abdominal wall [6]. Although the appearances overlapped with the reported appearances of many retroperitoneal tumours [18],no statistically significant differences were found in the stepwise multivariate logistic regression model in our study. One obvious specific feature of 3 schwannomas was smooth expansion of a nerve root exit foramen without showing bony destruction, which is highly suggestive of retroperitoneal schwannomas [19].

DCE-MRI has also been employed for tumour detection and characterization. In this study, 80% of retroperitoneal extra-adrenal paragangliomas exhibited strong initial signal increases during the arterial phase; however, 76.92% of schwannomas mostly demonstrated slow initial signal enhancement. These results are consistent with other studies [20, 21]. It should be noted that a pattern of continuous

Table 2 Quantitative characteristics of retroperitoneal extra-adrenal paragangliomas and schwannoma

Item	Reader 1			Reader 2		
	Paragangliomas ($n = 24$)	Schwannoma ($n = 26$)	P-value	Paragangliomas ($n = 24$)	Schwannoma ($n = 26$)	P-value
Tumor maximum size (cm)	5.61 ± 2.11	6.35 ± 3.24	0.350	5.70 ± 2.10	6.19 ± 3.04	0.521
Ratio of diameter (TD/LD)	0.878 ± 0.145	0.831 ± 0.148	0.175	0.855 ± 0.144	0.802 ± 0.151	0.212
Mean ADC value ($\times 10^{-3}$ mm^2/s)	1.541 ± 0.425	1.614 ± 0.345	0.508	1.565 ± 0.425	1.651 ± 0.322	0.421

Values are Mean values ± standard deviations. P values were calculated by using t test
Ratios of diameter = Mean TD(transverse diameter)/ Mean LD(longitudinal diameter). *ADC* Apparent Diffusion Coefficient

Table 3 Frequency of assessed imaging features in retroperitoneal extra-adrenal paragangliomas and schwannoma

Imaging Feature	Reader 1			Reader 2		
	Paragangliomas (*n* = 24)	Schwannoma (*n* = 26)	*P*-value	Paragangliomas (*n* = 24)	Schwannoma (*n* = 26)	*P*-value
Location						
Right paravertebral region	8.33(2/24)	50(13/26)	0.001	8.33(2/24)	50(13/26)	0.001
Left paravertebral region	37.5(9/24)	11.53(3/26)		41.67(10/24)	11.54(3/26)	
Prevertebral region	54.17(13/24)	23.08(6/26)		50(12/24)	23.08(6/26)	
Pelvic cavity	0(0)	15.38(4/26)		0(0)	15.38(4/26)	
Shape						
Round or oval	83.33(20/24)	92.31(24/26)	0.589	87.5(21/24)	84.62(22/26)	1.000
Irregular	16.67(4/24)	7.69(2/26)		12.5(3/24)	15.38(4/26)	
Boundaries						
Well-defined	66.67(16/24)	88.46(23/26)	0.063	70.83(17/24)	84.62(22/26)	0.240
Partly poorly defined	33.33(8/24)	11.54(3/26)		29.17(7/24)	15.38(4/26)	
Microscopic fat						
YES	12.5(3/24)	23.08(6/26)	0.546	16.67(4/24)	15.38(4/26)	1.000
NO	87.5(21/24)	76.92(20/26)		83.33(20/24)	84.62(22/26)	
Subacute hemorrhage						
YES	54.17(13/24)	34.62(9/26)	0.164	50(12/24)	34.62(9/26)	0.271
NO	45.83(11/24)	65.38(17/26)		50(12/24)	65.38(17/26)	
Necrosis						
YES	75(18/24)	34.62(9/26)	0.004	70.83(17/24)	34.62(9/26)	0.010
NO	25(6/24)	65.38(17/26)		29.17(7/24)	65.38(17/26)	
Cysts						
YES	62.5(15/24)	92.31(24/26)	0.011	66.67(16/24)	96.15(25/26)	0.019
NO	37.5(9/24)	7.69(2/26)		33.33(8/24)	3.85(1/26)	
Degree of tumor enhancemen						
Avid enhancement	41.67(10/24)	3.85(1/26)	<0.001	33.33(8/24)	7.69(2/26)	<0.001
Moderate enhancement	41.67(10/24)	19.23(5/26)		50(12/24)	15.38(4/26)	
Slight enhancement	16.67(4/24)	76.92(20/26)		16.67(4/24)	76.92(20/26)	

Data are percentages with raw numbers of patients (n) in parenthesis
P values were calculated by using x^2 test

Table 4 Comparison of concordance between readers for each assessed qualitative imaging feature

Attribute	Concordance
Location	98(49/50)
Shape	94(47/50)
Tumor boundaries	96(48/50)
Microscopic fat	94(47/50)
Subacute hemorrhage	92(46/50)
Necrosis	52(26/50)
Cystic degeneration	76(38/50)
Degree of tumor enhancement	94(47/50)

Values are percentages with raw numbers of patients (n) in parenthesis

Table 5 Stepwise multivariate logistic regression analysis relating statistically significant MR imaging features to retroperitoneal extra-adrenal paragangliomas

Readers and Features	Adjusted Odds Ratio
Radiologist 1	
Necrosis	0.101 (0.017, 0.595)
Degree of tumor enhancement	0.097 (0.026, 0.354)
Radiologist 2	
Necrosis	0.148 (0.032, 0.684)
Degree of tumor enhancement	0.150 (0.048, 0.472)

The model c statistic (Area Under Curve, AUC) was 0.893 (95%CI was 0.807–0.978) for reader 1, AUC = 0.853 (95%CI was 0.748–0.957) for reader 2. Numbers in parentheses are 95% confidence intervals signal increase of masses was common in these tumours in the venous and delayed phases and was not helpful to distinguish paragangliomas from schwannomas. Necrotic change was noted in more than 70% of retroperitoneal extra-adrenal paragangliomas but in only 34.62% of schwannomas in our study. Necrotic changes tend to occur as paragangliomas increase in size [18]. Further research showed that a combination of avid enhancement with necrosis provided diagnostic accuracies of 0.853 and 0.893 for the diagnosis of retroperitoneal extra-adrenal paragangliomas in our series. In other words, these findings allowed the differentiation of paragangliomas from schwannomas: avid enhancement and necrosis were predictive of paragangliomas, while slight enhancement was correlated with schwannomas. Paragangliomas are characteristically highly vascular neoplasms and an abundant capillarynetwork,and may have precarious microcirculation because of high levels of tissue vasoconstrictor substances. These histologic features can cause spontaneous massive intratumoural haemorrhage and necrotic degeneration, resulting in the formation of a pseudocyst, and exhibits marked and early enhancement in DCE-MRI [22, 23]. Further, Sahdev et al. reported that necrotic changes were observed in more than 70% of retroperitoneal extra-adrenal paragangliomas and tended to occur as paragangliomas increased in size [18]. However, many theories attempt to explain the degeneration cystic schwannoma. One theory involves the degeneration of Antoni B areas leading to cyst formation, while progressing in size; another theory holds that with increasing tumor central ischemic necrosis occurs that causes cysts within the tumor [24, 25]. On histopathological examination, Antoni B area is a myxoid component.

No significant differences were shown between the mean lesion sizes and mean ADC values of these two types of tumours in our study. This study suggested that the ADC quantitative assessment could not provide significant value for the differential diagnosis of both of the tumours. We found that the mean ADC values of these tumours were greater than the mean ADC values of neck paragangliomas and schwannomas [26, 27].

Evidence of degeneration, which includes cysts, subacute haemorrhage and microscopic fat, was common for retroperitoneal extra-adrenal paragangliomas and schwannomas, and all tended to be observed [28]. Takatera et al. [19] reported that 66% retroperitoneal schwannomas showed cystic degeneration, while schwannomas demonstrated an exceptional risk of degeneration [11, 29]. In this study, more than 90% of retroperitoneal schwannomas showed the same feature, which was only found in 62.5% of retroperitoneal extra-adrenal paragangliomas, highlighting that fact that this feature is helpful in the differential diagnosis. Literature studies have reported that haemorrhagic portions can be seen in paragangliomas and schwannomas [30, 16]; however, they did not report that the feature was able to distinguish these tumours. The feature of subacute haemorrhage was found in 50% of retroperitoneal extra-adrenal paragangliomas and 34.62% of schwannomas, and only one case showed a fluid-fluid sign in paragangliomas. In addition, microscopic fat was not reported in the literature, and there was no obvious specificity. Calcifications can occur in all types of neurogenic tumours. In our study, calcifications were seen in only 3 lesions, without showing any obvious specificity. However, some authors have reported that punctate calcifications can be seen in retroperitoneum extra-adrenal paragangliomas, along with punctuate or curvilinear calcifications along the walls of masses in schwannomas [31].

There are several limitations in our study. **First**, this was a retrospective study with a relatively small sample size for benign retroperitoneal extra-adrenal paragangliomas and schwannomas, reflecting the low incidence rates of these tumours. The imaging features of our patients were similar to those described in other radiological series, and the small number of cases reflected the rarity of the tumours. **Second**, due to the study's retrospective nature, two different field strengths of magnetic resonance scanners were used. Although we demonstrated that field strength had no effect on ADC measurements of renal tumours between 1.5 T and 3.0 T, we did not include many retroperitoneal tumours. In addition, ADCs of various kinds of retroperitoneal lesions should be compared between 1.5 T and 3.0 T. **Third**, lesions presented with predominantly cystic changes, haemorrhage and necrosis, which may affect ADC values or signal intensity measurements. **Finally**, there was only one malignant schwannoma and no malignant paragangliomas. We excluded these tumours from the analysis and did not perform any further studies of benign and malignant retroperitoneal tumours.

Conclusions

In summary, in this study, we present the largest series of radiological studies of benign retroperitoneal extra-adrenal paragangliomas and schwannomas. These tumours are often found incidentally or present with vague and nonspecific symptoms. They are rare retroperitoneal neoplasms, usually presenting as large ovoid or spherical masses with smooth, well-defined borders and do not invade or obstruct adjacent structures. The combination of avid enhancement with necrosis, clinical CA-related symptoms, positive VMA/24 h, positive CA/24 h and positive 131I–MIBG provided diagnostic accuracy for the diagnosis of retroperitoneal extra-adrenal paragangliomas in our series. When these features are correctly recognized, there should be a high level of suspicion for paragangliomas.

Abbreviations

ADC: Apparent diffusion coefficient; AUC: Area under the curve; CA: Catecholamine; DCE-MRI: Dynamic contrast-enhanced MRI; FOV: Field of view; LD: Longitudinal diameter; MIBG: Metaiodobenzylguanidine scintigraphy; MRI: Magnetic resonance imaging; ROI: Region of interest; T1WI: T1-weighted imaging; T2WI: T2-weighted imaging; TD: Transverse diameter; VMA: Vanilmandelic acid

Acknowledgements

The authors would like to thank Jingjing Pan for assistance with the preparation of this manuscript.

Funding

This study was supported by grants from the National Natural Science Foundation of China (No. 81271535) and the Health Care Special Project (14BJZ02). The funders took no part in the study design, data collection and analysis, decision to publish, or preparation of the manuscript.

Author contributions

YS and YZ carried out the studies. YS, YZ and ZS drafted the manuscript. HY, YS, LM, HW, YW and KZ participated in the design of the study and conceived of the study. YZ, YW, LM and YW contributed materials/analysis tools. YS, YZ and LM performed the statistical analysis. All authors read and approved the final manuscript.

Competing interests

The authors declare that there are no conflicts of interest in this study.

Author details

[1]Department of Radiology, Chinese PLA General Hospital, Fuxing Road 28, Box, Beijing 100853, China. [2]Department of Radiology, Chinese Navy General Hospital, Beijing, China. [3]Department of Medical Radiation Sciences, Curtin University, Perth 6102, Australia.

References

1. Neville A, Herts BRCT. Characteristics of primary retroperitoneal neoplasms. Crit Rev Comput Tomogr. 2004;45:247–70.
2. Nah YW, Suh JH, Choi DH, Ko BK, Nam CW, Kim GY, et al. Benign retroperitoneal schwannoma:surgical consideration. Hepato-Gastroenterology. 2005;52:1681–4.
3. Amparo EG. Where is the organ of Zuckerkandl? AJR Am J Roentgenol. 1993;160:662.
4. Song JY, Kim SY, Park EG, Kim CJ, Kim DG, Lee HK, et al. Schwannoma in the retroperitoneum. J Obstet Gynaecol Res. 2007;33:371–5.
5. Jansen JC, van den Berg R, Kuiper A, van der Mey AG, Zwinderman AH, Cornelisse CJ. Estimation of growth rate in patient with head and neck ganglioneuromas influence the treatment proposal. Cancer. 2000;88:2811–6.
6. Rajiah P, Sinha R, Cuevas C, Dubinsky TJ, Bush WH Jr, Kolokythas O. Imaging of uncommon retroperitoneal masses. Radiographics. 2011;31:949–76.
7. Wang H, Ye H, Guo A, Wei Z, Zhang X, Zhong Y, et al. Bladder paraganglioma in adults: MR appearance in four patients. Eur J Radiol. 2011;80:e217–20.
8. RRosenkrantz AB, Hindman N, Fitzgerald EF, Niver BE, Melamed J, Babb JSMRI. Features of renal oncocytoma and chromophobe renal cell carcinoma. AJR Am J Roentgenol. 2010;195:W421–7.
9. Hindman N, Ngo L, Genega EM, Melamed J, Wei J, Braza JM, et al. Angiomyolipoma with minimal fat: can it be differentiated from clear cell renal cell carcinoma by using standard MR techniques? Radiology. 2012;265:468–77.
10. Feinstein AR, Cicchetti DV. High agreement but low kappa. Part I. The problems of two paradoxes. J Clin Epidemiol. 1990;43:43–549.
11. Hoarau N, Slim K, Da Ines DCT. MR imaging of retroperitoneal schwannoma. Diagn Interv Imaging. 2013;94:1133–9.
12. Elsayes KM, Staveteig PT, Narra VR, Chen ZM, Moustafa YL, Brown J. Retroperitoneal masses: magnetic resonance imaging findings with pathologic correlation. Curr Probl Diagn Radiol. 2007;36:97–106.
13. Elsayes KM, Narra VR, Leyendecker JR, Francis IR, Lewis JS Jr, Brown JJMRI. Of adrenal and extraadrenal pheochromocytoma. AJR Am J Roentgenol. 2005; 184:860–7.
14. Varghese JC, Hahn PF, Papanicolaou N, Mayo-Smith WW, Gaa JA, Lee MJ. MR differentiation of pheochromocytome from other adrenal lesions based on qualitative analysis of T2 relaxation times. Chin Radial. 1997;52:603–6.
15. Cerofolini E, Landi A, DeSantis G, Maiorana A, Canossi G, Romagnoli RMR. Of benign peripheral nerve sheath tumors. J Comput Assist Tomogr. 1991;15:593.
16. Hayasaka K, Tanaka Y, Soeda S, Huppert P, Claussen CD. MRfindings in primary retroperitoneal schwannoma. Acta Radiol. 1999;40:78–82.
17. Scopsi L, Callini P, Muscolino GA. New observation of the Carney's triad, with long follow-up period and additional tumors. Cancer Detect Prev. 1999;23:435–43.
18. Sahdev A, Sohaib A, Monson JP, Grossman AB, Chew SL, Reznek RHCT. MR imaging of unusual locations of extra-adrenal paragangliomas (pheochromocytomas). Eur Radiol. 2005;15:85–92.
19. Takatera H, Takiuchi H, Namiki M, Takaha M, Ohnishi S, Sonoda T. Retroperitoneal schwannoma. Urology. 1986;28:529–31.
20. Arnold SM, Strecker R, Scheffler K, Spreer J, Schipper J, Neumann HP, et al. Dynamic contrast enhancement of paragangliomas of the head and neck: evaluation with time-resolved 2D MR projection angiography. Eur Radiol. 2003;13:1608–11.
21. Nakashima J, Ueno M, Nakamura K, Tachibana M, Baba S, Deguchi N, et al. Differential diagnosis of primary benign and malignant retroperitoneal tumors. Int J Urol. 1997;4:441–6.
22. Modlin IM, Farndon JR, Shepherd A, Johnston ID, Kennedy TL, Montgomery DA, et al. Phaeochromocytomas in 72 patients: clinical and diagnostic features, treatment and long term results. Br J Surg. 1979;66(7):456–65.
23. Suga K, Motoyama K, Hara A, Kume N, Ariga M, Matsunaga N. Tc-99m MIBG imaging in a huge clinically silent pheochromocytoma with cystic degeneration and massive hemorrhage. Clin Nucl Med. 2000;25:796–800.
24. Kim P, Ebersold MJ, Onofrio BM, Quast LM. Surgery of spinal nerve schwannoma. Risk of neurological deficit after resection of involved root. J Neurosurg. 1989;71:810–4.
25. Meşină C, Mogoantă SŞ, Cristian DA, Dumitrescu TV, Drăgoescu PO, Meşină-Botoran MI, et al. Retroperitoneal ancient schwannoma-case presentation. Romanian J Morphol Embryol. 2015;56:1517–22.
26. Yuan Y, Shi H, Tao X. Head and neck paragangliomas: diffusion weighted and dynamic contrast enhanced magnetic resonance imaging characteristics. BMC Med Imaging. 2016;16:12.
27. Das A, Bhalla AS, Sharma R, Kumar A, Thakar A, Goyal A. Diffusion-weighted imaging in extracranial head and neck schwannomas: a distinctive appearance. Indian J Radiol Imaging. 2016;26:231–6.
28. Donnal JF, Backer ME, Mahony MS, Leight GS. Benign retroperitoneal schwannoma. Urology. 1988;31:332–4.
29. Sangster GP, Migliaro M, Heldmann MG, Bhargava P, Hamidian A, Thomas-Ogunniyi J. The gamut of primary retroperitoneal masses: multimodality evaluation with pathologic correlation. Abdom Radiol (NY). 2016;41:1411–30.
30. Brennan C, Kajal D, Khalili K, Ghai S. Solid malignant retroperitoneal masses—a pictorial review. Insights Imaging. 2014;5:53–65.
31. Kitajima K, Kono A, Konishi J, Suenaga Y, Takahashi S, Sugimura K. 18F-FDG-PET/CT findings of retroperitoneal tumors: a pictorial essay. Jpn J Radiol. 2013;31:301–9.

15

Rationale and design of the CAROLINA® - cognition substudy: a randomised controlled trial on cognitive outcomes of linagliptin versus glimepiride in patients with type 2 diabetes mellitus

Geert Jan Biessels[1*], Jolien Janssen[1,2], Esther van den Berg[1,3], Bernard Zinman[4], Mark A. Espeland[5], Michaela Mattheus[6], Odd Erik Johansen[7] and on behalf of the CAROLINA® investigators

Abstract

Background: Type 2 diabetes mellitus is associated with cognitive dysfunction and an increased risk of dementia. Linagliptin is a glucose-lowering agent of the dipeptidyl peptidase-IV (DPP-IV) inhibitor class that is of particular interest for the prevention of accelerated cognitive decline, because it may potentially benefit the brain through pleiotropic effects, beyond glucose lowering. This paper presents the design of a study that aims to establish if linagliptin is superior to the sulfonylurea glimepiride in the prevention of accelerated cognitive decline in patients with type 2 diabetes mellitus.

Methods: The cognition substudy is an integral part of the ongoing event-driven, randomised, double blind CARdiOvascular safety of LINAgliptin (CAROLINA®) trial, which evaluates the effect of treatment with linagliptin versus glimepiride on cardiovascular outcomes. CAROLINA® includes patients with type 2 diabetes mellitus with sub-optimal glycaemic control at elevated cardiovascular risk. The substudy will evaluate patients randomised and treated who have a baseline Mini Mental State Examination (MMSE) score ≥ 24, documented years of formal education with at least one valid cognitive assessment at baseline and during follow-up. The primary cognitive outcome is the occurrence of accelerated cognitive decline at the end of follow-up. The two treatment groups will be compared by using a logistic regression. Accelerated cognitive decline is defined as a rate of cognitive decline that falls at or below the 16th percentile of decline for the whole cohort on either the MMSE or a combined score of the trail making and verbal fluency test. Potential confounders are taken into account at an individual patient level, using a regression based index.

Discussion: Between December 2010 and December 2012, 6042 patients were randomised and treated with either linagliptin (5 mg) or glimepiride (1-4 mg) once daily in CAROLINA®. Cognitive tests were conducted in nearly 4500 participants at baseline and are scheduled for two subsequent assessments, after 160 weeks of follow-up and end of follow-up. This substudy of the ongoing CAROLINA® trial will establish if linagliptin is superior to glimepiride in the prevention of accelerated cognitive decline in patients with type 2 diabetes mellitus. Final results are expected in 2019.

Keywords: Type 2 diabetes mellitus, Cognition, Dipeptidyl peptidase-IV inhibitor, Oral glucose-lowering agent, Dementia

* Correspondence: G.J.Biessels@umcutrecht.nl
[1]Department of Neurology, G03.232 Brain Center Rudolf Magnus, University Medical Center, PO Box 85500, 3508, GA, Utrecht, the Netherlands
Full list of author information is available at the end of the article

Background

Type 2 diabetes mellitus (T2DM) is a rising public health concern with over 400 million cases worldwide in 2015 and an estimated number of over 600 million cases by 2040 [1]. Prevention of long-term complications is a major focus of diabetes treatment. In this respect, cognitive dysfunction and dementia are diabetes-associated complications that receive increasing attention [2, 3]. It is well recognised that the risk of dementia is increased in people with T2DM [4]. A recent meta-analysis evaluated 20 studies reporting on the risk of any type of dementia, 20 on Alzheimer's disease and 13 on vascular dementia (VaD), including a total of 1,148,041 participants, of whom 89,708 had diabetes. The pooled relative risk (95% CI) for dementia in people with diabetes was 1.73 (1.65–1.82), for Alzheimer's disease 1.56 (1.41–1.73) and for VaD 2.27 (1.94–2.66) [5] as compared to people without. In addition, diabetes is associated with more subtle cognitive changes, that are referred to as diabetes-associated cognitive decrements [2, 3].

Accelerated cognitive decline is a cause for concern in patients with T2DM, yet no preventive treatment has been established. Lifestyle, vascular, and diabetes-specific risk factors present many promising targets for prevention and treatment [2, 6, 7]. These include management of glycaemic control and avoidance of severe hypoglycaemic events [8]. Previous observational studies that examined the effect of glucose-lowering treatments (including metformin, sulfonylureas, thiazolidinedione, insulin or a combination of these) on the risk of cognitive decline have not demonstrated consistent findings [2]. Because observational studies have a substantial risk of bias, randomised controlled trials (RCTs) are needed; unfortunately few have been performed. A recent meta-analysis summarised the results of five well conducted RCTs on the effect of intensive versus standard glycaemic control on cognitive decline in patients with T2DM, involving over 24,000 participants [9]. This pooled analysis showed that intensive glycaemic control was not associated with a slower rate of cognitive decline, compared with standard glycaemic control, although there was some heterogeneity among studies [9]. These previous RCTs have in common that they used mean cognitive performance as their primary outcome, which may include many participants with little or no cognitive decline. Although duration of follow-up of the studies ranged from 3 to 6 years [9], the actual average decline in mean cognitive performance was limited [10–13]. Over the past years it has become clear, also from observational studies, that the average decline in cognition over time associated with diabetes [2] is relatively slow, limiting the sensitivity of follow up studies to detect meaningful differences. Importantly however, among patients with T2DM there is heterogeneity in the rate of cognitive decline, where some have accelerated decline which in some cases progress to dementia. For example, in a large cohort of patients with T2DM over the age of 60 years, annual incidence of dementia of 2.6% was reported [14]. It might therefore be more appropriate - and clinically meaningful with regards to establishing interventions - to focus on occurrence of accelerated cognitive decline in individual patients. Such an approach is chosen in the CAROLINA®-cognition substudy. Interestingly, the ORIGIN study (which studied effects on outcomes of intensive glucose lowering with insulin glargine) did a post-hoc analysis using this approach in the ORIGIN MIND substudy and observed a modest, albeit statistically non-significant, benefit of intensive glycaemic control [10] versus standard care.

Dipeptidyl peptidase-IV (DPP-IV) inhibitors improve glycaemic control by inhibiting the enzyme DPP-IV thereby enhancing the incretin effects, i.e., increasing the availability of active glucagon-like peptide (GLP)-1 and glucose-dependent insulinotropic polypeptide (GIP), which are secreted from the intestine after a meal. In the presence of hyperglycaemia, these hormones promote glucose-dependent insulin secretion and reduce glucagon secretion [15]. Beyond their effects on DPP-IV activity and glucose, several preclinical studies suggest anti-inflammatory, anti-atherosclerotic and neuroprotective effects that might be relevant in the context of preventing accelerated cognitive decline [15–19]. Experimental studies also show promising results of incretin-based therapies in models of Alzheimer's disease and stroke [17]. These potential pleiotropic modes of action make DPP-IV inhibitors attractive candidate drugs to prevent accelerated cognitive decline in T2DM. Recently, an observational study found that increased plasma DPP-IV activity was associated with a high risk of mild cognitive impairment in elderly patients with T2DM [20], providing further support to test a strategy of modulating DPP-IV activity in T2DM to prevent cognitive impairment. The international, randomised, double blinded CARdiOvascular safety of LINAgliptin (CAROLINA®) trial is designed to provide a long-term evaluation of treatment durability and cardiovascular safety of treatment with the DPP-IV inhibitor linagliptin compared to the currently widely used sulfonylurea (SU) glimepiride [21, 22]. Linagliptin is a once-daily, DPP-IV inhibitor with a xanthine-based structure that is characterised by a pharmacological profile distinct from other drugs in this class [23] largely due to its non-renal route of elimination (80% hepatic versus 5% renal) [24]. The cognition substudy is an integrated part of CAROLINA®.

Objectives

The primary objective of the CAROLINA®-cognition substudy is to investigate if the proportion of participants with accelerated cognitive decline is lower in the group randomised to treatment with linagliptin compared to the group randomised to glimepiride after 160 weeks, or at end of follow-up.

Secondary objectives

Unravelling the processes that underlie cognitive decline in T2DM is important to support future prevention strategies. Secondary objectives are therefore:

1) At baseline: to explore associations between characteristic features of T2DM (i.e., glycaemic and anthropometric parameters), cardiovascular risk factors (i.e., blood pressure and lipid levels) and cognitive performance
2) Longitudinal: to explore associations between baseline characteristic features of T2DM, cardiovascular risk factors – and changes in these factors over time – and cognitive decline during follow-up
3) Longitudinal: to explore the associations between baseline mood – and changes in mood over time - and cognitive decline during follow-up

Methods

Design and sample

The CAROLINA® trial is a randomised, active comparator, double blind study to evaluate the cardiovascular safety of linagliptin versus glimepiride in patients with T2DM at elevated cardiovascular risk. Patients were randomised between 2010 and 2012 from approximately 600 trial centres in 43 different countries. Key inclusion criteria are shown in Table 1.

CAROLINA® is an event driven study. It is planned to run until a minimum of 631 confirmed Major Adverse Cardiovascular Events (MACE) have been accrued. MACE include cardiovascular death (including fatal stroke and fatal myocardial infarction (MI)), non-fatal MI (excluding silent MI) and non-fatal stroke. The estimated study duration is about 432 weeks. For more detailed information about the CAROLINA® main study see the Boehringer Ingelheim trial protocol (1218.74, Clintrial.gov id NCT01243424) and the previously published paper on the design and baseline characteristics [21].

CAROLINA cognition substudy

Cognitive tests are conducted at baseline, after 160 weeks and at planned end of follow-up (or at permanent treatment-discontinuation). To be eligible for cognitive testing in this substudy, participants need to live in a country that have a native language built on the Latin alphabet, due to psychometric test-battery validation. Participants are included in the analysis data-set of the CAROLINA®-cognition substudy of baseline data if they are randomised and treated with at least one dose of study drug and have at least one valid cognitive assessment at baseline and documented years of formal education. For the analyses of follow-up data in addition at least one valid cognitive assessment during follow-up

Table 1 Key inclusion criteria CAROLINA®

Insufficient glycaemic control defined as one of the criteria (A or B)	AND	Elevated risk of cardiovascular events defined as any (one or more) of the criteria (A, B, C or D)
(A) HbA1c 6.5 - 8.5% (48–69 mmol/mol) while patient is treatment naïve or treated with: (I) Metformin monotherapy (II) α-Glucosidase inhibitor monotherapy (e.g. acarbose, voglibose) (III) Metformin plus α-glucosidase inhibitor (e.g. acarbose, voglibose) **(B) HbA1c 6.5 - 7.5% (48–58 mmol/mol) while patient is treated with:** (I) SU monotherapy (II) Glinide monotherapy (e.g. repaglinide, nateglinide) (III) Metformin plus SU (for a maximum of 5 years) (IV) Metformin plus glinide (for a maximum of 5 years) (V) α-Glucosidase inhibitor plus SU (for a maximum of 5 years) (VI) α-Glucosidase inhibitor plus glinide (for a maximum of 5 years)		**(A) Previous vascular disease:** (I) MI (>6 weeks prior to informed consent IC) (II) Documented coronary artery disease (≥50% luminal diameter narrowing of left main coronary artery or in at least two major coronary arteries in angiogram) (III) Percutaneous coronary intervention (>6 weeks prior to IC) (IV) Coronary artery bypass grafting (>4 years prior to IC) or with recurrent angina following surgery (V) Ischaemic or haemorrhagic stroke (>3 months prior to IC) (VI) Peripheral occlusive arterial disease **(B) Evidence of vascular-related end-organ damage:** (I) Moderately impaired renal function (as defined by MDRD formula) with eGFR 30–59 ml/min/1.73 m2 (II) Random spot urinary albumin:creatinine ratio ≥30 μg/mg in two of three unrelated specimens in the previous 12 months. (III) Proliferative retinopathy defined as retinal neovascularization or previous retinal laser coagulation therapy **(C) Age ≥ 70 years** **(D) At least two of the following cardiovascular risk factors:** (I) T2DM duration >10 years (II) Systolic BP > 140 mmHg (or on at least 1 BP-lowering treatment) <6 months prior to IC (III) Current daily cigarette smoking (IV) LDL-cholesterol ≥ 135 mg/dL (3.5 mmol/L) (or specific current treatment for this lipid abnormality) <6 months prior to IC

Table adapted from Marx et al. 2015 [21]. CAROLINA: CARdiovascular Outcome Trial of LINAgliptin Versus Glimepiride in Type 2 Diabetes; IC: informed consent; T2DM: type 2 diabetes mellitus; BP: blood pressure; SU: sulphonylurea; MI: myocardial infarction; MDRD: modified diet in renal disease; eGFR: estimated glomerular filtration rate and baseline Mini Mental State Examination (MMSE) score ≥ 24 is required as illustrated in Fig. 1. An overview of the CAROLINA cognition substudy according to the "SPIRIT checklist" is provided in Additional file 1.

Cognitive assessment and psychometric tests

This cognitive assessment included a cognitive paper based test battery that is brief and easy to administer in a standardised way. The tests are sensitive to relatively mild cognitive changes in T2DM, well standardised and validated, and available in multiple languages (using the modern Latin alphabet). The specific tests selected were:

1. Mini Mental State Examination (MMSE). The MMSE is a screening instrument that was developed to determine whether older adults have cognitive impairments [25]. It consists of a range of items assessing orientation, memory for words, drawing, backward counting and semantic knowledge, with a maximum score of 30. The MMSE takes approximately five minutes to administer and participating centres use country-specific validated questionnaires of the MMSE. A cut-off of <24 is widely used, and has been accepted, as indicating the presence of cognitive impairment [26]. A limitation of the MMSE is that it is insensitive to cognitive decrements in domains affected by vascular-related cognitive impairment, in particular attention, executive functioning and information processing speed [27]. Therefore two additional tests that tap into these domains were included - the Trail Making Test (TMT) and the verbal fluency test (VFT). Although the TMT and the VFT measure different cognitive processes, there is a clear consensus in cognitive theory and clinical practice that both tests assess important aspects of speed, attention and executive functioning [28].
2. TMT. The TMT is a test of scanning, visuomotor tracking, divided attention and cognitive flexibility [29]. The test requires a subject to 'connect-the-dots' of 25 consecutive targets on a sheet of paper. Two versions are available: A, in which the targets are all numbers (1,2,3, etc.), and B, in which the subject alternates between numbers and letters (1, A, 2, B, etc.). The goal is to finish the test as quickly as

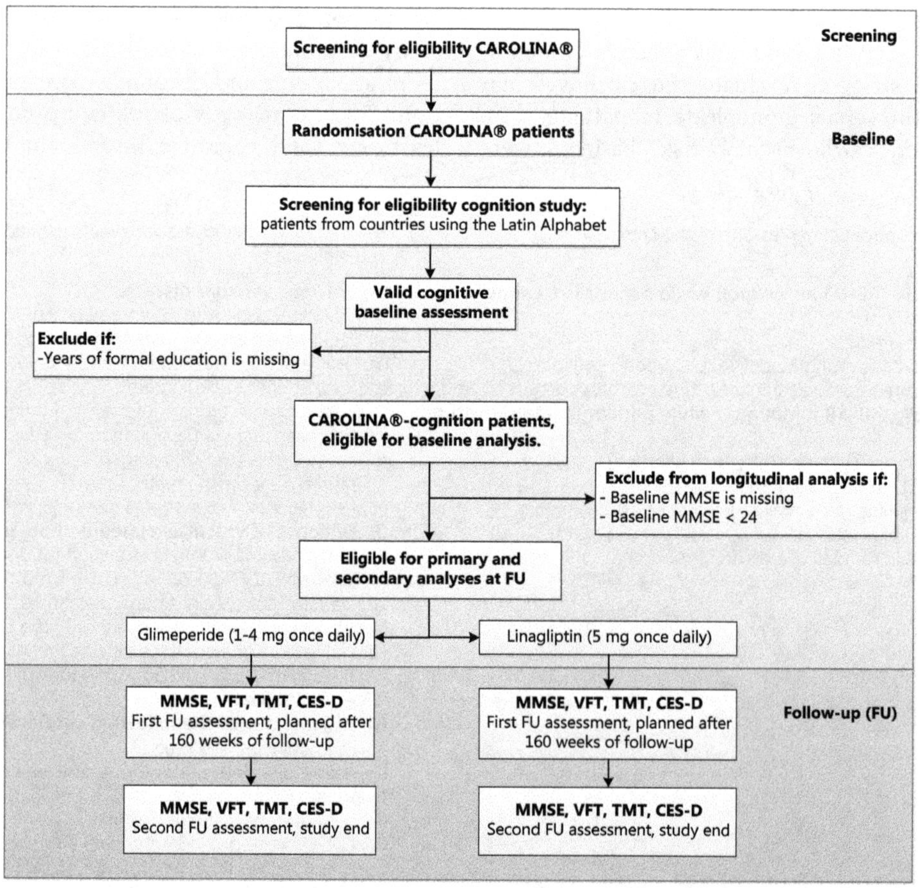

Fig. 1 overview design CAROLINA®-cognition substudy. Abbreviations: FU: follow-up, A&E score: Attention and Executive functioning score, MMSE: Mini Mental State Examination, VFT: Verbal Fluency Test, TMT: Trail Making Test, CES-D: Centre for Epidemiologic Studies Depression Scale

possible, and the time taken to complete the test is recorded. The maximum score (i.e. 300 s) is assigned to patients who are unable to complete the test within five minutes. The TMT is highly sensitive to the presence of cognitive impairment [30]. The TMT B is sensitive to T2DM-associated cognitive decrements, and in older individuals test performance clearly decreases over time [31–33]. The English versions of the TMT test instructions were translated into the local languages. Potential effects of translation of the test instructions on test difficulty, although unlikely, cannot be ruled out a priori and therefore will be tested (see sensitivity analyses, Table 2).

3. VFT. The VFT requires a subject to generate as many words as possible in 60 s. The category version (semantic fluency) requires generation of words from a certain category (e.g. animals), the letter version (phonemic fluency) requires generation of words starting with a specific letter. The tests are sensitive to the effects of ageing and performance is clearly affected in T2DM [27, 32, 33]. It is viewed as a sensitive indicator of (even mild) cognitive dysfunction. In CAROLINA, the category animals and the letters F, A and S are used for all languages. The number of words/animals after 15 s and after 60 s are recorded. The test takes approximately five minutes to complete. The English versions of the test instructions were translated into the local languages. Because of word-frequency differences between different Latin-based languages the letters FAS will not yield identical performance in different languages. However, FAS-equivalent letter combinations were available in a minority of languages only. Therefore, we chose to calculate a language-specific correction score (see analysis).

For the purpose of assessing effects on Attention and Executive functioning, the TMT and the VFT are combined to one composite score for Attention and Executive functioning (the A&E score). The A&E score is calculated as follows:

1) The VFT scores for the letters F, A and S in 60 s are averaged to one VFT letter fluency score.
2) The VFT is corrected for language influences by calculating least square (LS) means in an analysis of covariance (ANCOVA) model including age, gender, years of formal education, race and language as independent variables. The LS means for language are derived and then compared to one reference language (English), i.e. correction factors are calculated for each language separately (LSmean language/ LSmean English). Correction factors will be calculated for the three letters F, A and S taken together, and for the category fluency (i.e. animals) separately. The VFT scores of each participant are then corrected by multiplying the score with the corresponding correction factor. After correction, the scores are converted into z-scores. Z-scores are used to standardise raw test scores and make them directly comparable, z-scores are calculated as follows: (individual raw test score – mean baseline test score study population)/ baseline standard deviation.
3) The corrected VFT letter fluency and the VFT category fluency z-scores (both after 60 s) are averaged to one VFT overall score, where the letter fluency and the category fluency each account for 50%.
4) The TMT ratio is calculated, providing an index for executive functioning: (TMT B –TMTA) / TMT A.
5) The TMT ratio and VFT overall score are converted into z-scores.
6) The mean of the TMT ratio and VFT overall z-scores is used to generate one composite score for attention and executive functioning. In secondary analysis the TMT and VFT will be analysed separately to control for potential test-specific effects.

Table 2 Sensitivity analyses for the primary outcome

Reason sensitivity analysis	How is the sensitivity analysis performed?
Check the influence of inappropriate inclusion, potentially confounding co-morbid conditions and trial medication use	Participants will be excluded from the analysis if: • major inclusion or exclusion criteria are violated • incorrect trial medication is taken • major neurological or psychiatric disease was present at baseline
Check the influence of classifying participants who did not understand the instructions at follow-up as having accelerated cognitive decline	The last observation carried forward method will be used for patients with missing MMSE and A&E RBI-scores at follow-up if the reason for missing is the inability of the patient to understand the instructions (instead of classifying them as having accelerated cognitive decline)
Check for bias by differential lost to follow-up (worst case scenario)	All patients with missing MMSE and A&E RBI-scores at follow-up will be considered to have accelerated cognitive decline
Investigate the impact of further baseline variables on the RBI score result, Check for confounding by depression symptoms	Age, gender, years of formal education, race, ethnicity and language and CES-D (score < 16, ≥ 16) are included as covariates in the logistic regression analysis

As depression is a confounder to cognitive performance, participants also complete a depression questionnaire. In the CAROLINA® cognition substudy, we use the Centre for Epidemiologic Studies Depression Scale (CES-D), a widely used and validated 20-item questionnaire on depressive symptoms over the past week [34]. A score of ≥16 is indicative of a depression [35]. Whenever available in a county, the validated version of the CES-D was used. For languages were no validated version was available, a back translation was created and verified.

As both too high or too low blood glucose values can affect cognitive performance, self-monitoring of blood glucose (SMBG) values levels are to be measured (finger prick) prior to each cognitive assessment. Whenever the SMBGis not within 4 – 13 mmol/L the cognitive assessment is postponed. If values >3 or <18 mmol/L the finger prick could be repeated after at least one hour provided that the SMBGis within the 4–13 mmol/L range. In case glucose values ≤3 or ≥18 mmol/L glycemic management should be reviewed and the assessment postponed 1–7 days.

To optimise the quality of the cognitive outcomes, face-to-face meetings including training for examiners were organised in conjunction with the study start-up meetings. In addition, written step-by-step instructions for the (preparation of the) test assessment were provided. All tests were administered by the investigator or designated site-personnel who were all fluent in the language of test administration. The language in which the tests are performed is captured in the CRF. It is also recorded whether this language is the native language of the patient. If the tests are not performed in patient's native language the VFT scores are considered to be invalid and are set to missing.

The investigator or designated site-personnel can add a comment to the test score if they doubt the validity of the test. All those comments are independently reviewed by two members of the analysis team and categorised into whether those have an impact on the test score results ("valid" or "not valid" test score results). Discrepancies are resolved by means of discussion and before unblinding of the study. All test scores considered as not valid are set to missing. If the comments indicate that all tests of the patient are invalid (e.g. patient is illiterate) the patient is excluded from CAROLINA®-cognition analysis. Furthermore impossible scores (e.g. VFT score after 60 s which is less than after 15 s) are also set to missing.

When baseline VFT and TMT scores are very low, deterioration over time cannot be reliably assessed due to floor effects. Therefore, patients with a baseline VFT score below 3 will not be considered for longitudinal analysis on the VFT and patients with a TMT ratio z-score of 2 or higher at baseline not for the longitudinal analyses on the TMT. In this case the composite score for attention and executive functioning is just based on the valid data.

Cognitive outcomes

The primary outcome of CAROLINA®-cognition is the occurrence of accelerated cognitive decline at end of follow-up (a dichotomous outcome measure; presence or absence of accelerated cognitive decline).

Secondary cognitive outcomes are assessed as follows:

- The actual change in cognitive performance at end of follow-up (i.e. a continuous outcome measure; change in performance from baseline).
- The proportion of participants with accelerated cognitive decline after 160 weeks of follow-up.
- The actual change in cognitive performance after 160 weeks of follow-up (i.e. a continuous outcome measure; change in performance from baseline).

Primary outcome considerations

Conceptually, there are different ways to define accelerated cognitive decline. A fixed cut-off (e.g. occurrence of MMSE <24 at time point of assessment) or a minimal amount of decline (e.g. occurrence of >4 points of decline from baseline) can be used. However, a fixed cut-off does not take baseline performance into account and an absolute decline does not account for important individual factors influencing cognitive decline, such as education. We therefore choose to use a regression based index score (RBI score) of cognitive change over time. This RBI score adjusts for potential confounders as age, language, education, baseline performance, and regression to the mean on an individual participant basis [36]. In addition, the RBI also reduces the impact of learning effects: repeated neuropsychological assessment can cause practice effects, both material-specific effects and the fact that a person is no longer "test-naïve" after the first neuropsychological assessment. While the latter cannot be prevented, the former is countered by the use of RBI. Accelerated cognitive decline in the CAROLINA® cognition substudy is defined as a score at or below the 16th percentile (the equivalent of approximately one standard deviation below the mean) on the MMSE- or the A&E RBI z-score.

To convert MMSE and A&E z-scores into RBI scores, predicted follow-up scores (FUpredict) are calculated for each individual by means of an ANCOVA model. This model includes the following covariates: the individual's baseline test performance, age, years of formal education, gender, race, and test–retest interval. Subsequently the RBI scores are calculated for each individual by comparing his/her actual observed cognitive (FUobserved) score to his/her predicted cognitive score (RBI-score = (FUobserved – FUpredict)/ standard deviation (SD) of residuals). Hence, a negative RBI-score reflects a decline in cognitive function (relative to the other study participants) faster than expected (based on the adjusted covariates).

Clearly, dichotomizing the cognitive test results for the primary outcome measure does have implications for the analyses. It is also different from the approach of previous studies in the field [10–13]. Of note, our rationale for the dichotomy is that it has become apparent that cognitive decline in older individuals with T2DM is clearly not a unitary construct [2]. On average – at the group level - cognition declines only very slowly over time [10–13]. Yet, there is a subset of individuals with accelerated decline [2]. While ideally this accelerated cognitive decline would be defined in terms of incident dementia or mild cognitive impairment, this was not deemed to be feasible in the present multinational, multicenter study, because of variability in diagnostic approaches. We therefore choose the pragmatic approach as described above, which is likely to capture the patients with the worst cognitive outcome, although not in terms of a fixed diagnostic construct. Dichotomizing the cognitive test results based on the RBI could result in an underestimation of the standard error of the primary estimate of group difference in rate of cognitive decline. It also comes at the expense of information loss and power. Yet, it was decided to sacrifice some statistical power in order to enable the possibility of having a more powerful statement at the end of the trial. Moreover, the actual change in cognitive performance at end of follow-up (i.e. change in performance from baseline as a continuous measure) is an additional predefined outcome measure to confirm the results of the primary analysis.

Time windows

The time from baseline to end of follow-up cognitive assessment will vary between participants as patients were recruited over a period of two years. Furthermore, as visits may be rescheduled and each patient is followed up for a different time interval as per study design time windows were defined to assign each cognitive assessment to either baseline, week 160 or end of follow-up.

Baseline cognitive assessments were planned to be conducted at the day of randomisation, prior to intake of the first dose of study drug. The first follow-up assessment is scheduled after 160 weeks of follow-up (a time window up to 166 weeks is accepted) and the final cognitive assessment is scheduled within seven days after the last intake of study medication.

In practice the baseline test was conducted between Dec 2010 – Dec 2012 and the planned week 160 test was conducted between Dec 2013 – Jan 2016. The formal end of the trial will be determined in time, by reaching the predefined number of patients with primary endpoint events in the mother-trial, estimated to occur in Q2 2018. All patients that are still on treatment by then have their end of follow-up assessment at that time point. Patients that stop their treatment before the end of the trial will have their end of follow-up assessment at that moment. For all participants with a cognitive assessment after week 166, this assessment will be assigned to the second time interval (end of follow-up).

Other study parameters

Demographics at baseline (full definitions listed in Additional file 2)

Demographic information is collected at baseline and include age, gender, years of formal education, race (Black/African American, White, Asian, American Indian/Alaska Native, Hawaiian/Pacific Islander), ethnicity (Latino/Hispanic, non-Latino/Hispanic), medication use, medical history, and alcohol use.

Diabetes-related variables

Blood samples are drawn at baseline and at the day of the first and second cognitive follow-up assessments and include, HbA1c, FBG, and C-peptide. Samples are always taken after an overnight fast (at least 10 h after the last meal) and all blood samples are analysed at a central laboratory using validated assays. Medical history is recorded in the case report form (CRF) and includes duration of diabetes and presence of diabetic complications (diabetic neuropathy, diabetic foot and proliferative retinopathy; full definitions listed in Additional file 2). Previous medication use, including SU or glinide is recorded. Episodes of hypoglycaemia, including severe hypoglycaemic episodes, are recorded prospectively.

Cardiovascular risk profile (full definitions listed in Additional file 2)

Cardiovascular risk factors are assessed at baseline and at the day of the first and second cognitive follow-up assessments. They include: smoking habits, systolic and diastolic blood pressure, body mass index (BMI), waist circumference, a lipid panel (total cholesterol, high density lipoprotein (HDL) cholesterol, low density lipoprotein (LDL) cholesterol, triglycerides), and assessment of renal function/albuminuria. Blood pressure is measured using either a standard mercury sphygmomanometer or an electronic device after five minutes of rest. Weight measurements are standardised and similar scales are used at each visit. Waist circumference is measured in the midpoint between the lowest rib and the iliac crest using a non-elastic tape, after the patient exhaled. Estimated glomerular filtration rate is calculated using the Modification of Diet in Renal Disease (MDRD) formula.

History of macrovascular disease includes: ischemic heart disease, cerebrovascular disease and peripheral arterial occlusive disease. Cardiovascular events are recorded prospectively.

Statistical analysis

Sample size considerations

Accelerated decline is defined as an RBI score within the lowest 16% for the MMSE and/*or* the A&E RBI score. It is expected that an estimated of 20-22% will meet this criterion for the primary cognitive outcome measure of CAROLINA®. There were no formal power calculations performed for this substudy. However with 4500 participants, approximately 900–1000 participants will thus meet this primary cognitive outcome measure, which will allow, at a reasonable power, a detection of a hypothesised relative risk reduction with linagliptin for accelerated cognitive decline of approximately 20% (power 0.8; alpha 0.05, two-sided testing).

Primary analysis

The primary analysis will be performed in all patients randomised and treated with at least one dose of study drug, who have a baseline assessment and at least one follow-up cognitive assessment available (of which at least one of the two RBI scores can be calculated). In this modified intention to treat analysis the proportion of participants with accelerated cognitive decline will be compared between the two treatment groups at end of follow-up using a logistic regression analysis with factor for treatment. The odds ratio (OR) along with the 95% Wald confidence interval (CI) and the two-sided *p*-value for treatment comparison will be presented.

Predefined subgroup analyses

The primary outcome will be analysed in the following subgroups to explore the consistency of the treatment effect: gender (male, female), age (<70, ≥70 years), race (black, white), ethnicity (Latino/Hispanic, non-Latino/Hispanic), CES-D (score < 16, ≥ 16 and median split), cardiovascular risk groups (based on inclusion criterion groups A, B, C, D; see Table 1) and duration of diabetes (<=1 year, >1 to <=5 years, >5 to <=10 years, >10 years).

Handling of missing cognitive data

Missing baseline cognitive data will not be imputed. For missing data due to incomplete testing, the remaining test scores will be used to judge if accelerated cognitive decline is present. If one of the VFT subscores is missing, the remaining scores will be used to calculate the overall score. If either the TMT A or the TMT B is missing no TMT ratio will be calculated. If either the VFT overall z-score or the TMT ratio is missing the remaining score will be used to calculate the A&E score at baseline and follow-up.

If one follow-up assessment is completely missing it will be replaced by her/his last observed post-randomization measurement or linearly intrapolated in case of a missing assessment in between assessments.

If a cognitive test is not done or not completed, the investigator or research assistant should indicate whether this was due to the inability of the patient to understand the instructions. If this is the case at an follow-up visit and neither the MMSE nor the A&E RBI-score can be calculated due to missing values, the patient is classified as having accelerated cognitive decline.

Sensitivity analyses for the primary outcome

To test the robustness of the results, sensitivity analyses will be performed for the primary outcome (for the second FU assessment), as shown in Table 2.

Secondary analyses

To investigate potential early treatment effect, we will also look into the occurrence of accelerated cognitive decline at week 160, i.e., the first cognitive assessment post baseline.

In addition, to determine whether the definition we used for accelerated cognitive decline influenced the results, we will investigate the following alternative definitions for accelerated cognitive decline at week 160 and end of follow-up:

- having a score at or below the 16th percentile on the MMSE- or the A&E z-score (i.e. without using RBI scores).
- having a score at or below the 10th (instead of the 16th) percentile on the MMSE- or the A&E RBI-score
- having a follow-up MMSE score of <24 or a decline of >4 points in MMSE relative to baseline

To investigate the actual change in cognitive performance over time, the change in z-scores for all individual test scores (from baseline to first and second follow-up assessment) will be analysed. This will be done using a restricted maximum likelihood (REML) based mixed model repeated measures (MMRM) approach. The primary comparison will be the difference in adjusted LS means between the two treatment groups.

Finally, to investigate the effect of treatment on the occurrence of depression, the occurrence of a CES-D score of ≥16 will be analysed for the first and second follow-up assessments. This will be done using a logistic regression analyses, as for the primary outcome.

Exploratory analyses of risk factors for cognitive dysfunction

Additional analyses are planned to investigate the association between mood, diabetes-related factors, and cardiovascular factors and cognitive dysfunction. Cross-sectional baseline analyses will be conducted aimed at answering etiologic questions. Longitudinal analyses will be performed exploring both etiologic and prognostic questions in relation to cognitive decline.

Linear regression analyses will be used for the baseline analysis including the MMSE score and the A&E z-score as the cognitive outcome measures. These analyses will be adjusted for age, gender, years of formal education and race. If a significant association is found for a certain variable (e.g. HbA1c levels) other covariates may be added stepwise to the model to investigate this relation further. Non-linear associations will also be considered. We will perform subgroup analyses stratified by age (<70, ≥70 years) and gender (male, female). Similar approaches will be taken for etiologic longitudinal analyses, using a restricted maximum likelihood based mixed model repeated measures approach.

Since all of these secondary analyses are considered of exploratory nature, no correction for multiple testing will be made.

Discussion

The CAROLINA® trial provides a unique opportunity to investigate the effect of treatment with linagliptin compared to the SU glimepiride on the occurrence of accelerated cognitive decline in patients with T2DM. The large sample size, the long follow-up period and the study population of middle aged and older (mean age 64.7 ± 9.4 years) individuals at elevated cardiovascular risk, offer an excellent cohort to study cognitive outcomes. With the primary outcome measure occurrence of accelerated cognitive decline the cognition study focuses on those individuals who suffer from cognitive problems; a novel and very clinically meaningful approach.

CAROLINA®-cognition, a substudy of the CAROLINA® trial, is the first large RCT that will yield important information regarding DPP-IV inhibitor versus SU treatment in the reduction of accelerated cognitive decline in patients with T2DM. A positive result in CAROLINA®-cognition could provide important leads towards a new prevention strategy for dementia in T2DM and as such have major clinical T2DM treatment ramifications.

Abbreviations

A&E: Attention and Executive functioning; ANCOVA: Analysis of covariance; BMI: Body mass index; BP: Blood pressure; CABG: Coronary Artery Bypass Graft; CAROLINA: Cardiovascular Outcome Study of Linagliptin Versus Glimepiride in Patients With Type 2 diabetes mellitus; CES-D: Centre for Epidemiologic Studies Depression Scale; CI: Confidence interval; DPP-IV: Dipeptidyl peptidase-IV; GIP: Glucose-dependent insulinotropic polypeptide; GLP-1: Glucagon-like-peptide-1; HbA1c: Glycated hemoglobin; HDL: High Density Lipoprotein; LDL: Low Density Lipoprotein; MACE: Major Adverse Cardiovascular Event; MDRD: Modification of Diet in Renal Disease; MI: Myocardial Infarction; MMRM: Mixed model repeated measures; MMSE: Mini mental state examination; OR: Odds ratio; ORIGIN: Outcome Reduction With Initial Glargine Intervention; PCI: Percutaneous Coronary Intervention; RBI: Regression Based Index; RCT: Randomised controlled trial; REML: Restricted maximum likelihood; SMBG: Self-monitoring of blood glucose; SU: Sulfonylurea; T2DM: Type 2 Diabetes Mellitus; TMT: Trail Making Test; VFT: Verbal Fluency Test

Acknowledgements

Not applicable.

Funding

The CAROLINA®-cognition study is funded by the pharmaceutical company Boehringer Ingelheim GmBH & Co.KG and Eli Lilly and company.

Authors' contributions

GJB and JJ drafted the manuscript. EB, OEJ and GJB participated in the design of the study. JJ, MM and GJB drafted the statistical analysis plan. OEJ participated in the study coordination. EB, BZ, MAE, MM and OEJ reviewed the manuscript and were involved in its critical revision before submission. All authors read and approved the final manuscript.

Competing interests

We have read and understood BMC policy on declaration of interests and declare the following interests: Odd Erik Johansen is a clinical program leader employeed by Boehringer Ingelheim, Asker, Norway. Michaela Mattheus is the responsible trial statistician at Boehringer Ingelheim, Ingelheim, Germany. Prof Bernie Zinman, Toronto, Canada and Prof Mark Espeland, Winston-Salem, US, are members of the CAROLINA® executive steering committee and receive consultancy support from Boehringer Ingelheim. Prof. dr. GJ Biessels, neurologist at the University Medical Centre Utrecht receives research support from Boehringer Ingelheim.

Author details

[1]Department of Neurology, G03.232 Brain Center Rudolf Magnus, University Medical Center, PO Box 85500, 3508, GA, Utrecht, the Netherlands. [2]Julius Center for Health Sciences and Primary Care, University Medical Center Utrecht, Utrecht, the Netherlands. [3]Department of Neurology, Erasmus MC - University Medical Center, Rotterdam, the Netherlands. [4]Lunenfeld-Tanenbaum Research Institute, Mount Sinai Hospital, Toronto, Canada, Division of Endocrinology, University of Toronto, Toronto, Canada. [5]Department of Biostatistical Sciences, Wake Forest School of Medicine, Winston-Salem, NC, USA. [6]Global biometrics and datamanagement, Boehringer Ingelheim, Ingelheim, Germany. [7]Clinical development, Therapeutic Area Metabolism, Boehringer Ingelheim, Asker, Norway.

References

1. International Diabetes Federation. IDF diabetes atlas - 7th edition. http://www.diabetesatlas.org. 2015. Accessed 3 octobre 2016.
2. Biessels GJ, Strachan MW, Visseren FL, Kappelle LJ, Whitmer RA. Dementia and cognitive decline in type 2 diabetes and prediabetic stages: towards targeted interventions. Lancet Diabetes Endocrinol. 2014;2:246–55.
3. Koekkoek PS, Kappelle LJ, van den Berg E, Rutten GE, Biessels GJ. Cognitive function in patients with diabetes mellitus: guidance for daily care. Lancet Neurol. 2015;14:329–40.
4. Biessels GJ, Staekenborg S, Brunner E, Brayne C, Scheltens P. Risk of dementia in diabetes mellitus: a systematic review. Lancet Neurol. 2006;5:64–74.
5. Gudala K, Bansal D, Schifano F, Bhansali A. Diabetes mellitus and risk of dementia: a meta-analysis of prospective observational studies. J Diabetes Investig. 2013;4:640–50.
6. Feinkohl I, Price JF, Strachan MW, Frier BM. The impact of diabetes on cognitive decline: potential vascular, metabolic, and psychosocial risk factors. Alzheimers Res Ther. 2015;7:46.

7. Feinkohl I, Keller M, Robertson CM, Morling JR, McLachlan S, Frier BM, et al. Cardiovascular risk factors and cognitive decline in older people with type 2 diabetes. Diabetologia. 2015;58:1637–45.
8. Geijselaers SL, Sep SJ, Stehouwer CD, Biessels GJ. Glucose regulation, cognition, and brain MRI in type 2 diabetes: a systematic review. Lancet Diabetes Endocrinol. 2015;3:75–89.
9. Tuligenga RH. Intensive glycaemic control and cognitive decline in patients with type 2 diabetes: a meta-analysis. Endocr Connect. 2015;4:R16–24.
10. Cukierman-Yaffe T, Bosch J, Diaz R, Dyal L, Hancu N, Hildebrandt P, et al. Effects of basal insulin glargine and omega-3 fatty acid on cognitive decline and probable cognitive impairment in people with dysglycaemia: a substudy of the ORIGIN trial. Lancet Diabetes Endocrinol. 2014;2:562–72.
11. Koekkoek PS, Ruis C, van den Donk M, Biessels GJ, Gorter KJ, Kappelle LJ, et al. Intensive multifactorial treatment and cognitive functioning in screen-detected type 2 diabetes–the ADDITION-Netherlands study: a cluster-randomized trial. J Neurol Sci. 2012;314:71–7.
12. Launer LJ, Miller ME, Williamson JD, Lazar RM, Gerstein HC, Murray AM, et al. Effects of intensive glucose lowering on brain structure and function in people with type 2 diabetes (ACCORD MIND): a randomised open-label substudy. Lancet Neurol. 2011;10:969–77.
13. Luchsinger JA, Palmas W, Teresi JA, Silver S, Kong J, Eimicke JP, et al. Improved diabetes control in the elderly delays global cognitive decline. J Nutr Health Aging. 2011;15:445–9.
14. Exalto LG, Biessels GJ, Karter AJ, Huang ES, Katon WJ, Minkoff JR, et al. Risk score for prediction of 10 year dementia risk in individuals with type 2 diabetes: a cohort study. Lancet Diabetes Endocrinol. 2013;1:183–90.
15. Phillips LK, Prins JB. Update on incretin hormones. Ann N Y Acad Sci. 2011; 1243:E55–74.
16. Chen S, Liu AR, An FM, Yao WB, Gao XD. Amelioration of neurodegenerative changes in cellular and rat models of diabetes-related Alzheimer's disease by exendin-4. Age (Dordr). 2012;34:1211–24.
17. Groeneveld ON, Kappelle LJ, Biessels GJ. Potentials of incretin-based therapies in dementia and stroke in type 2 diabetes mellitus. J Diabetes Investig. 2016;7:5–16.
18. Porter DW, Irwin N, Flatt PR, Holscher C, Gault VA. Prolonged GIP receptor activation improves cognitive function, hippocampal synaptic plasticity and glucose homeostasis in high-fat fed mice. Eur J Pharmacol. 2011;650:688–93.
19. Satoh-Asahara N, Sasaki Y, Wada H, Tochiya M, Iguchi A, Nakagawachi R, et al. A dipeptidyl peptidase-4 inhibitor, sitagliptin, exerts anti-inflammatory effects in type 2 diabetic patients. Metabolism. 2013;62:347–51.
20. Zheng T, Qin L, Chen B, Hu X, Zhang X, Liu Y, et al. Association of Plasma DPP4 activity with mild cognitive impairment in elderly patients with type 2 diabetes: results from the GDMD study in China. Diabetes Care. 2016;39:1594–601.
21. Marx N, Rosenstock J, Kahn SE, Zinman B, Kastelein JJ, Lachin JM, et al. Design and baseline characteristics of the CARdiovascular outcome trial of LINAgliptin versus Glimepiride in type 2 diabetes (CAROLINA(R)). Diab Vasc Dis Res. 2015;12:164–74.
22. Rosenstock J. Rationale and design of the CAROLINA trial. An active comparator CARdiOvascular outcome study of the DPP-4 inhibitor LINAgliptin in patients with type 2 diabetes at high cardiovascular risk. Diabetes. 2011;60:A303.
23. Deacon CF, Holst JJ. Linagliptin, a xanthine-based dipeptidyl peptidase-4 inhibitor with an unusual profile for the treatment of type 2 diabetes. Expert Opin Investig Drugs. 2010;19:133–40.
24. Blech S, Ludwig-Schwellinger E, Grafe-Mody EU, Withopf B, Wagner K. The metabolism and disposition of the oral dipeptidyl peptidase-4 inhibitor, linagliptin, in humans. Drug Metab Dispos. 2010;38:667–78.
25. Folstein MF, Folstein SE, McHugh PR. "mini-mental state". A practical method for grading the cognitive state of patients for the clinician. JPsychiatr Res. 1975;12:189–98.
26. Tombaugh TN, McIntyre N. The mini-mental state examination: a comprehensive review. J Am Geriatr Soc. 1992;40:922–35.
27. Hachinski V, Iadecola C, Petersen RC, Breteler MM, Nyenhuis DL, Black SE, et al. National Institute of Neurological Disorders and Stroke-Canadian stroke network vascular cognitive impairment harmonization standards. Stroke. 2006;37:2220–41.
28. Lezak MD, Howieson BD, Bigler ED, Tranel D. Neuropsychological assessment. 5th ed. Oxford: Oxford University Press Inc; 2012.
29. Corrigan JD, Hinkeldey NS. Relationships between parts a and B of the trail making test. J Clin Psychol. 1987;43:402–9.
30. Reitan RM, Wolfson D. A selective and critical review of neuropsychological deficits and the frontal lobes. Neuropsychol Rev. 1994;4:161–98.
31. Gregg EW, Yaffe K, Cauley JA, Rolka DB, Blackwell TL, Narayan KM, et al. Is diabetes associated with cognitive impairment and cognitive decline among older women? Study of osteoporotic fractures research group. Arch Intern Med. 2000;160:174–80.
32. Kanaya AM, Barrett-Connor E, Gildengorin G, Yaffe K. Change in cognitive function by glucose tolerance status in older adults: a 4-year prospective study of the rancho Bernardo study cohort. Arch Intern Med. 2004;164:1327–33.
33. van den Berg E, Reijmer YD, de BJ KRP, Kappelle LJ, Biessels GJ. A 4 year follow-up study of cognitive functioning in patients with type 2 diabetes mellitus. Diabetologia. 2010;53:58–65.
34. Radloff LS. The CES-D Scale. A Self-Report Depression Scale for Research in the General Population. Appl Psychol Measurem. 1977;1:385–401.
35. Smarr KL, Keefer AL. Measures of depression and depressive symptoms: Beck depression inventory-II (BDI-II), Center for Epidemiologic Studies Depression Scale (CES-D), geriatric depression scale (GDS), hospital anxiety and depression scale (HADS), and patient health Questionnaire-9 (PHQ-9). Arthritis Care Res (Hoboken). 2011;63(Suppl 11):S454–66.
36. Temkin NR, Heaton RK, Grant I, Dikmen SS. Detecting significant change in neuropsychological test performance: a comparison of four models. J Int Neuropsychol Soc. 1999;5:357–69.

16

Low incidence of multidrug-resistant bacteria and nosocomial infection due to a preventive multimodal nosocomial infection control

Vera Spatenkova[1*], Ondrej Bradac[2], Daniela Fackova[3], Zdenka Bohunova[3] and Petr Suchomel[4]

Abstract

Background: Nosocomial infection (NI) control is an important issue in neurocritical care due to secondary brain damage and the increased morbidity and mortality of primary acute neurocritical care patients. The primary aim of this study was to determine incidence of nosocomial infections and multidrug-resistant bacteria and seek predictors of nosocomial infections in a preventive multimodal nosocomial infection protocol in the neurointensive care unit (NICU). The secondary aim focused on their impact on stay, mortality and cost in the NICU.

Methods: A10-year, single-centre prospective observational cohort study was conducted on 3464 acute brain disease patients. There were 198 (5.7%) patients with nosocomial infection (wound 2.1%, respiratory 1.8%, urinary 1. 0%, bloodstream 0.7% and other 0.1%); 67 (1.9%) with Extended spectrum beta-lactamase (ESBL); 52 (1.5%) with Methicillin-resistant Staphylococcus aureus (MRSA), nobody with Vancomycin-resistant enterococcus (VRE). The protocol included hygienic, epidemiological status and antibiotic policy. Univariate and multivarite logistic regression analysis was used for identifying predictors of nosocomial infection.

Results: From 198 NI patients, 153 had onset of NI during their NICU stay (4.4%; wound 1.0%, respiratory 1.7%, urinary 0. 9%, bloodstream 0.6%, other 0.1%); ESBL in 31 (0.9%) patients, MRSA in 30 (0.9%) patients. Antibiotics in prophylaxis was given to 63.0% patients (59.2 % for operations), in therapy to 9.7% patients. Predictors of NI in multivariate logistic regression analysis were airways (OR 2.69, 95% CI 1.81-3.99, $p<0.001$), urine catheters (OR 2.77, 95% CI 1.00-7.70, $p=0.050$), NICU stay (OR 1.14, 95% CI 1.12-1.16, $p<0.001$), transfusions (OR 1.79, 95% CI 1.07-2.97, $p=0.025$) antibiotic prophylaxis (OR 0.50, 95% CI 0.34-0.74, $p<0.001$), wound complications (OR 2.30, 95% CI 1.33-3.97, $p=0.003$). NI patients had longer stay ($p<0.001$), higher mortality ($p<0.001$) and higher TISS sums ($p<0.001$) in the NICU.

Conclusions: The presented preventive multimodal nosocomial infection control management was efficient; it gave low rates of nosocomial infections (4.2%) and multidrug-resistant bacteria (ESBL 0.9%, MRSA 0.9% and no VRE). Strong predictors for onset of nosocomial infection were accesses such as airways and urine catheters, NICU stay, antibiotic prophylaxis, wound complications and transfusion. This study confirmed nosocomial infection is associated with worse outcome, higher cost and longer NICU stay.

Keywords: Neurocritical care, Nosocomial infections, Multidrug-resistant bacteria, Outcome, Preventive protocol

* Correspondence: vera.spatenkova@nemlib.cz
[1]Neurocenter, Neurointensive Care Unit, Regional Hospital, Husova 357/10, Regional Hospital, 46063 Liberec, Czech Republic
Full list of author information is available at the end of the article

Background

Nosocomial infections (NI) are still an important issue in neurocritical care due to secondary brain damage and the increased morbidity and mortality of primary acute neurocritical care patients [1–5]. NI is associated with higher antibiotic consumption, thereby worsening the epidemiological situation in the intensive care unit by increasing the occurrence of multidrug-resistant bacteria [6]. For these reasons, they have a significant economic impact because they prolong stay [7–10] in the neurointensive care unit (NICU) and the higher frequency of diagnostic and therapeutic processing significantly raises healthcare costs.

Nosocomial infections can be caused by many risk factors, not all of which have been fully investigated. However, keeping a hygienic and epidemiological regime of critical care [11–13] and the rational use of antibiotics makes a significant impact [14, 15].

The primary aim of this study was to determine incidence of nosocomial infections and multidrug-resistant bacteria and seek predictors of nosocomial infections in a preventive multimodal nosocomial infection protocol in our neurocritical care. The secondary aim focused on their impact on stay, mortality and cost in the NICU.

Method

Study design and setting

A monocentric 10-year observation prospective cohort study was conducted in the entire population of 3464 patients with acute brain disease, admitted to an eight-bed, adult neurological and neurosurgical intensive care unit in the Neurocenter of the 900-bed Regional Hospital with a catchment area of approximately half a million people. The study was performed in the NICU, which consists of four different rooms: one room with one bed, two rooms with two beds and one room with three beds. The study was approved by the Liberec hospital Ethics Committees for Multicentric Clinical Trials.

We prospectively examined the following determined demographic and clinical parameters in our local NICU: brain diagnosis, type of admission (primary, secondary to 24 hours and after 24 hours; acute or planned; rehospitalisation), admission and overall Therapeutic Intervention Scoring System (TISS), admission Glasgow Coma Scale (GCS), admission Acute Physiology and Chronic Health Evaluation (APACHE) II score, length of stay in the NICU, mortality in the NICU, Glasgow Outcome Scale (GOS) upon discharge from the NICU, C-reactive protein (CRP), operations (amount, day of hospital and NICU hospitalisation, acute or planned, reoperation, time and type of operation), American Society of Anesthesiologists (ASA) Score, drainage, airways, mechanical ventilation, catheters (artery, central venous, urine) and tubes, administration of corticoids, transfusions, ulcer prophylaxis and diabetes mellitus.

Preventive multimodal nosocomial infection protocol

In the preventive multimodal nosocomial infection protocol, we categorised hygienic and epidemiological status and antibiotic policy.

Hygienic and epidemiological regime

The basis of the hygienic and epidemiological regime in our preventive multimodal protocol consisted of cleanliness, disinfection, sterilisation, barrier patient care techniques, the separation of clean and contaminated procedures and the regular monthly exchange of disinfectants. We categorised principles for staff, patients and facilities.

1/Staff and visitors

The foremost part of this protocol was maintaining the hygiene and disinfection of all staff members' hands before and after care for each patient, enabled by the bottled disinfectant provided at each entrance and each bed. This rule was also required for visitors. Staff members were not allowed to wear jewellery or watches on their hands and had to keep their fingernails cut short. Internal staff had to wear new, clean, special NICU clothing every day, a protective coat when outside the NICU, and masks, surgical caps and gowns when caring for isolated patients or during invasive medical procedures. Aprons were worn while washing patients. External staff as well as visitors wore surgical gowns, but not overshoes, and only 2 family members were allowed in the patient's room at a time.

2/Patients

Care of the patient was performed on the principle of barrier care techniques. Tools for individual patients including disinfection, stethoscopes, thermometers and washing aids were available by each bed. Patients were washed twice a day with liquid soap. Disinfection soap was used only before entering the operating theatre. Oral hygiene included cleaning teeth with our special toothbrushes with chlorhexidine and subglottic secretion drainage, after washing, the patient's body was rubbed with a non-allergic cream. Patients' clothes and bedding were changed twice a day. Dirty laundry was put in special sacks rather than dropped freely on the floor.

Basic principles of care for drainage, catheters, infusion, suction from the airway, breathing circuit sets, tubes included: 1/single-use products, 2/closed systems, 3/the minimum necessary duration, 4/minimal and only necessary disconnection, using the port system, 5/the regular (peripheral venous catheters, all infusion sets, connecting tubes and ports) and irregular (central venous catheters, endotracheal tubes and tracheostomy) exchange of all these tubes and catheters was made according to the exchange protocol. Invasive procedures included the sterile insertion of systems and regularly exchanged, fully covering and

Table 1 Demographic and clinical data of population of patients with acute brain disease, with or without nosocomial infection

Parameter	Unit	Total population	NI group	Control group	*p* value
Number total	pts	3464 (100%)	198 (5.7%)	3266 (94.3%)	
January	pts	327 (9.4%)	7 (3.6%)	310 (9.5%)	
February	pts	249 (7.2%)	19 (9.6%)	230 (7.0%)	
March	pts	267 (7.7%)	19 (9.6%)	248 (7.6%)	
April	pts	305 (8.8%)	13 (6.6%)	292 (8.9%)	
May	pts	269 (7.8%)	21 (10.6%)	248 (7.6%)	
June	pts	290 (8.4%)	17 (8.6%)	273 (8.4%)	0.660
July	pts	310 (8.9%)	19 (9.6%)	291 (8.9%)	
August	pts	274 (7.98%)	12 (6.1%)	262 (8.0%)	
September	pts	307 (8.9%)	14 (7.1%)	293 (9.0%)	
October	pts	280 (8.1%)	13 (6.6%)	267 (8.2%)	
November	pts	291 (8.4%)	17 (8.6%)	274 (8.4%)	
December	pts	295 (8.5%)	17 (8.6%)	278 (8.5%)	
Age	pts		57.2±15.6	56.3±15.6	0.416
Male	pts	2004 (57.9%)	117 (59.1%)	1887 (57.8%)	0.716
Weight	kg		78.7±17.1	77.6±15.8	0.423
BMI			26.8±5.0	26.8±4.9	0.966
NICU stay	day		15.3±11.7	4.8±5.4	<0.001
Admission					
Primary	pts	746 (21.5%)	47 (23.7%)	699 (21.4%)	
Secondary to 24 h	pts	739 (21.3%)	51 (25.8%)	688 (21.1%)	0.134
Secondary after 24 h	pts	1979 (57.1%)	100 (50.5%)	1879 (57.5%)	
Acute admission	pts	1020 (29.4%)	70 (35.4%)	950 (29.1%)	<0.001
Rehospitalisation	pts	40 (1.22%)	4 (2.0%)	44 (1.3%)	0.331
Diagnoses					
Stroke	pts	1498 (43.2%)	110 (55.6%)	1388 (42.5%)	
Trauma	pts	472 (13.6%)	27 (13.6%)	445 (13.6%)	
Tumour	pts	1078 (31.1%)	33 (16.7%)	1045 (32.0%)	<0.001
Epilepsy	pts	133 (3.8%)	3 (1.5%)	130 (4.0%)	
Hydrocephalus	pts	119 (3.4%)	13 (6.6%)	106 (3.2%)	
Infection	pts	88 (2.5%)	11 (5.6%)	77 (2.4%)	
Others	pts	75 (2.2%)	1 (0.5%)	74 (2.3%)	
Stroke	pts				<0.001
Ischemic	pts	580 (16.7%)	21 (10.6%)	559 (17.1%)	
ICH	pts	471 (13.6%)	49 (24.7%)	422 (12.9%)	
SAH	pts	447 (12.9%)	40 (20.2%)	407 (12.5%)	
TISS on admission			54.7±1.9	56.0±1.7	<0.001
TISS total			270632.8±231533.1	60415.1±92140..3	<0.001
GCS on admission			11.5±3.5	13.1±3.0	<0.001
APACHE II on admission			15.1±5.5	11.8±5.8	<0.001
GOS on NICU discharge			3.1±1.1	3.9±1.1	<0.001
Mortality in NICU	pts	152 (4.4%)	21 (10.6%)	131 (4.0%)	<0.001
Mortality in NICU	day		16.2±10.4	7.5±5.7	<0.001

Table 1 Demographic and clinical data of population of patients with acute brain disease, with or without nosocomial infection *(Continued)*

Parameter	Unit	Total population	NI group	Control group	*p* value
CRP on admission			31.7±45.6	17.5±39.1	<0.001
CRP postoperative			30.0±44.4	14.0±33.0	<0.001
CRP 1 day after operation			59.8±56.9	31.6±39.6	<0.001
CRP highest in NICU stay			228.0±122.5	66.1±80.3	<0.001

BMI body mass index, *NICU* neurointensive care unit, *ICH* intracerebral haemorrhage, *SAH* subarachnoid haemorrhage, *TISS* Therapeutic Intervention Scoring System, *GCS* Glasgow Coma Scale, *APACHE* Acute Physiology and Chronic Health Evaluation, *GOS* Glasgow Outcome Scale, *CRP* C-reactive protein

constantly dry sterile wound covers. Furthermore, the protocol included the hourly monitoring of residual gastric volume.

The protocol included the regular microbiological screening of nose, throat, trachea, skin, urine and rectum from admission and then every three days, as well as every catheter except the peripheral venous for the timely detection of multidrug-resistant bacteria extended spectrum beta-lactamases (ESBL) or methicillin-resistant Staphylococcus aureus (MRSA) or Vancomycin-resistant enterococcus (VRE).

Patients with an infection or with multidrug-resistant bacteria ESBL and MRSA were completely isolated.

3/Facilities

Daily cleaning with disinfection of surfaces including the bed, monitors, and other equipment around the bed, door handles and floors was conducted three times a day. Walls were cleaned once a day for the isolated patients, otherwise once a week. Each room had its own bucket for surfaces and walls. The floors were mopped using a system of two buckets and a cloth, with each room having its own. All cupboards containing materials and medical equipment were cleaned with disinfectant once a week. Waste was sorted and disposed of using specially marked plastic containers and sacks. After the patient was discharged, the bed was completely disinfected. The room was painted with a washable coating once a year.

Antibiotic policy

The protocol included the monitoring of antibiotics in a local computer database. Antibiotic policy was implemented in close cooperation with the antibiotic centre and intended to keep the rational antibiotic policy aim of eliminating the overuse of antibiotics, especially those not used during bacterial pathogeny colonisation. The indications for using prophylactic antibiotics were surgical procedures (operation, external ventricular and lumbar drainage, intracranial sensors), liquorrhoea and aspiration. The protocol required maintaining dose and timing before the operation, perioperative administration for lengthy operations, and the non-prolongation of antibiotic administration after the operation or drainage or implantation of sensors. Empiric antibiotic therapy was to start after samples were taken for microbiological examination to enable their administration according to culture and sensitivity.

Nosocomial infection

Infections were identified according to clinical symptoms such as fever, bacterial pathogens from secretions, liquor, urine, wounds, catheters, haemoculture with a defined microbiology colony count, imaging methods, biochemical and haematological laboratory tests. Nosocomial infections were defined as infections starting after two calendar days in the hospital. We identified nosocomial infections in 198 patients (5.7%). There were more wound infections (2.1%), than respiratory (1.8%), urinary (1.0%), bloodstream (0.7%) and others (0.1%).

Statistical analysis

Parametric *t*-tests or non-parametric Mann-Whitney U tests were used for comparison of continuous variables. Comparison of categorical parameters was carried out using Chi-square or Fisher tests as appropriate. Univariate logistic regression was used for identifying prognostic factors of NI. Factors from univarite analysis with level of significance defined as $p < 0.1$ were used for multivarite regression analysis, factors with p value <0.1 were left in the model. *P*–values of less than 0.05 were considered significant. STATISTICA 13.2 (TIBCO Software Inc., Palo Alto, CA, USA) software was used for statistical analyses. The control group was defined as patients without nosocomial infections.

Results

We did not find any demographic differences such as age, gender, weight or body mass index between the NI group and the control group, as can be seen in Table 1. However, there was a difference in diagnosis, more patients with stroke and hydrocephalus had more NI than those with other diagnoses. According to the scoring system, patients with nosocomial infection upon admission had significantly lower GCS scale and higher APACHE II. Prognostic parameters were also significantly higher in the NI patients group. They stayed in the NICU longer, had higher mortality and worse Glasgow Coma Scale upon discharge.

Table 2 Characteristics of brain operations

Operation	Unit	Total population N=2231	NI group N=151	Control group N=2080	p value
Operation	pts	2231(64.4%)	151(76.3%)	2080 (63.7%)	<0.001
More than 1 operation	pts	214(9.6%)	42(27.8%)	172(8.3%)	<0.001
ASA score			3.8±1.0	3.1±1.1	<0.001
Day of hospitalisation	day		5.5±9.8	7.1±17.1	0.430
Day of NICU			1.6±1.3	1.3±1.1	0.535
Acute operation	pts	905(40.6%)	106(70.2%)	799(38.4%)	<0.001
Reoperation	pts	479(21.5%)	58(38.4%)	421(20.2%)	<0.001
Time of operation	minutes		151.9±108.4	137.7±89.4	0.080
Craniotomy	pts	1361(61.0%)	82(54.3%)	1279(61.5%)	0.080
Craniectomy	pts	363(16.3%)	50(33.1%)	313(15.0%)	<0.001
Trepanation	pts	227(10.2%)	23(15.2%)	204(9.8%)	0.033
Hypophysis	pts	85(3.8%)	0(0.0%)	85(4.1%)	0.011
Shunt	pts	108(4.8%)	12(7.9%)	96(4.6%)	0.066
Others	pts	99(4.4%)	9(6.0%)	90(4.3%)	0.347
Drainage	pts	1678(75.2%)	131(86.8%)	1547(74.4%)	<0.001
Redon	pts	858(38.5%)	49(32.5%)	809(38.9%)	0.001
Time overall	day		2.0±0.9	1.8±1.3	0.395
Gravity drainage	pts	807(36.2%)	75(49.7%)	732(35.2%)	0.029
Time overall	day		3.5±2.1	2.7±2.2	0.004
Lumbar	pts	218(9.8%)	36(23.8%)	182(8.8%)	<0.001
Day overall	day		7.7±5.5	5.1±3.2	<0.001
Ventricular	pts	138(6.2%)	21(13.9%)	117(5.6%)	<0.001
Day overall	day		13.4±9.9	5.9±4.3	<0.001

ASA American Society of Anesthesiologists, *NICU* neurointensive care unit

Table 3 Characteristics of respiratory procedures

Parameter	Unit	Total population N=3646	NI group N=198	Control group N=3266	p value
Airways	pts	710 (20.5%)	112 (56.6%)	598 (18.3%)	<0.001
ETT	pts	327(46.1%)	15(13.4%)	312(52.2%)	
TSK	pts	161(22.7%)	29(25.9%)	132(22.1%)	<0.001
ETT/TST	pts	222(31.3%)	68(60.7%)	154(25.8%)	
ETK time NICU	day		4.2±2.1	2.9±2.2	<0.001
ETK time	day		4.4±2.1	2.9±2.3	<0.001
TSK time NICU	day		14.2±10.2	8.4±7.8	<0.001
TSK time	day		21.8±34.6	21.6±62.2	0.980
TSK type Classic	pts	43(11.2%)	9(9.3%)	34(11.9%)	0.456
TSK NICU made	pts	250(65.3%)	75(77.3%)	175(61.2%)	0.006
Mechanical ventilation	pts	543(15.7%)	87(43.9%)	456(14.0%)	<0.001
Invasive	pts	539(99.3%)	87(100.0%)	452(99.1%)	<0.001
Time	day		14.1±9.9	5.6±5.9	<0.001
Indication					
Neuro	pts	414(76.2%)	54(62.1%)	360(78.9%)	0.161
Respiratory	pts	32(5.9%)	7(8.0%)	25(5.5%)	

ETT endotracheal tube, *TST* tracheostomy tube, *NICU* neurointensive care unit

They were also more expensive economically, and had significantly higher total TISS.

Characteristics of brain operations can be seen in Table 2. Patients who had undergone operations and drainage had significantly higher nosocomial infection. These patients had more endotracheal tubes and tracheostomies, mechanical ventilations (Table 3), artery and central venous catheters (Table 4), urine and gastrointestinal tubes (Table 5).

We confirmed transfusions ($p<0.001$), ulcer prophylaxis ($p<0.001$) and corticoids ($p=0.002$) as further parameters influencing nosocomial infection, but we did not see more

Table 4 Characteristics of vascular catheters

Parameter	Unit	Total population *N*=3464	NI group *N*=198	Control group *N*=3266	*p* value
Artery catheter	pts	907(26.2%)	90(45.5%)	817(25.0%)	<0.001
Time	day		9.5±6.6	7.5±3.7	0.018
Number of artery catheters		923(100.0%)	91(100.0%)	832(100.0%)	
Radialis	pts	873(94.6%)	89(97.8%)	784(94.2%)	0.165
Brachialis	pts	14(1.5%)	0(0.0%)	14(1.7%)	0.211
Femoralis	pts	36(3.9%)	2(2.2%)	34(4.1%)	0.371
Left	pts	598(64.8%)	64(70.3%)	534(64.2%)	0.275
Time in NICU	day		8.27±5.45	4.10±3.36	0.094
Time all	day		8.41±5.40	4.41±3.43	0.377
Made in NICU	pts	216(23.4%)	47(51.6%)	169(20.3%)	<0.001
Made in operation theatre	pts	607(65.8%)	46(50.5%)	561(67.4%)	0.001
Cultivation of catheter	pts	691(74.9%)	74(81.3%)	617(74.2%)	0.157
Positive	pts	113(16.4%)	18(24.3%)	95(15.4%)	0.050
STSP	pts	100(88.5%)	13(72.2%)	87(91.6%)	0.018
Haemoculture cultivation	pts	164(17.8%)	31(34.1%)	133(16.0%)	<0.001
Positive	pts	34(20.7%)	9(29.0%)	25(18.8%)	0.206
STSP	pts	18(52.9%)	3(33.3%)	15(60.0%)	0.169
Central venous catheter	pts	372(10.7%)	64(32.3%)	308(9.4%)	<0.001
Time overall	day		9.9±7.4	7.5±3.7	0.077
Number of venous catheter		378(100%)	66(100%)	312(100%)	
Subclavia	pts	336(88.9%)	60(90.9%)	276(88.5%)	0.308
Jugularis	pts	19(5.0%)	1(1.5%)	18(5.8%)	0.157
Femoralis	pts	16(4.2%)	4(6.1%)	12(3.8%)	0.398
Axilaris	pts	7(1.9%)	1(1.5%)	6(1.9%)	0.836
Right	pts	323(85.4%)	59(89.4%)	264(84.6%)	0.164
Type one-line	pts	75(19.8%)	10(15.2%)	65(20.8%)	
Type two-line	pts	192(50.8%)	39(59.1%)	153(49.0%)	0.214
Type three-line	pts	64(16.9%)	8(12.1%)	56(17.9%)	
Time in NICU	day		8.20±7.31	4.70±4.92	<0.001
Time all	day		11.19±8.70	7.24±5.50	<0.001
Made in NICU	pts	162(42.9%)	41(62.1%)	121(38.8%)	<0.001
Made in operation theatre	pts	14(3.7%)	1(1.5%)	13(4.2%)	0.309
Cultivation of catheter	pts	261(69.0%)	45(68.2%)	216(69.2%)	0.977
Positive	pts	52(19.9%)	16(35.6%)	36(16.7%)	0.004
STSP	pts	40(76.9%)	10(62.5%)	30(83.3%)	0.010
Haemoculture cultivation	pts	72(19.0%)	16(24.2%)	56(17.9%)	0.090
Positive	pts	15(20.8%)	2(12.5%)	13(23.2%)	0.352
STSP	pts	13(86.7%)	2(100.0%)	11(84.6%)	0.551

NICU neurointensive care unit, *STSP* Staphylococcus species

Table 5 Characteristics of urine and gastrointestinal procedures

Parameter	Unit	Total population *N*=3464	NI group *N*=198	Control group *N*=3266	*p* value
Urine catheter	pts	3166(91.4%)	189(95.5%)	2927(89.6%)	0.008
Epicystostomy	pts	6(0.2%)	1(0.5%)	5(0.2%)	0.247
Time	day		15.5±11.6	4.7±5.5	<0.001
Time overall	day		22.6±13.1	12.8±9.7	<0.001
Gastrointestinal tube	pts	904(26.1%)	128(64.6%)	776(23.8%)	<0.001
Nasogastric tube	pts	882(25.5%)	125(63.1%)	757(23.2%)	<0.001
Time	day		15.4±11.2	6.2±6.9	<0.001
Time overall	day		19.6±12.6	10.7±9.4	<0.001

nosocomial infection in patients with diabetes mellitus (*p*=0.203), (Table 6).

ESBL occurred in 1.9% and MRSA in 1.5% of the total population, without differences between NI group patients and the control group (Table 7). We did not have any case of vancomycin-resistant enterococcus.

Antibiotics policy is shown in Table 8. Antibiotic prophylaxis was given to 63% of the total population, mostly (59.2%) in association with operations. In 33.4% of the patients it was only administered in the operating theatre. Prolonged administration in the NICU was associated with more NIs (*p*=0.017). Antibiotic therapy was given to 9.7% of the total population.

We compared patients with NI onset in the NICU (77.3%) with NI present on admission (22.7%), (Table 9). We identified 153 (4.4%; wound 1.0%, respiratory 1.7%, urinary 0.9%, bloodstream 0.6% and other 0.1%) patients with NI onset in the NICU. Patients with NI onset in the NICU stayed in the NICU significantly longer, and were more expensive, but these patients did not have higher mortality. Multivariate logistic regression analysis seeking significant predictors for onset of NI in the NICU can be seen in Table 10. Our results showed that strong predictors on onset of NI in our neurocritical care were accesses such as airways and urine catheters, NICU stay, antibiotic prophylaxis, wound complications and transfusion. This analysis did not find the multidrug-resistant bacteria as ESBL and MRSA to be a predictor of NI.

Discussion

Maintaining nosocomial infection control management is one marker of quality in neurocritical care. Its target is to improve clinical outcomes and decrease costs in the neurocritical care unit. Preventions of nosocomial infections are an important issue in all medical or surgical critical care units, but in neurocritical care they have

Table 6 Further monitored parameters influencing onset of nosocomial infection

Parameter	Unit	Total population *N*=3464	NI group *N*=198	Control group *N*=3266	*p* value
Corticoids	pts	1172(33.8%)	47(23.7%)	1125(34.4%)	0.002
Dexamethasone	pts	944(27.3%)	31(15.7%)	913(28.0)	<0.001
Methylprednisolone	pts	35(1.0%)	5(2.5%)	30(0.9%)	0.028
Hydrocortisone	pts	241(7.0%)	12(6.1%)	229(7.0%)	0.610
Time	day		6.37±8.78	3.58±2.56	<0.001
Transfusions	pts	176(5.1%)	41(20.7%)	135(4.1%)	<0.001
Number			2.46±8.78	2.57±2.56	0.695
Blood loss	ml		523.77±668.07	380.74±478.76	0.019
Haemoglobin			93.35±21.03	115.34±21.62	<0.001
Ulcer prophylaxis	pts	1838(53.1%)	134(67.7%)	1704(52.2%)	<0.001
One medicine	pts	1669(48.2%)	119(60.1%)	1550(47.5%)	0.406
Sucralfate	pts	758(21.9%)	26(13.1%)	732(22.4%)	0.002
H2 antagonist	pts	196(5.7%)	27(13.6%)	169(5.2%)	<0.001
Omeprazole	pts	1062(30.7%)	97(49.0%)	965(29.5%)	<0.001
Diabetes Mellitus	pts	491(14.2%)	22(11.1%)	469(14.4%)	0.203
Op. wound complication	pts	133(3.8%)	35(17.7%)	98(3.0%)	<0.001
Liquorrhoea	pts	81(2.3%)	23(11.6%)	58(1.8%)	<0.001

Table 7 Multidrug-resistant bacteria ESBL and MRSA in NICU

Parameter	Unit	Total population *N*=3464	NI group *N*=198	Control group *N*=3266	*p* value
Multidrug-resistant	pts	116(3.3%)	12(6.1%)	104(3.2%)	0.029
ESBL	pts	67(1.9%)	6(3.0%)	61(1.9%)	0.566
On admission	pts	36(1.0%)	4(2.0%)	32(1.0%)	0.249
Nose	pts	11(0.3%)	1(0.5%)	10(0.3%)	0.986
Throat	pts	21(0.6%)	4(2.0%)	17(0.5%)	0.051
Trachea	pts	15(0.4%)	1(0.5%)	14(0.4%)	0.725
Urine	pts	19(0.5%)	0(0.0%)	19(0.6%)	0.106
Rectum	pts	31(0.9%)	3(1.5%)	28(0.9%)	0.848
Brain	pts	2(0.1%)	1(0.5%)	1(0.0%)	0.039
Others	pts	5(0.1%)	1(0.5%)	4(0.1%)	0.369
MRSA	pts	52(1.5%)	7(3.5%)	45(1.4%)	0.320
On admission	pts	22(0.6%)	0(0.0%)	22(0.7%)	0.015
Nose	pts	27(0.8%)	4(2.0%)	23(0.7%)	0.766
Throat	pts	11(0.3%)	1(0.5%)	10(0.3%)	0.632
Trachea	pts	14(0.4%)	2(1.0%)	12(0.4%)	0.916
Brain	pts	5(0.1%)	1(0.5%)	4(0.1%)	0.652
Haemoculture	pts	1(0.0%)	0(0.0%)	1(0.0%)	0.690
Others	pts	5(0.1%)	0(0.0%)	5(0.2%)	0.354

NICU neurointensive care unit, *ESBL* Extended spectrum beta-lactamase, *MRSA* Methicillin-resistant Staphylococcus aureus

an additional risk as a cause of secondary brain damage, which affects the morbidity and mortality of primary brain diseases [1–5]. As the aim of neurocritical care is to avoid all insults causing secondary brain damage, preventive management of nosocomial infections is a challenge for neurointensivists. Incidence of nosocomial infections can be reduced by keeping a hygienic and epidemiological regime and rational antibiotic policy. Nosocomial infection management demands constant maintenance and stable teamwork while maintaining standard procedures. We present our preventive multimodal nosocomial infection protocol, which we implemented in our NICU. The first phase involves imposing hygienic principles and the antibiotics policy. The second phase, actually keeping to this protocol, is a much more difficult task in our experience, as a vital component for its success is the participation of the whole team, from doctors and nurses to cleaners working in the neurocritical care unit and even visitors. The use of standard procedures and meticulous checks are an important part of the regime.

Here we present the impact of our preventive nosocomial infection management on the incidence of nosocomial infections in all the patients admitted to our NICU with acute brain disease. The results show that our preventive protocol was not sufficient to completely eliminate all nosocomial infections, but it did lead to a relatively low nosocomial infection incidence of 4.4%. We did not observe differences between various seasons of the year, either among primary or secondary admissions, but we did among acute admissions, acute operations and reoperations. Infections were more frequently associated with strokes than other brain diagnoses. There were significantly more infections in airways, mechanical ventilations and catheters, but only airways and urine catheters were strong predictors in multivariate logistic regression analysis. These are still risk factors which remained despite the maintenance of the preventive strategy. Further predictors were confirmed to be the well-known factors of NICU stay, wound complications, antibiotic prophylaxis and transfusion.

The increasing colonisation of multidrug-resistant bacteria ESBL and MRSA is a big problem among critically ill patients and this situation is getting worse. At present, many patients already have these bacteria on admission and this colonization constitutes a risk of nosocomial infections [16–18]. We deal with this by completely isolating these patients using barrier care techniques in order to prevent the transmission of these multidrug-resistant ESBL and MRSA to other, uncolonised patients. This was reflected in our results, which showed that we had newly occurred ESBL in only in 31 (0.9%) patients and MRSA in 30 (0.9%) patients. In this study we did not find that multidrug-resistant bacteria were a predictor of nosocomial infections.

Antibiotics policy, predominantly the overuse of antibiotics, is another big issue in preventive multimodal nosocomial infection protocol. From our results, we see

Table 8 Administration of antibiotics in NICU

Parameter	Unit	Total population *N*=3464	NI group *N*=198	Control group *N*=3266	*p* value
Antibiotic prophylaxis	pts	2183(63.0%)	127(64.1%)	2056(63.0%)	0.736
One prophylaxis	pts	1931(55.7%)	91(46.0%)	1840(56.3%)	<0.001
Operation	pts	2049(59.2%)	116(58.6%)	1933(59.2%)	0.222
Only operation theatre	pts	1157(33.4%)	61(30.8%)	1096(33.6%)	
Operation 1 dose	pts	924(26.7%)	42(21.2%)	882(27.0%)	
Operation 2 doses	pts	191(5.5%)	14(7.1%)	177(5.4%)	0.006
Operation 3 doses	pts	40(1.2%)	4(2.0%)	36(1.1%)	
Operation 4 doses	pts	2(0.1%)	1(0.5%)	1(0.0%)	
NICU	day		4.96±5.69	3.31±2.88	0.017
Others					
Aspiration	pts	51(1.5%)	5(2.5%)	46(1.4%)	0.218
Suspected infection	pts	49(1.0%)	2(1.0%)	47(1.4%)	0.600
Trauma	pts	30(1.4%)	2(1.0%)	28(0.9%)	0.844
Liquorrhoea	pts	46(0.9%)	6(3.0%)	40(1.2%)	0.034
Drainage	pts	35(1.3%)	6(3.0%)	29(0.9%)	0.004
Others	pts	31(1.0%)	4(2.0%)	27(0.8%)	0.090
NICU	Day		7.75±4.61	4.54±3.33	<0.001
Type of antibiotic					
Cefazolin	pts	1733(50.0%)	106(53.5%)	1627(49.8%)	0.242
Amoxicillin clavulanate	pts	362(10.5%)	30(15.2%)	332(10.2%)	0.028
Clindamycin	pts	127(3.7%)	5(2.5%)	122(3.7%)	0.351
Antibiotic therapy	pts	335(9.7%)	169(85.4%)	166(5.1%)	<0.001
One infection	pts	326(9.4%)	161(81.3%)	165(5.1%)	0.019
One antibiotic	pts	220(6.4%)	100(50.5%)	120(3.7%)	0.061
Two antibiotics	pts	78(2.3%)	44(22.2%)	34(1.0%)	
NICU start	pts	224(6.5%)	151(76.3%)	73(2.2%)	<0.001
Empirical therapy	pts	201(5.8%)	101(51.0%)	100(3.1%)	0.929
According to cultivation	pts	189(5.5%)	106(53.5%)	83(2.5%)	0.019
Days of ATB all	day		8.82±6.89	6.09±4.95	<0.001
Type of antibiotic					
Ceftriaxone	pts	34(1.0%)	9(4.5%)	25(0.8%)	0.003
Ceftazidime	pts	6(0.2%)	3(1.5%)	3(0.1%)	0.982
Meropenem	pts	75(2.2%)	48(24.2%)	27(0.8%)	0.008
Penicillin	pts	13(0.4%)	5(2.5%)	8(0.2%)	0.378
Oxacillin	pts	23(0.7%)	17(8.6%)	6(0.2%)	0.020
Ciprofloxacin	day	84(2.4%)	57(28.8%)	27(0.8%)	<0.001
Trimethoprim	pts	17(0.5%)	10(5.1%)	7(0.2%)	0.478
Gentamicin	pts	25(0.7%)	15(7.6%)	10(0.3%)	0.321
Others	pts	71(2.0%)	29(14.6%)	42(1.3%)	0.068

NICU neurointensive care unit, *ATB* antibiotic

that antibiotic prophylaxis is mainly used in association with operations and only 9.7% of the total population received antibiotic therapy. Unindicated use of antibiotics contributes to the emergence and spread of multidrug-resistant bacteria, which are becoming a growing problem in healthcare facilities. Antibiotics should only be given during operations and their administration should not be prolonged in the NICU. During the prophylactic use of

Table 9 Nosocomial infections on admission and onset in the NICU

Parameter	Unit	NI total	NI on admission	NI onset in NICU	*p* value
Number total	pts	198 (100%)	45 (22.7%)	153 (77.3%)	
Age	pts	57.2±15.6	53.7±16.9	58.3±15.1	0.086
Male	pts	117(59.1%)	18(40.0%)	63(41.2%)	<0.001
NICU stay	day	15.3±11.7	6.9±7.2	17.7±11.6	<0.001
Diagnoses					
Stroke	pts	110(55.6%)	13(28.9%)	97(63.4%)	
Trauma	pts	27(13.6%)	3(6.7%)	24(15.7%)	
Tumour	pts	33(16.7%)	13(28.9%)	20(13.1%)	
Epilepsy	pts	3(1.5%)	0(0.0%)	3(2.0%)	<0.001
Hydrocephalus	pts	13(6.6%)	7(15.6%)	6(3.9%)	
Infection	pts	11(5.6%)	9(20.0%)	2(1.3%)	
Others	pts	1(0.5%)	0(0.0%)	1(0.7%)	
TISS on admission		54.7±1.9	56.0±179	54.3±1.8	<0.001
TISS total		270632.8±231533.1	111173.7±231533.1	309492.6±234698.9	<0.001
GCS on admission		11.5±3.5	12.0±3.3	11.3±3.5	0.234
APACHE II on admission		15.1±5.5	13.6±5.4	15.4±5.5	0.099
GOS on NICU discharge		3.1±1.1	3.5±1.2	3.0±1.1	0.015
Mortality in NICU	pts	21(10.6%)	3(6.7%)	18(11.8%)	0.329
Operation	pts	151(76.3%)	37(82.2%)	114(74.5%)	0.285
Airways	pts	112(56.6%)	16(35.6%)	96(62.7%)	0.001
Mechanical ventilation	pts	87(43.9%)	7(15.6%)	80(52.3%)	<0.001
Artery catheter	pts	90(45.5%)	6(13.3%)	84(54.9%)	<0.001
Central venous catheter	pts	64(32.3%)	11(24.4%)	53(34.6%)	0.199
Lumbar drainage	pts	36(18.2%)	5(11.1%)	31(20.3%)	0.162
Ventricular drainage	pts	21(10.6%)	3(6.7%)	18(11.8%)	0.329
Corticoids	pts	47(23.7%)	11(24.4%)	36(23.5%)	0.899
Transfusions	pts	41(20.7%)	5(11.1%)	36(23.5%)	0.071
Ulcer prophylaxis	pts	134(67.7%)	27(60.0%)	107(69.9%)	0.210
Diabetes Mellitus	pts	22(11.1%)	3(6.7%)	19(12.4%)	0.280
Antibiotic prophylaxis	pts	127(64.1%)	23(51.1%)	104(68.0%)	0.038
Antibiotic therapy	pts	169(85.4%)	28(62.2%)	141(92.2%)	<0.001
ESBL	pts	6(3.0%)	1(2.2%)	5(3.3%)	0.719
MRSA	pts	7(3.5%)	1(2.2%)	6(3.9%)	0.587
One infection	pts	189(95.5%)	45(100.0%)	144(94.1%)	
Two infections	pts	8(4.0%)	0(0.0%)	8(5.2%)	0.250
Three infections	pts	1(0.5%)	0(0.0%)	1(0.7%)	
Bloodstream	pts	23(11.6%)	1(2.2%)	22(14.4%)	0.025
Vascular catheter	pts	14(7.1%)	1(2.2%)	13(8.5%)	0.149
Respiratory	pts	63(31.8%)	3(6.7%)	60(39.2%)	< 0.001
VAP	pts	34(17.2%)	1(2.2%)	33(21.6%)	0.002
Urinary	pts	35(17.7%)	5(11.1%)	30(19.6%)	0.189
Urinary catheter	pts	33(16.7%)	5(11.1%)	25(16.3%)	0.255
Wound without operation	pts	2(1.0%)	1(2.2%)	1(0.7%)	0.355
Wound with operation	pts	70(35.4%)	35(77.8%)	35(22.9%)	<0.001

Table 9 Nosocomial infections on admission and onset in the NICU *(Continued)*

Parameter	Unit	NI total	NI on admission	NI onset in NICU	*p* value
Wound complication					
Liquorrhoea	pts	14(7.1%)	7(15.6%)	7(4.6%)	0.012
Dehiscence	pts	11(5.6%)	9(20.0%)	2(1.3%)	<0.001
Fistula	pts	6(3.6%)	3(6.7%)	3(2.0%)	0.105

NICU neurointensive care unit, *TISS* Therapeutic Intervention Scoring System, *GCS* Glasgow Coma Scale, *APACHE* Acute Physiology and Chronic Health Evaluation, *GOS* Glasgow Outcome Scale, *ESBL* Extended spectrum beta-lactamase, *MRSA* Methicillin-resistant Staphylococcus aureus, *VAP* ventilator associated pneumonia

antibiotics it is essential not only to keep to the indication, but also to maintain the time of administration. However, this study confirmed that antibiotic prophylaxis policy is an important task, because antibiotic prophylaxis was found to be a predictor of nosocomial infection in the neurocritical care population. While using antibiotics, it is essential to maintain the correct administration and not use antibiotics during the colonisation of the patient, but only for the infection. Timing, dosage and tissue penetration are important in their administration.

Our microbiological screening was the same for all patients, who can therefore be compared easily. The unified system included nose, throat, trachea, skin, urine and rectum tests from admission, so that we would know what the patient was admitted with, and then regularly every three days. This means that this microbiological screening sometimes fell on the weekend, which at first was difficult to implement in the microbiological department. Regular microbiological screening from admission took place every three days, giving us an overview of the microbiological state of the patient and allowing us to find colonization of multidrug-resistant bacteria [18] and further perform the targeted antibiotic treatment of nosocomial infections.

Although it would be better to have single-patient boxes, the lay-out of four divided rooms provides some of the benefits and enables the isolation of patients with multidrug-resistant bacteria ESBL and MRSA, as it is very important to isolate these patients so that these bacteria do not spread to the rest of the NICU and the other patients. Our results show that over a ten-year period we did not have a large incidence of the multidrug-resistant bacteria ESBL and MRSA, while there was not a single case of VRE. This is in contrast to the Minhas [19] study, where he mentioned 2.5% of VRE in the neurosurgical and neurological intensive care unit.

This study confirmed that accesses are still a risk factor for nosocomial infection. Due to increasing numbers of invasive medical procedures in neurocritical care, local preventive infection control management has an important task. Although preventive multimodal strategy is widely known to reduce nosocomial infection and multidrug resistant bacteria, it is sometimes difficult to maintain. Nonetheless, the results of this study show the importance of this maintenance. We present our 10 year prospective infection control management, which was efficient, as it led to a rate of 4.4% nosocomial infections in acute neurological and neurosurgical care patients. Due to multiple testing, there is a higher probability of family-wise error. On the other hand, the results must be read in context, not every p-value below 0.05 is commented on as a finding.

This study showed prospective infection control management in 3464 neurocritically care patients. Although they all came from a single neurocentre, which is a limitation of this study, there are already many more epidemiologic studies regarding nosocomial infection control and multi-drug resistant bacteria from the medical and surgery intensive care units than from neurocritical care units, whether neurosurgical or neurological, and very few studies concerned with neurological-neurosurgical critical care units [19, 20]. In this area, more studies focus on specific diagnoses [1, 2, 7, 21, 22] than whole neurocritical care populations.

Table 10 Multivariate logistic regression analysis of nosocomial infection onset in NICU

Multivariate analysis				
Nosocomial infections predictors	Odds Ratio	Lower CL 95%	Upper CL 95%	*p* value
NICU stay (per day)	1.14	1.12	1.16	< 0.001
Airways	2.69	1.81	3.99	< 0.001
Urine catheter	2.77	1.00	7.70	0.050
Transfusions	1.79	1.07	2.97	0.025
Wound complications	2.30	1.33	3.97	0.003
Antibiotic prophylaxis	0.50	0.34	0.74	< 0.001

NICU neurointensive care unit, *CL* confidence limit

Conclusions

This study showed that this preventive multimodal nosocomial infection control management was efficient, because it gave low rates of nosocomial infections (4.2%), both ESBL and MRSA in a mere 0.9% of patients each and not a single case of VRE. Strong predictors for the onset of nosocomial infections were accesses such as airways and urine catheters, NICU stay, antibiotic prophylaxis, wound complications and transfusion. This study confirmed the well-known fact that nosocomial infections are associated with worse outcome, higher cost and longer NICU stay.

Abbreviations

APACHE: Acute Physiology and Chronic Health Evaluation; ASA: American Society of Anesthesiologists; ATB: antibiotic; BMI: body mass index; CRP: C-reactive protein; ESBL: Extended spectrum beta-lactamase; ETT: endotracheal tube; GCS: Glasgow Coma Scale; GOS: Glasgow Outcome Scale; ICH: intracerebral haemorrhage; MRSA: Methicillin-resistant Staphylococcus aureus; NI: nosocomial infection; NICU: neurointensive care unit; SAH: subarachnoid haemorrhage; STSP: *Staphylococcus species*; TISS: Therapeutic Intervention Scoring System; TST: tracheostomy tube; VRE: Vancomycin-resistant enterococcus

Acknowledgement

We thank the translator and native English speaker Henry Morgan (BA honours) for the correction of the English text. This study was published as an abstract of the 23rd annual congress of the European Society of Intensive Care Med Experimental 2016;4(S1):426.

Funding

This study was supported by grants from the Scientific Board of the hospital, number VR 140312.

Authors' contributions

VS, OB, DF, ZB, PS: revising it critically for important intellectual content, final approval of the manuscript, read and agreed to be accountable for all aspects of the work in ensuring that questions related to the accuracy or integrity of any part of the work are appropriately investigated and resolved. VS: conception and design, acquisition of data, interpretation of data; drafting the manuscript, OB: statistical analysis, interpretation of data, DF, ZB: acquisition of data, interpretation of data. PS: conception.

Competing interests

The authors declare that they have no competing interests.

Author details

[1]Neurocenter, Neurointensive Care Unit, Regional Hospital, Husova 357/10, Regional Hospital, 46063 Liberec, Czech Republic. [2]Department of Neurosurgery, Military University Hospital and First Medical School, Charles University, Prague, Czech Republic. [3]Department of Clinical microbiology and immunology, Antibiotic Centre, Regional Hospital, Liberec, Czech Republic. [4]Neurocenter, Department of Neurosurgery, Regional Hospital, Liberec, Czech Republic.

References

1. Zygun DA, Zuege DJ, Boiteau PJ, Laupland KB, Henderson EA, Kortbeek JB, Doig CJ. Ventilator-associated pneumonia in severe traumatic brain injury. Neurocrit Care. 2006;5:108–14.
2. Murthy SB, Moradiya Y, Shah J, Merkler AE, Mangat HS, Iadacola C, et al. Nosocomial Infections and Outcomes after Intracerebral Hemorrhage: A Population-Based Study. Neurocrit Care. 2016;25:178–84.
3. Foreman PM, Chua M, Harrigan MR, Fisher WS 3rd, Vyas NA, Lipsky RH, Walters BC, Tubbs RS, Shoja MM, Griessenauer CJ. Association of nosocomial infections with delayed cerebral ischemia in aneurysmal subarachnoid hemorrhage. J Neurosurg. 2016;125:1383–9.
4. Westendorp WF, Nederkoorn PJ, Vermeij JD, Dijkgraaf MG, van de Beek D. Post-stroke infection: a systematic review and meta-analysis. BMC Neurol. 2011;11:110.
5. Bronchard R, Albaladejo P, Brezac G, Geffroy A, Seince PF, Morris W, et al. Early onset pneumonia: risk factors and consequences in head trauma patients. Anesthesiology. 2004;100:234–9.
6. Bassetti M, De Waele JJ, Eggimann P, Garnacho-Montero J, Kahlmeter G, Menichetti F, et al. Preventive and therapeutic strategies in critically ill patients with highly resistant bacteria. Intensive Care Med. 2015;41:776–95.
7. Ohwaki K, Yano E, Nagashima H, Nakagomi T, Tamura A. Impact of infection on length of intensive care unit stay after intracerebral hemorrhage. Neurocrit Care. 2008;8:271–5.
8. Josephson SA, Moheet AM, Gropper MA, Nichols AD, Smith WS. Ventilator-associated pneumonia in a neurologic intensive care unit does not lead to increased mortality. Neurocrit Care. 2010;12:155–8.
9. Chen YY, Chou YC, Chou P. Impact of nosocomial infection on cost of illness and length of stay in intensive care units. Infect Control Hosp Epidemiol. 2005;26:281–7.
10. Higgins TL, McGee WT, Steingrub JS, Rapoport J, Lemeshow S, Teres D. Early indicators of prolonged intensive care unit stay: impact of illness severity, physician staffing, and pre-intensive care unit length of stay. Crit Care Med. 2003;31:45–51.
11. Halperin JJ, Moran S, Prasek D, Richards A, Ruggiero C, Maund C. Reducing Hospital-Acquired Infections Among the Neurologically Critically Ill. Neurocrit Care. 2016;25:170–7.
12. Traa MX, Barboza L, Doron S, Snydman DR, Noubary F, Nasraway SA Jr. Horizontal infection control strategy decreases methicillin-resistant Staphylococcus aureus infection and eliminates bacteremia in a surgical ICU without active surveillance. Crit Care Med. 2014;42:2151–7.
13. Morgan DJ, Rogawski E, Thom KA, Johnson JK, Perencevich EN, Shardell M, et al. Transfer of multidrug-resistant bacteria to healthcare workers' gloves and gowns after patient contact increases with environmental contamination. Crit Care Med. 2012;40:1045–51.
14. Kollef MH, Micek ST. Antimicrobial stewardship programs: mandatory for all ICUs. Crit Care. 2012;16:179.
15. Rimawi RH. Just Say "Stop": Avoiding Prolonged Empiric Antibiotics. Crit Care Med. 2015;43:2675–6.
16. Ziakas PD, Anagnostou T, Mylonakis E. The prevalence and significance of methicillin-resistant Staphylococcus aureus colonization at admission in the general ICU Setting: a meta-analysis of published studies. Crit Care Med. 2014;42:433–44.
17. Ziakas PD, Zacharioudakis IM, Zervou FN, Mylonakis E. Methicillin-resistant Staphylococcus aureus prevention strategies in the ICU: a clinical decision analysis*. Crit Care Med. 2015;43:382–93.
18. Sarikonda KV, Micek ST, Doherty JA, Reichley RM, Warren D, Kollef MH. Methicillin-resistant Staphylococcus aureus nasal colonization is a poor predictor of intensive care unit-acquired methicillin-resistant Staphylococcus aureus infections requiring antibiotic treatment. Crit Care Med. 2010;38: 1991–5.
19. Minhas P, Perl TM, Carroll KC, Shepard JW, Shangraw KA, Fellerman D, et al. Risk factors for positive admission surveillance cultures for methicillin-resistant Staphylococcus aureus and vancomycin-resistant enterococci in a neurocritical care unit. Crit Care Med. 2011;39:2322–9.
20. Dettenkofer M, Ebner W, Els T, Babikir R, Lucking C, Pelz K, et al. Surveillance of nosocomial infections in a neurology intensive care unit. J Neurol. 2001;248:959–64.
21. Divani AA, Hevesi M, Pulivarthi S, Luo X, Souslian F, Suarez JI, et al. Predictors of nosocomial pneumonia in intracerebral hemorrhage patients: a multi-center observational study. Neurocrit Care. 2015;22:234–42.

17

Celiac disease and risk of myasthenia gravis

Sujata P. Thawani[1], Thomas H. Brannagan[2], Benjamin Lebwohl[3,4], Peter H. R. Green[3] and Jonas F. Ludvigsson[4,5,6*]

Abstract

Background: Case reports suggest there may be an association between celiac disease (CD) and myasthenia gravis (MG).

Methods: We identified 29,086 individuals with CD in Sweden from 1969 to 2008. We compared these individuals with 144,480 matched controls. Hazard ratios (HRs) for future MG (identified through ICD codes) were estimated using Cox regression.

Results: During 326,376 person-years of follow-up in CD patients, there were 7 MG cases (21/million person-years) compared to 22 MG cases in controls during 1,642,273 years of follow-up (14/million person-years) corresponding to a HR of 1.48 (95% CI = 0.64–3.41). HRs did not differ when stratifying for age, sex or calendar period. HRs were highest in the first year after follow-up, though insignificant. Individuals with CD were at no increased risk of MG more than 5 years after CD diagnosis (HR = 0.70; 95% CI = 0.16–3.09).

Conclusion: This study found no increased risk of MG in patients with CD.

Keywords: Autoimmune, Celiac, Gluten, Myasthenia gravis

Background

Celiac disease (CD) is an immune mediated chronic disease that affects the proximal small intestine [1]. An increased susceptibility to other immune mediated diseases such as type 1 diabetes (T1D), rheumatoid arthritis, and Sjogren's disease has been well described in association with CD [2]. Myasthenia Gravis (MG) is a rare immune mediated disease involving the neuromuscular junction with a prevalence estimate of 11.71 to 32/100,000, which also includes cases of mild or pure ocular MG [3–6]. CD is common with a 1% prevalence estimate [7–9]. Reports of fatigue and muscle weakness may suggest that MG is also present in CD as described in several case reports [10–12]. CD has also been found to precede a documented diagnosis of MG in the population based Swedish Patient Register with a 1.7 odds ratio of developing MG after a diagnosis of CD, [13] This analysis did however utilize hospital-based CD diagnoses with the subsequent risk of overestimating the association between CD and MG. In Sweden, like in the United States, many patients with CD are never admitted to the hospital [14].

Serological markers associated with MG have been reported in CD cases [15]. A retrospective analysis of 23 acetylcholine receptor (AChR) antibody patients, revealed one patient with both IgA-endomysial and IgA tissue transglutaminase antibodies. This single patient had a subsequent endoscopic evaluation that was consistent with CD [15]. In another series, one out of 70 CD patients and one out of ten control patients with systemic lupus erythromatosus had elevated muscle AChR antibody levels [16]. In addition, human leukocyte antigen (HLA) types B8 and DR3 appear to be associated with both MG and CD suggesting a shared immune origin [17, 18].

The objective of our study was to examine the relative risk and absolute risk of developing MG in a nationwide population-based sample of patients with biopsy-verified CD.

Methods

We used nationwide biopsy data from Sweden's 28 pathology departments to identify CD cases. These data were

* Correspondence: jonasludvigsson@yahoo.com
[4]Department Medical Epidemiology and Biostatistics, Karolinska Institutet, 171 77 Stockholm, Sweden
[5]Department of Pediatrics, Örebro University Hospital, Örebro University, Örebro, Sweden
Full list of author information is available at the end of the article

then linked to the Swedish Patient Register containing both inpatient and hospital-based outpatient data to ascertain the risk of MG [19].

Study participants

Between October 2006 and February 2008 we collected data from small intestinal biopsy reports from all 28 Swedish pathology departments. Biopsies had been conducted between 1969 and 2008 (Table 1). We obtained data on date of biopsy, topography (duodenum or jejunum), morphology codes consistent with villous atrophy (VA) which was used as our definition for CD) and personal identity number [20]. For each patient with CD, the government agency Statistics Sweden identified up to five reference individuals from the Total Population Register. Matching criteria were age, sex, calendar year and county. We then removed individuals with data irregularities, and thereafter had data on 29,096 individuals with CD and 144,520 reference individuals (identical to the cohort used in our earlier paper on CD and mortality) [21].

Celiac disease

CD was defined as VA (Marsh stage 3) according to biopsy report [22]. Having a positive CD serologic test result was not a prerequisite for CD diagnosis although 88% of individuals in a random subset of individuals with VA and available data on serology had positive CD serology at the time of biopsy [23]. Additional details on the data collection has been published elsewhere [23].

Table 1 Characteristics of participants presented as n (%)

Characteristics	Reference individuals	Celiac disease
Total	144,480	29,086
Age at study entry (years)		
0–19	58,851 (40.7)	11,802 (40.6)
20–39	26,378 (18.3)	5311 (18.3)
40–59	32,237 (22.3)	6471 (22.2)
60-	27,014 (18.7)	5502 (18.9)
Sex		
Female	89,523 (62.0)	17,999 (61.9)
Male	54,957 (28.0)	11,087 (38.1)
Calendar Period		
-1989	20,371 (14.1)	4104 (14.1)
1990–1999	59,860 (41.4)	12,055 (41.4)
2000-	64,249 (44.5)	12,947 (44.4)
Nordic	136,242 (94.3)	28,129 (96.7)
Type 1 diabetes	596 (0.4)	956 (3.3)
Autoimmune thyroid diseases	2502 (1.7)	1435 (4.9)

Autoimmune thyroid disease, for definitions

On average, three tissue specimens were examined for each biopsy report.

Myasthenia gravis (MG)

MG was defined according to relevant international classification of disease (ICD) codes in the Swedish National Patient Register: ICD7: 744.00; ICD8: 733.00; ICD9: 358A; ICD10: G70.0. The Patient Register started in 1964 and contains diagnoses from ICD-7 through ICD-10. The Patient Register included inpatient care but since 2001, hospital-based outpatient care has also been included. We did not have access to data on acetylcholine receptor antibody results, but National Patient Register-based MG diagnosis has been validated against the Stockholm MG Cohort. This analysis found that 147/177 diagnoses in the Patient Register could be confirmed against the Stockholm MG Cohort and the positive predictive value of MG is 83% [13].

Individuals with MG before CD diagnosis and corresponding controls based on dates were excluded from all prospective analyses ($n = 8$ and $n = 22$ respectively). We then excluded another 2 CD patients and 2 controls due to data irregularities (uncertainties regarding date of death) and another 18 reference individuals since their index individual with CD had been excluded and analyses were performed retaining strata. Hence, there remained 29,086 individuals with CD and 144,480 matched controls.

Other covariates

Data on the following potential confounding factors were collected from the government agency *Statistics Sweden*: country of birth (Nordic vs. not Nordic), educational level (≤9 years of primary school, 2 years of high school, 3–4 years of high school, college/university) and socioeconomic status according to six categories (according to the European Socioeconomic Classification, ESeC: levels 1, 2, 3 + 6, 7, 8, and 9) [24]. Missing data on education and socioeconomic status (4 and 31% respectively) were fitted into separate categories for the statistics. We also identified individuals with T1D and autoimmune thyroid disease defined according to relevant ICD codes.

Statistical analyses

We estimated hazard ratios (HR) for MG using Cox regression. We used an internal stratification system and each stratum (consisting of one CD patient and up to five controls) was analyzed separately and a summary HR was calculated. Through visual inspection of log-minus-log curves we found that the proportional hazard assumption was valid. The attributable risk percent (the proportion of MG in patients with CD that could be explained by the underlying CD) was estimated by 1–1/HR.

Table 2 Risk of myasthenia gravis in patients with celiac disease according to follow-up

Follow-up	HR; 95% CI	*P*-value	Observed vs. Expected	Person-years	Incidence rate[a]	Excess risk[a]	Attributable percentage
All	1.48; 0.64–3.41	0.356	7 vs 5	326,376	21	7	32
< 1 year	8.09; 0.70–94.04	0.095	1 vs 0	28,773	35	30	88
1–5 years	2.19 0.69–6.91	0.182	4 vs 2	108,012	37	20	54
> 5 years	0.70; 0.16–3.09	0.640	2 vs 3	189,591	10	−4	−42

Beyond 1 year of follow-up
[a]Myasthenia gravis cases per 1,000,000 person-years in patients with celiac disease

Follow-up started at first biopsy with CD diagnosis and at the same time in matched controls. Follow-up ended when one of the following occurred: death, emigration, first MG diagnosis, or end of study (December 31, 2009).

In a priori analyses, we examined the time-dependent risk of MG (time since CD diagnosis: < 1 year, 1–4.99 years; and > 5 years). We also performed analyses stratified by age at diagnosis of CD (≤19, 20–39, 40–59 and ≥60 years), sex, and calendar period (– 1989, 1990–99, 2000-). In a separate analysis we adjusted for country of birth, education, socioeconomic status, T1D, and autoimmune thyroid disease.

In order to examine the temporal association between CD and MG, we also calculated the odds ratios (ORs) for having a diagnosis of MG prior to the first biopsy for CD. For this analysis, we used conditional logistic regression comparing each individual with CD with his or her matched control.

A post-hoc power analysis found that we had an 80% power at a significance level of 0.05 to detect a HR of 3.1 for MG.

We used SPSS 22 to calculate statistics. *P*-values < 0.05 were considered statistically significant.

Ethics

This study was approved by the Regional Ethical Review Board in Stockholm (2006/633–31/4). Because this was a register-based study, none of the participants was contacted and all data were anonymized prior to data analysis [25].

Results

From our prior paper

The median age of CD diagnosis was 30 years (range 0–95 years). Median year of diagnosis and first biopsy was 1998 (range 1969–2008). Median age at first diagnosis with MG was 44 years in CD patients and 48 years in controls. Most study participants were women (Table 1), and were diagnosed in the 1990s or later.

Risk of future MG in patients with CD

During 326,376 person-years of follow-up in CD patients, there were seven cases of MG (21 per million person-years). This compares with 22 MG cases in controls during 1,642,273 person-years of follow-up (14 per million person-years). This corresponded to a HR of 1.48 (95% CI = 0.64–3.41).

Adjusting for socioeconomic status, education, and country of birth, had a marginal influence on the HR

Table 3 Risk of MG myasthenia gravis in patients with celiac disease. Stratified analyses

Follow-up	HR; 95% CI	*P*-value	Observed vs. Expected	Person-years	Person-years Incidence rate[a]	Excess risk[a]	Attributable percentage
Age (yrs)							
< 20	2.60; 0.50–13.60	0.257	2 vs 1	147,218	14	8	62
20–39	1.99; 0.40–9.92	0.402	2 vs 1	60,204	33	16	50
40–59	0.58; 0.07–4.58	0.602	1 vs 2	75,119	13	−10	−74
> =60	1.55; 0.33–7.37	0.581	2 vs 1	43,835	46	16	36
Sex							
Female	2.28; 0.82–6.37	0.166	5 vs 2	204,000	24	14	56
Male	0.79; 0.18–3.52	0.760	2 vs 3	122,376	16	−4	−26
Calendar period							
-1989	1.33; 0.27–6.48	0.726	1 vs 1	85,893	12	3	25
1990–99	1.16; 0.26–5.29	0.848	2 vs 2	161,814	12	2	14
2000-	2.10; 0.57–7.66	0.264	3 vs 1	78,669	38	20	52

[a]Myasthenia gravis cases per 1,000,000 person-years in patients with celiac disease

(HR = 1.68; 95% CI = 0.71–3.94). Excluding the first year of follow-up, the HR decreased somewhat (HR = 1.29; 5% CI = 0.53–3.14; Table 2). The lower risk estimate beyond the first year signaled a higher risk in the immediate year after CD diagnosis, although the HR in the first year failed to attain statistical significance (HR = 8.09; 95% CI = 0.70–94.04; $p = 0.095$).

The difference in risk estimates between men and women was not statistically significant (Table 3)(p for interaction = 0.290).There was also no difference in risk estimates according to age groups (p for interaction = 0.629) or calendar period (p for interaction = 0.863).

Prior MG in patients with CD

Conditional logistic regression found no increased risk for earlier MG in CD (OR = 1.70; 95% CI = 0.79–3.66).

Discussion

This nationwide population-based study found no association between CD and future MG. The high HR in the first year of follow-up (8.09) compared to the HR after more than 5 years (0.70) suggests surveillance bias just after MG diagnosis.

Recently, Fang et al. also using Swedish data, examined the autoimmune spectrum in MG and found an OR of 1.7 for earlier CD in MG [13]. The authors however ascertained CD using the Patient Register. Until the year 2000, the Patient Register only contained inpatient data. CD rarely requires hospital admission and is primarily managed and diagnosed in the outpatient setting [14, 26]. Therefore, this earlier study may have identified a larger proportion of cases with severe CD or severe comorbidities, thereby pushing the risk estimate upwards.

Previous case reports and retrospective analyses of the association between CD and MG have examined serological markers shared between patients with both CD and MG [12, 15, 16]. Although serological markers could not be specifically examined in this analysis, validation studies of CD diagnoses with serological studies was performed in a subset of CD patients undergoing small intestinal biopsy, yielding a positive predictive value of 95% [23]. The diagnosis of MG has also been previously validated in the Patient Register [13, 27]. In addition to its population-based setting, another strength of this analysis is that the CD diagnoses were based on small intestinal biopsy reports [23], which was the gold standard for diagnosis of CD in Sweden throughout the study period.

Although our study used nationwide population based data, this analysis lacked statistical power. MG is rare in the general population with prevalence estimates ranging from 15 to 179 cases per million [7, 8]. The diagnosis of MG was determined by diagnosis codes in this study, and should be corroborated by electrophysiological and serum studies. This information was not available in the Patient Register thus some cases may have been missed. Some data suggest that, among patients with CD, adherence to a gluten free diet is associated with protection against other autoimmune diseases [28, 29]. However, we did not have information on dietary adherence amongst participants diagnosed with CD to assess if this had any effect on a later diagnosis of MG.

Conclusions

In conclusion, in this population-based cohort study we did not demonstrate an increased risk of MG in CD. This could partly be due to insufficient power since our power analysis suggested that we could only demonstrate a 3.1-fold increased risk of MG in CD. However, our study shows that the absolute risk of MG is low in CD and we therefore discourage routine testing for acetylcholine receptor (AChR) antibodies in CD.

Abbreviations

CD: Celiac disease; CI: Confidence Interval; HR: Hazard ratio; ICD: International Classification of Disease (codes; MG: Myasthenia Gravis; OR: Odds ratio; VA: Villous atrophy

Acknowledgements

Not applicable.

Funding

BL was supported by The National Center for Advancing Translational Sciences, National Institutes of Health (UL1 TR000040).

JFL was supported by grants from the Swedish Society of Medicine and the Swedish Research Council.

Authors' contributions

SPT contributed to analysis, interpretation of the data, study design, and drafting the manuscript. THB, BL, PHRG, and JFL contributed to study concept and design, interpretation of data and revision of manuscript. All authors read and approved the final version of the manuscript submitted. We warrant that the article is the Authors' original work. On behalf of all Co-Authors, the corresponding Author shall bear full responsibility for the submission.

Competing interests

The authors declare that they have no competing interests.

Author details

[1]Department of Neurology, New York University School of Medicine, New York, NY, USA. [2]Peripheral Neuropathy Center, Neurological Institute, Columbia University, College of Physicians and Surgeons, New York, NY, USA.

[3]Celiac Disease Center, Department of Medicine, Columbia University College of Physicians and Surgeons, New York, NY, USA. [4]Department Medical Epidemiology and Biostatistics, Karolinska Institutet, 171 77 Stockholm, Sweden. [5]Department of Pediatrics, Örebro University Hospital, Örebro University, Örebro, Sweden. [6]Division of Epidemiology and Public Health, School of Medicine, University of Nottingham, Nottingham, UK.

References

1. Ludvigsson JF, Green PH. Clinical management of coeliac disease. J Intern Med. 2011;269(6):560–71.
2. Green PH, Jabri B. Celiac disease. Annu Rev Med. 2006;57:207–21.
3. Breiner A, Widdifield J, Katzberg HD, Barnett C, Bril V, Tu K. Epidemiology of myasthenia gravis in Ontario, Canada. Neuromuscul Disord. 2016;26(1):41-6. https://doi.org/10.1016/j.nmd.2015.10.009. Epub 2015 Oct 27.
4. Gattellari M, Goumas C, Worthington JM. A national epidemiological study of myasthenia gravis in Australia. Eur J Neurol. 2012;19(11):1413–20.
5. Lai CH, Tseng HF. Nationwide population-based epidemiological study of myasthenia gravis in Taiwan. Neuroepidemiology. 2010;35(1):66–71.
6. Andersen JB, Engeland A, Owe JF, Gilhus NE. Myasthenia gravis requiring pyridostigmine treatment in a national population cohort. Eur J Neurol. 2010;17(12):1445–50.
7. Somnier FE, Keiding N, Paulson OB. Epidemiology of myasthenia gravis in Denmark. A longitudinal and comprehensive population survey. Arch Neurol. 1991;48(7):733–9.
8. Carr AS, Cardwell CR, McCarron PO, McConville J. A systematic review of population based epidemiological studies in myasthenia gravis. BMC Neurol. 2010;10:46.
9. Dube C, Rostom A, Sy R, Cranney A, Saloojee N, Garritty C, et al. The prevalence of celiac disease in average-risk and at-risk western European populations: a systematic review. Gastroenterology 2005;128(4 Suppl 1):S57–67.
10. Edwards JH. Letter: Gluten and myasthenia gravis. Lancet. 1975;2(7923):41.
11. Kuzin MI, Vinogradova MA, Smakov GM. Syndrome of inadequate digestion of fats in patients with myasthenia before and after thymectomy. Klin Med (Mosk). 1971;49(10):73–9.
12. Csaplar M, Juhasz M, Muzes G, Jakab C, Aranyi Z, Rozsa C, et al. Association of coeliac disease and myasthenia gravis. Orv Hetil. 2006;147(18):841–4.
13. Fang F, Sveinsson O, Thormar G, Granqvist M, Askling J, Lundberg IE, et al. The autoimmune spectrum of myasthenia gravis: a Swedish population-based study. J Intern Med. 2015;277(5):594–604.
14. Rampertab SD, Pooran N, Brar P, Singh P, Green PH. Trends in the presentation of celiac disease. Am J Med. 2006;119(4):355 e9–14.
15. Freeman HJ, Gillett HR, Gillett PM, Oger J. Adult celiac disease with acetylcholine receptor antibody positive myasthenia gravis. World J Gastroenterol. 2009;15(38): 4741–4.
16. Briani C, Doria A, Ruggero S, Toffanin E, Luca M, Albergoni MP, et al. Antibodies to muscle and ganglionic acetylcholine receptors (AchR) in celiac disease. Autoimmunity. 2008;41(1):100–4.
17. Louka AS, Sollid LM. HLA in coeliac disease: unravelling the complex genetics of a complex disorder. Tissue Antigens. 2003;61(2):105–17.
18. Price P, Witt C, Allcock R, Sayer D, Garlepp M, Kok CC, et al. The genetic basis for the association of the 8.1 ancestral haplotype (A1, B8, DR3) with multiple immunopathological diseases. Immunol Rev. 1999;167:257–74.
19. Ludvigsson JF, Andersson E, Ekbom A, Feychting M, Kim JL, Reuterwall C, et al. External review and validation of the Swedish national inpatient register. BMC Public Health. 2011;11:450.
20. Ludvigsson JF, Otterblad-Olausson P, Pettersson BU, Ekbom A. The Swedish personal identity number: possibilities and pitfalls in healthcare and medical research. Eur J Epidemiol. 2009;24(11):659–67.
21. Ludvigsson JF, Montgomery SM, Ekbom A, Brandt L, Granath F. Small-intestinal histopathology and mortality risk in celiac disease. JAMA. 2009;302(11):1171–8.
22. Marsh MN. Gluten, major histocompatibility complex, and the small intestine. A molecular and immunobiologic approach to the spectrum of gluten sensitivity ('celiac sprue'). Gastroenterology. 1992;102(1):330–54.
23. Ludvigsson JF, Brandt L, Montgomery SM, Granath F, Ekbom A. Validation study of villous atrophy and small intestinal inflammation in Swedish biopsy registers. BMC Gastroenterol. 2009;9:19.
24. Olen O, Bihagen E, Rasmussen F, Ludvigsson JF. Socioeconomic position and education in patients with coeliac disease. Dig Liver Dis. 2012;44(6):471–6.
25. Ludvigsson JF, Haberg SE, Knudsen GP, Lafolie P, Zoega H, Sarkkola C, et al. Ethical aspects of registry-based research in the Nordic countries. Clin Epidemiol. 2015;7:491–508.
26. Violato M, Gray A, Papanicolas I, Ouellet M. Resource use and costs associated with coeliac disease before and after diagnosis in 3,646 cases: results of a UK primary care database analysis. PLoS One. 2012;7(7):e41308.
27. Kalb B, Matell G, Pirskanen R, Lambe M. Epidemiology of myasthenia gravis: a population-based study in Stockholm, Sweden. Neuroepidemiology. 2002; 21(5):221–5.
28. Cosnes J, Cellier C, Viola S, Colombel JF, Michaud L, Sarles J, et al. Incidence of autoimmune diseases in celiac disease: protective effect of the gluten-free diet. Clin Gastroenterol Hepatol. 2008;6(7):753–8.
29. Mones RL. Incidence of autoimmune diseases in celiac disease: protective effect of the gluten-free diet. J Pediatr Gastroenterol Nutr. 2009;48(5):645–6.

18

Characteristics of a newly diagnosed Polish cohort of patients with neurological manifestations of Wilson disease evaluated with the Unified Wilson's Disease Rating Scale

Anna Członkowska[1,2*], Tomasz Litwin[1], Karolina Dzieżyc[1], Michal Karliński[1], Johan Bring[3] and Carl Bjartmar[4]

Abstract

Background: Wilson disease is a rare genetic disorder in which impaired copper excretion results in toxic copper levels and tissue damage. Manifestations are primarily hepatic and/or neuropsychiatric, with a variety of neurological phenotypes. The aim of this study was to characterize neurological signs of Wilson disease in newly diagnosed patients and to determine whether they correlated with disability, liver function, and copper metabolism.

Methods: Fifty-three treatment-naïve patients recently diagnosed with Wilson disease who exhibited neurological symptoms were included. Neurological manifestations were characterized by examination in terms of symptom type and degree of neurological impairment (Unified Wilson's Disease Rating Scale [UWDRS] Part III) and correlated with degree of disability (UWDRS Part II), abnormalities in copper parameters and hepatic status.

Results: Most patients (62.3%) exhibited tremor and ataxia, whereas 15.1% were dystonic, and 11.3% had parkinsonism. Discrete or unclassified signs only were observed in 11.3% of patients. A good correlation between disability (UWDRS Part II) and neurological impairment (UWDRS Part III) was observed (Pearson $r = 0.84$). However, there was a lack of correlation when either disability or neurological impairment were analyzed with copper parameters or liver impairment.

Conclusions: The predominant neurological manifestations in this cohort of newly diagnosed Wilson disease patients were ataxia and tremor. Neurological impairment measured was highly correlated with the level of disability. However, hepatic manifestations of Wilson disease and copper levels did not appear to be correlated with neurological status and disability. These results highlight the challenges faced when assessing Wilson disease with its highly variable symptomatology.

Keywords: Wilson disease, Disability evaluation, Neurological manifestations, Unified Wilson's Disease Rating Scale (UWDRS)

* Correspondence: czlonkow@ipin.edu.pl
[1]2nd Department of Neurology, Institute of Psychiatry and Neurology, 02 957 Warsaw, Poland
[2]Department of Experimental and Clinical Pharmacology, Medical University of Warsaw, Warsaw, Poland
Full list of author information is available at the end of the article

Background

Wilson disease (WD) is a rare autosomal recessive genetic disorder caused by mutations in the *ATP7B* gene located on chromosome 13 [1]. ATP7B is a P-type adenosine triphosphatase (ATPase) expressed mainly in hepatocytes that is involved in the transmembrane transport of copper. Decreased function of the ATP7B protein reduces the incorporation of copper into ceruloplasmin and leads to copper accumulation in the liver, brain, and other organs [2, 3].

It has previously been estimated that approximately 1 in 30,000 people worldwide have WD, with a heterozygote carrier frequency of 1 in 90. However, results from biochemical and genetic prevalence studies suggest that WD may be more common than previously estimated and the disease may be unrecognized in a substantial number of individuals [4, 5].

Typical presentation of WD is in adolescence to early adulthood, but it may occur at any age [6, 7]. Clinical presentation can vary widely in terms of type and severity, but the key features are various degrees of liver disease, neuropsychiatric manifestations and Kayser-Fleischer rings [2, 8, 9]. Although the initial signs and symptoms of WD can be classed as primarily hepatic (40%), neurological (40%), and psychiatric or asymptomatic (20%), it should be noted that patients often develop combined hepatic and neurological, or psychiatric disease [8, 9]. Untreated WD is universally fatal, commonly due to liver disease, or progressive neurological deterioration although the prognosis has improved due to available treatments [6, 9].

The neurological abnormalities of WD show marked variation in both type of presentation and severity, but can generally be classified into syndrome types based on predominant symptoms, such as tremor and ataxia, bradykinesia (parkinsonism-like), and dystonia. In many cases, classification of neurological features is challenging as patients can have various signs and more than one abnormality, each with a different level of severity [8, 9].

The Unified Wilson's Disease Rating Scale (UWDRS) was developed as a tool for the comprehensive evaluation of neurological signs and symptoms in patients with WD. The scale is based on partly modified elements from well-established and validated scales assessing neurological status, such as the Barthel index, the Unified Parkinson's Disease Rating Scale (UPDRS), and the Unified Huntington's Disease Rating Scale (UHDRS) [8, 10]. Part I of UWDRS concerns consciousness, while Part II evaluates disability. UWDRS Part III involves a neurological examination and uses clinical rating scales e.g., for tremor and cerebellar disorders to measure neurological signs [8, 10].

Data regarding correlation of the neurological phenotype with disability, hepatic status, as well as copper metabolism, are sparse [11–13]. In the current study, we analyzed a cohort of newly diagnosed and previously untreated WD patients with neurological symptoms who were consecutively admitted to our center. The aim was to characterize the neurological manifestations in terms of symptom type and degree of neurological impairment (UWDRS Part III) and correlate these features with degree of disability (UWDRS Part II), abnormalities in copper metabolism, and hepatic status.

Methods

The study was conducted at a single center, the 2nd Department of Neurology, Institute of Psychiatry and Neurology, Warsaw, Poland. Treatment naïve patients were consecutively enrolled as they were seen at the hospital over a period from 2005 to 2014. Neurologically asymptomatic patients with WD who presented with hepatic, psychiatric or preclinical forms of the disease, or patients previously receiving any WD therapy, were excluded. All patients were diagnosed with WD based on a combination of abnormal copper results, presence of a Kayser-Fleisher ring and genetic testing results, performed in our center, as previously described [14, 15]. Ethics committee approval was obtained from the local bioethics committee and all patients provided written informed consent prior to participation.

Neurological assessments

The main outcome variable of the study was the UWDRS Parts II and III. The UWDRS consists of three parts including consciousness (Part I, single item), activities of daily living (based on the Barthel Scale) as reported by the patient or their proxy and verified by the neurologist if possible (Part II, items 2–11), and a detailed neurological examination (Part III, items 12–34) [8, 10].

In addition, patients were further classified based on the predominant neurological syndrome type at diagnosis by experienced neurologists using best clinical judgement and based on classifications described by Marsden [16] and Oder et al. [17], i.e., tremor (including patients with predominant tremor and ataxia), parkinsonism (including rigidity, rest tremor and hypokinesia), dystonia (including choreoathetosis), or discrete neurological/unclassified signs not encompassed by these classifications, such as slight dysarthria, drooling, hypomimia, occasional mild tremor etc.

Copper measurements and other assessments

Serum ceruloplasmin was measured using the improved colorimetric enzymatic assay developed by Ravin in 1961 [18]. Total serum copper concentration and 24-h urinary copper excretion were measured by flame atomic absorption spectrometry. The levels of free copper, measured as non-ceruloplasmin bound copper (NCC), were calculated according to previously described formula [19–21].

Basic laboratory liver tests (i.e., enzymatic, synthetic, and bilirubin) were performed in the hospital laboratory using standard methods.

Statistical analysis

Categorical variables are presented as a number of valid observations and proportions calculated with exclusion of unknown values from the denominator. Continuous variables are presented as a mean with standard deviation (SD).

Pearson's correlation coefficient (r) was used to express correlations between UWDRS Part II score and UWDRS Part III score in the whole cohort and according to predominant clinical manifestation. Additionally, similar correlations were calculated between UWDRS score and baseline copper levels, hepatic parameters, age at onset of symptoms and age at the diagnosis. Calculations were carried out using STATISTICA 12.0 software package (Stat Soft Inc., Tulsa, USA, 2013). P-values < 0.05 were considered statistically significant.

Results

A total of 53 newly diagnosed WD patients (30 males, 23 females) with neurological manifestations were included in the analysis (Table 1). Most patients had liver test results that were in the normal range or only slightly/moderately elevated as shown in Table 1. In the majority of patients, compared with the normal range, ceruloplasmin, and total serum copper concentrations were low (mean 13.7 mg/dL and 62.0 mg/dL, respectively), whilst urinary copper excretion was elevated (mean 128 μg/dL/24 h) (Table 1). Mean NCC levels were elevated (3.4 μmol/L; SD 2.0, range 0.6 to 10.9).

The most common individual neurological signs were dysarthria (73.6%), arms postural tremor (69.8–71.7%), impaired finger tapping (66.0%), impaired posture (66.0%), and reduced facial expression (66.0%) (Table 2). The syndrome of highest prevalence was ataxia/tremor (62.3%) followed by dystonia (15.1%) and parkinsonism (11.3%). A small proportion of patients (11.3%) had only discrete signs or were considered as unclassified.

Mean Part II UWDRS score was 5.0 (SD 8.5, range 0 to 37) and mean Part III UWDRS score was 24.4 (SD 22. 3, range 1 to 87) (Table 3). Overall individual scores in UWDRS Part III (neurological signs) were found to strongly correlate with Part II individual scores (disease-related disability; $r = 0.84$, $p < 0.001$) (Fig. 1, Table 3). In addition, there was a strong correlation between Part III and Part II scores in subgroups according to the predominant neurological syndrome, ataxia/tremor, dystonia, or parkinsonism (Table 3).

When we evaluated correlations with laboratory parameters, there was no significant correlation between UWDRS Part II scores or UWDRS Part III scores and

Table 1 Characteristics and laboratory values at baseline

	n	Study population Mean (SD) unless otherwise stated	Normal range
Female gender (*n* [%])	53	23 (43.4)	
Age (years)	53	36.2 (11.3)	
Age at onset (years)	52	30.4 (12.5)	
Onset to diagnosis (years)	52	5.6 (6.6)	
Presence of Kayser-Fleischer ring (*n* [%])	53	44 (83.0)	
Ceruloplasmin (mg/dL)	53	13.7 (6.3)	25–45
Serum copper (μg/dL)	53	62.0 (17.8)	70–140
Urinary copper (μg/24 h)	53	128 (142)	< 50
Non-ceruloplasmin-bound copper (μmol/L)	53	3.4 (2.0)	a
Alanine aminotransferase (IU/L)	53	38 (43)	< 41
Aspartate aminotransferase (IU/L)	53	36 (21)	< 40
Gamma-glutamyltransferase (IU/L)	52	70 (57)	< 42
International normalized ratio	52	1.3 (0.2)	0.8–1.2
Bilirubin (mg/dL)	53	1.1 (0.6)	< 1
Serum albumin (g/dL)	47	4.0 (0.7)	3.5–5.0

SD standard deviation

[a]Non-ceruloplasmin-bound copper (NCC) is not commonly used in clinical practice in healthy individuals as approximately 80% have negative values. NCC has been reported to be above 4 μmol/L in most patients with Wilson disease [21]

Table 2 Most common neurological signs and symptoms (present in > 50% of patients)

Symptom	*n*	Any abnormality, %	Mean score in UWDRS item
Speech impairment (dysarthria)	53	73.6	1.17
Postural tremor in left arm	53	71.7	1.11
Postural tremor in right arm	53	69.8	1.23
Impaired left finger tapping	53	66.0	1.11
Impaired right finger tapping	53	66.0	1.13
Impaired posture	53	66.0	0.66
Reduced facial expression (hypomimia)	50	66.0	1.02
Impaired handwriting	51	56.9	1.24
Impaired rapid alternating movements of left hand	53	54.7	0.92
Impaired rapid alternating movements of right hand	53	50.9	0.89

UWDRS United Wilson's Disease Rating Scale

Table 3 Correlations between UWDRS Part II and UWDRS Part III scores according to predominant clinical manifestation of Wilson disease

Predominant clinical manifestation	UWDRS II score Mean (SD) [range]	UWDRS III score Mean (SD) [range]	Pearson's correlation coefficient, *r* (*p*-value)
Overall ($n = 53$)	5.0 (8.5) [0–37]	24.4 (22.3) [1–87]	0.84 ($p < 0.001$)
Ataxia/tremor ($n = 33$)	3.8 (6.4) [0–27]	23.5 (21.1) [1–79]	0.81 ($p < 0.001$)
Dystonia ($n = 8$)	11.1 (12.7) [1–37]	36.6 (18.5) [15–67]	0.90 ($p = 0.002$)
Parkinsonism ($n = 6$)	7.8 (12.6) [0–31]	34.0 (30.8) [6–87]	0.97 ($p = 0.001$)
Discrete signs or unclassified ($n = 6$)	0.3 (0.8) [0–2]	3.7 (3.7) [0–11]	0.04 ($p = 0.934$)

SD standard deviation, *UWDRS* United Wilson's Disease Rating Scale

the serum levels of ceruloplasmin, copper, NCC, or any of the liver tests (Additional file 1: Table S1). However, UWDRS Part III scores showed a weak but statistically significant positive correlation with age at onset of symptoms ($r = 0.34$, $p = 0.014$) and age at diagnosis ($r = 0.28$, $p = 0.039$) (Additional file 1: Table S1).

Discussion

In our study of 53 newly diagnosed and previously untreated patients with WD, most (62.3%) were classified as having primary ataxia/tremor syndrome, which generally concurs with the available literature [10, 17, 22], although comparisons between studies of neurological signs and levels of disability in WD are challenging due to the complexity of the clinical manifestations.

There are numerous scales available for parkinsonism, dystonia and ataxia, but there has been a lack of specific instruments for measuring the severity of impairment and disability associated with WD [8]. A specific rating scale for WD must be able to capture its multi-systemic impairment, be easily administered, yet be sensitive to small clinical change. There has been a reliance on the use of proxy scales, such as the Hoehn and Yahr scale, the Unified Parkinson's Disease Rating Scale (UPDRS), the Unified Huntington's Disease Rating Scale (UHDRS), the International Co-Operative Ataxia Rating Scale (ICARS) and the Rating Scale for Dystonia (RSD). However, these scales are not capable of capturing the distinctive and complex multi-systemic spectrum of WD and tend to include irrelevant features [23]. Also, focusing on tremor, ataxia, parkinsonism, or dystonia in isolation is insufficient to accurately reflect the neurological impairment experienced by patients with WD [10, 23]. For these reasons, Członkowska et al. developed the UWDRS [8]. It is a novel rating scale specific for WD, which was designed to accurately document the neurological and functional impairment suffered by patients with WD [8]. The UWDRS was found to capture the complex impairment seen in patients with WD and was widely used by the EuroWilson consortium and GeNeMove [8, 10] and has been used in a multicenter clinical trial in WD [24].

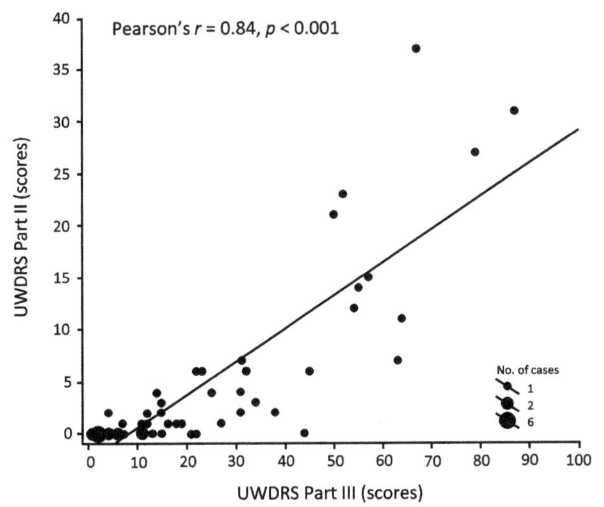

Fig. 1 Correlation between UWDRS Part II and UWDRS Part III Score (total cohort). *UWDRS* United Wilson's Disease Rating Scale

The current study demonstrated a significant correlation between disease-related disability (UWDRS Part II) and objective neurological examination (UWDRS Part III). This is consistent with the findings by Oder et al. demonstrating a clear-cut correlation between the severity of neurological impairment and the restriction in functional capacity [25]. In addition, Volpert et al. recently published a study demonstrating a strong correlation between "minimal UWDRS" (UWDRS Part II without one item) and total as well as neurological UWDRS scores [26]. In our study, we also demonstrated the correlation separately in all three major WD neurological subtypes. There was no correlation in subtype with discrete or unclassified signs, but the group was small and UWDRS scores by definition were low.

The management of patients with neurological WD is associated with therapeutic challenges, particularly for patients with tremor, parkinsonism, and dystonia, which are key factors contributing to the UWDRS score [10, 27]. Recommended initial pharmacological treatment for WD comprises chelating agents such as D-penicillamine or trientine, and zinc salts that reduce intestinal copper absorption. Despite these therapies, a considerable proportion of patients still experience neurological symptoms (50.5% [$n = 106$]) [28]. In particular, dysarthria/dysphagia, bradykinesia and postural tremor persist, highlighting the need for improved therapies for patients with WD [10].

To evaluate the efficacy of available WD therapies, more knowledge is needed regarding the natural course of WD, neurological features and liver impairment, as well as changes in copper parameters. The UWDRS has been shown to correlate with exchangeable copper (CuEXC) [13] and optical coherence tomography of the retina in WD patients [29], and it seems to be a useful tool to follow patients with neurological symptoms in WD. We also used this scale to evaluate treatment effects of D-penicillamine compared with zinc in our center [14].

In the current study, patients who were relatively older at diagnosis had more severe neurological impairment but without significant impact on disability. It is probable that the mild disability, even in the presence of neurological signs, led to a delay in diagnosis on the part of both the patient and physician. We found a lack of correlation between hepatic status at diagnosis and neurological impairment. Patients with acute and severe liver symptoms are usually managed by hepatology departments, and patients are generally referred to neurologists when they present with mild hepatic disease. However, most patients have some evidence of liver injury consistent with previous data [30]. Many patients who develop neurological signs as the first WD manifestation have compensated liver cirrhosis that develops insidiously [1, 2, 30].

In the current study, ceruloplasmin, urinary copper excretion, NCC, and total copper did not correlate with severity of neurological symptoms. This is consistent with previous data [11, 31], but in contrast to the results of Poujois et al. who found a correlation between UWDRS score at diagnosis and determination of CuEXC [13]. A single NCC value largely represents a snapshot of copper levels at the time of sampling, whereas the UWDRS score also represents accumulated long-term neurological manifestations resulting from chronically elevated free copper levels. Therefore, a strict correlation between these two parameters may not necessarily be expected. Regarding NCC determination, there are known differences between laboratories using different methods for measuring ceruloplasmin [32, 33]; however, all measurements of ceruloplasmin and copper in our patients were performed in the same laboratory. We found that NCC was detectable in all our patients and was in a range reported in the literature as typical for WD [21].

There were some limitations associated with our study. The analysis is based on a relatively small group of 53 patients. However, it is important to note that WD is a rare disease and the recruitment of treatment-naïve patients is challenging, even in a nationwide referral center. Many of our patients are referred from other hospitals early after treatment initiation to confirm the diagnosis and they remain under long-term outpatient care. Due to the rapid effect of D-penicillamine on copper metabolism, we decided not to include these previously treated patients in this study, which limited our sample size. Furthermore, the sample size did not allow meaningful analyses for all subgroups.

Conclusions

The results of this study confirm a strong correlation between the degree of neurological impairment and the level of disability captured with the UWDRS. However, there was no clear association between neurological status and serum markers of hepatic status, or copper parameters. These results confirm the highly heterogeneous symptomatology of WD and emphasize the challenges of applying single tools only for assessment of patients with WD.

Abbreviations

CuEXC: Exchangeable copper; ICARS: International Co-Operative Ataxia Rating Scale; NCC: Non-ceruloplasmin bound copper; RSD: Rating Scale for Dystonia; SD: Standard deviation; UHDRS: Unified Huntington's Disease Rating Scale; UPDRS: Unified Parkinson's Disease Rating Scale; UWDRS: Unified Wilson's Disease Rating Scale; WD: Wilson disease

Acknowledgements

We wish to thank all participants in this study. We thank Debbie Jordan and Emma Marshman who provided medical writing services, funded by Wilson Therapeutics AB.

Funding

Statistical analysis, performed by Johan Bring (Statisticon AB), was funded by Wilson Therapeutics AB. CB is an employee of Wilson Therapeutics AB. Wilson Therapeutics AB funded the article-processing charge.

Authors' contributions

AC: Study design, data acquisition and interpretation, drafting of manuscript, manuscript revision; TL: Data acquisition and interpretation, manuscript revision; KD: Data acquisition and interpretation, manuscript revision; MK: Data acquisition and interpretation, statistical analysis, manuscript revision; JB: Statistical analysis; CB: Study design, data analysis and interpretation, manuscript revision. All authors have approved the final article.

Competing interests

AC reports grants and personal fees from Wilson Therapeutics AB and the Polish government, and reports grants from USF Davies, outside the submitted work.

Author details

[1]2nd Department of Neurology, Institute of Psychiatry and Neurology, 02 957 Warsaw, Poland. [2]Department of Experimental and Clinical Pharmacology, Medical University of Warsaw, Warsaw, Poland. [3]Statisticon AB i Uppsala, Uppsala, Sweden. [4]Wilson Therapeutics AB, Stockholm, Sweden.

References

1. Gitlin JD. Wilson disease. Gastroenterology. 2003;125:1868–77.
2. Roberts EA, Schilsky ML. American Association for Study of Liver Diseases (AASLD). Diagnosis and treatment of Wilson disease: an update. Hepatology. 2008;47:2089–111.
3. Dhawan A, Taylor RM, Cheeseman P, De Silva P, Katsiyiannakis L, Mieli-Vergani G. Wilson's disease in children: 37-year experience and revised King's score for liver transplantation. Liver Transpl. 2005;11:441–8.
4. Bandmann O, Weiss KH, Kaler SG. Wilson's disease and other neurological copper disorders. Lancet Neurol. 2015;14:103–13.
5. Dzieżyc K, Litwin T, Chabik G, Gramza K, Członkowska A. Families with Wilson's disease in subsequent generations: clinical and genetic analysis. Mov Disord. 2014;29:1828–32.
6. Dziezyc K, Karlinski M, Litwin T, Członkowska A. Compliant treatment with anti-copper agents prevents clinically overt Wilson's disease in pre-symptomatic patients. Eur J Neurol. 2014;21:332–7.
7. Ferenci P, Członkowska A, Merle U, Ferenc S, Gromadzka G, Yurdaydin C, Vogel W, Bruha R, Schmidt HT, Stremmel W. Late-onset Wilson'disease. Gastroenterology. 2007;132:1294–8.
8. Członkowska A, Tarnacka B, Möller JC, Leinweber B, Bandmann O, Woimant F, Oertel WH. Unified Wilson's Disease Rating Scale – a proposal for the neurological scoring of Wilson's disease patients. Neurol Neurochir Pol. 2007;41:1–12.
9. European Association for Study of Liver. EASL clinical practice guidelines: Wilson's disease. J Hepatol. 2012;56:671–85.
10. Leinweber B, Möller JC, Scherag A, Reuner U, Günther P, Lang CJ, Schmidt HH, Schrader C, Bandmann O, Członkowska A, et al. Evaluation of the Unified Wilson's Disease Rating Scale (UWDRS) in German patients with treated Wilson's disease. Mov Disord. 2008;23:54–62.
11. Gromadzka G, Schmidt HH, Genschel J, Bochow B, Rodo M, Tarnacka B, Litwin T, Chabik G, Członkowska A. p.H1069Q mutation in ATP7B and biochemical parameters of copper metabolism and clinical manifestation of Wilson's disease. Mov Disord. 2006;21:245–8.
12. Litwin T, Członkowska A. Wilson disease – factors affecting clinical presentation. Neurol Neurochir Pol. 2013;47:161–9.
13. Poujois A, Trocello JM, Djebrani-Oussedik N, Poupon J, Collet C, Girardot-Tinant N, Sobesky R, Habès D, Debray D, Vanlemmens C, et al. Exchangeable copper: reflection of the neurological severity in Wilson's disease. Eur J Neurol. 2017;24:154–60.
14. Członkowska A, Litwin T, Karlinski M, Dziezyc K, Chabik G, Czerska M. D-penicillamine versus zinc sulfate as first-line therapy for Wilson's disease. Eur J Neurol. 2014;21:599–606.
15. Członkowska A, Gajda J, Rodo M. Effects of long-term treatment in Wilson's disease with D-penicillamine and zinc sulphate. J Neurol. 1996;243:269–73.
16. Marsden CD. Wilson's disease. Q J Med. 1987;65:959–66.
17. Oder W, Prayer L, Grimm G, Spatt J, Ferenci P, Kollegger H, Schneider B, Gangl A, Deecke L. Wilson's disease: evidence of subgroups derived from clinical findings and brain lesions. Neurology. 1993;43:120–4.
18. Ravin HA. An improved colorimetric enzymatic assay of ceruloplasmin. J Lab Clin Med. 1961;58:161–8.
19. Ferenci P, Steindl-Munda P, Vogel W, Jessner W, Gschwantler M, Stauber R, Datz C, Hackl F, Wrba F, Bauer P, et al. Diagnostic value of quantitative hepatic copper determination in patients with Wilson's disease. Clin Gastroenterol Hepatol. 2005;3:811–8.
20. Walshe JM. Serum 'free' copper in Wilson's disease. QJM. 2012;105:419–23.
21. Hedera P. Update on the clinical management of Wilson's disease. Appl Clin Genet. 2017;10:9–19.
22. Machado A, Chien HF, Deguti MM, Cançado E, Azevedo RS, Scaff M, Barbosa ER. Neurological manifestations in Wilson's disease: report of 119 cases. Mov Disord. 2006;21:2192–6.
23. Aggarwal A, Aggarwal N, Nagral A, Jankharia G, Bhatt M. A novel global assessment scale for Wilson's disease (GAS for WD). Mov Disord. 2009; 24:509–18.
24. Weiss KH, Askari FK, Czlonkowska A, Ferenci P, Bronstein JM, Bega D, Ala A, Nicholl D, Flint S, Olsson L, Plitz T, Bjartmar C, Schilsky ML. Bis-choline tetrathiomolybdate in patients with Wilson's disease: an open-label, multicentre, phase 2 study. Lancet Gastroenterol Hepatol. 2017;2:869–76.
25. Oder W, Grimm G, Kollegger H, Ferenci P, Schneider B, Deecke L. Neurological and neuropsychiatric spectrum of Wilson's disease: a prospective study of 45 cases. J Neurol. 1991;238:281–7.
26. Volpert HM, Pfeiffenberger J, Gröner JB, Stremmel W, Gotthardt DN, Schäfer M, Weiss KH, Weiler M. Comparative assessment of clinical rating scales in Wilson's disease. BMC Neurol. 2017;17:140.
27. Litwin T, Dusek P, Członkowska A. Neurological manifestations in Wilson's disease – possible treatment options for symptoms. Expert Opin Orphan Drugs. 2016;4:719–28.
28. Hölscher S, Leinweber B, Hefter H, Reuner U, Günther P, Weiss KH, Oertel WH, Möller JC. Evaluation of the symptomatic treatment of residual neurological symptoms in Wilson disease. Eur Neurol. 2010;64:83–7.
29. Langwinska-Wosko E, Litwin T, Dziezyc K, Karlinski M, Członkowska A. Optical coherence tomography as a marker of neurodegeneration in patients with Wilson's disease. Acta Neurol Belg. 2017;117:867–71.
30. Przybyłkowski A, Gromadzka G, Chabik G, Wierzchowska A, Litwin T, Członkowska A. Liver cirrhosis in patients newly diagnosed with neurological phenotype of Wilson's disease. Funct Neurol. 2014;29:23–9.
31. Litwin T, Gromadzka G, Członkowska A. Gender differences in Wilson's disease. J Neurol Sci. 2012;312:31–5.
32. Twomey PJ, Viljoen A, House IM, Reynolds TM, Wierzbicki AS. Limitations of non-ceruloplasmin-bound copper in routine clinical practice. Gut. 2007;56:154.
33. Duncan A, Yacoubian C, Beetham R, Catchpole A, Bullock D. The role of calculated non-caeruloplasmin-bound copper in Wilson's disease. Ann Clin Biochem. 2017;54:649–54.

19

Comparison of electroencephalographic changes in response to acute electrical and thermal stimuli with the tail flick and hot plate test in rats administered with opiorphin

Preet Singh[1*], Kavitha Kongara[1], David Harding[2], Neil Ward[1], Venkata Sayoji Rao Dukkipati[1], Craig Johnson[1] and Paul Chambers[1]

Abstract

Background: The objective of this study was to compare the changes in the electroencephalogram (EEG) in response to noxious stimuli with tail flick and hot plate responses of rats administered opiorphin.

Methods: Female Sprague -Dawley rats ($n = 8$ per group) randomly received intravenous (IV) injection of morphine (1 mg/kg,) or opiorphin (2 mg/kg,) or saline (0.5 ml,) in each of the three testing methods (EEG, tail flick and hot plate). Each type of test ($n = 24$ per test) was conducted in different population of rats on separate occasions. The tail flick and hot plate latencies were recorded until 5 min after test drug administration to conscious rats. The EEG was recorded in anaesthetised rats subjected to noxious thermal and electrical stimuli after test drug administration. At the end of 5 min in each of the testing methods rats were administered naloxone subcutaneously (SC) (1 mg/kg) and the test procedure was repeated.

Results: There was no significant increase in the median frequency and spectral edge frequency (F50 & F95) of EEG, indicators of nociception, of morphine and opiorphin groups after noxious stimulation. Noxious stimuli caused a significant increase in both F50 and F95 of the saline group. An injection of naloxone significantly increased the F50, thus blocking the action of both opiorphin and morphine. There was a significant increase in the tail flick latency after administration of opiorphin and morphine as compared to the baseline values. Rats of morphine group spent significantly longer on the hot plate when compared to those of the opiorphin and saline groups. There was no significant difference in the hot plate latencies of opiorphin and saline groups.

Conclusion: The results of this study suggest that the analgesic effect of opiorphin occurs at the spinal level and it is not as effective as morphine at supraspinal level. It may be due to rapid degradation of opiorphin or limited ability of opiorphin to cross the blood brain barrier or a higher dose of opiorphin is required for its action in the brain. Pharmacokinetic/pharmacodynamics studies along with in vivo penetration of opiorphin in the cerebrospinal fluid are required for further evaluation of opiorphin analgesia.

Keywords: Opiorphin, EEG, Hot plate test, Tail flick test

* Correspondence: P.M.Singh@massey.ac.nz
[1]Massey University, Institute of Veterinary, Animal and Biomedical Sciences, Palmerston North, New Zealand
Full list of author information is available at the end of the article

Background

Opiorphin (QRFSR) is one of the analgesic human peptides whose effects have been investigated in rats. It has the potential to be a treatment for chronic pain including neuropathic pain [1]. Opiorphin is a penta-peptide (Gln-Arg-Phe-Ser-Arg) which has similar analgesic efficacy to morphine with fewer side effects in rats. It is a dual endogenous ectopeptidase enkephalinase inhibitor; inhibits both neutral endopeptidase (NEP) and amino-peptidase N (AP-N) [2, 3]. IC50 for NEP and APN were 8 and 30 μM, respectively [4]. These enkephalinases inactivate endogenous opioids, and blocking this inactivation has similar effects to administration of exogenous **opioids peptides** such as morphine [1, 5]. Opiorphin is produced from the PRL1 precursor in response to pain, stress and emotional state [6] both in brain and in peripheral tissue such as kidneys, digestive tract, reproductive tract (both in males and females), tears and saliva [7]. It is rapidly metabolised to RFSR-peptide by plasma exo-aminopeptidases resulting in a short half-life of only 5 min [8].

Rougeot et al. [2] demonstrated a similar analgesic efficacy of opiorphin after intravenous administration to morphine in rats using tail flick and formalin tests, but the duration of action was short. The action of opiorphin can also be prolonged by using liposomal formulations instead of conventional opiorphin formulation [1, 9]. Benyhe et al. [10] and Bogeas et al. [8] used peptidomimetic products of opiorphin which were metabolically more stable than opiorphin. The analgesic efficacy of opiorphin has been demonstrated by using "the spinally controlled thermal acute nociception, tail flick test; the supraspinally controlled mechanical acute nociception, pin pain test and the chemically-induced inflammation causing chronic pain and the formalin test [2, 3, 11]. The tail flick test works at spinal level while formalin injection test mimics chronic peripheral pain. It can be argued that both these tests do not effectively assess the brain activity and rely only on the behavioural observations. The hot plate, a supraspinally controlled thermal acute pain test has less ethical cost as compared to the formalin test. It is easy to use, highly repeatable and causes pain of only a short duration [12].

Electroencephalography (EEG) has been used to evaluate antinociception objectively in anaesthetized animals [13–15]. It is a representation of the spontaneous electrical activity of the cerebral cortex. It is well established that the cerebral cortex participates in the processing of afferent nociceptive input that results in the conscious perception of pain. Supporting evidence has been provided from human and animal studies that showed correlation of behavioural responses with EEG spectral frequency changes due to noxious stimuli [13, 14]. Changes in the EEG power spectrum, specifically, median frequency (F50), spectral edge frequency (F95) and total power of the EEG (Ptot), have been used to evaluate the anti-nociceptive efficacy of analgesics in different species of animals in response to a variety of noxious stimuli [15, 16]. To date, there have been no reports on either the effect of opiorphin on the EEG of rats subjected to noxious stimuli or the use of hot plate test to demonstrate its analgesic efficacy. A thermal supraspinal test might show different results as compared to chemical nociception induced by formalin injection.

The aim of this study was to measure and compare the changes in the electroencephalogram (EEG) in response to noxious stimuli with tail flick and hot plate responses of rats administered opiorphin or morphine.

Methods

Study design

This study was approved by the Massey University Animal Ethics Committee (protocols 14/86 and 15/106). Female Sprague Dawley rats ($n = 72$) were randomly selected by coin toss from a population of 500. The animals were obtained from the Small Animal Production Unit, Massey University, Palmerston North, New Zealand. Female rats were used for this study because concerns about the priapism associated with opiorphin administration in male rats [17]. The average body weight of the selected rats was 250 g. The sample size was determined by use of power calculation using ranges derived from Wisner et al. [3]. The rats were raised under standard husbandry conditions with ad libitum feed and water. The rats were kept in plastic rat cages in pairs. They were accustomed to handling for a month prior to start of the actual experiment. The person conducting the experiment was unaware of the treatment groups. The rats were randomly selected by coin toss as receiving morphine or opiorphin or normal saline.

Tail flick and hot plate tests

The tail flick and the hot plate tests were conducted on 24 female rats for each test. These rats were divided into three groups; placebo, morphine and opiorphin, with 8 rats in each group. The drugs were injected intravenously into the tail vein. The rats were manually restrained using a perforated perspex tube exposing the tail of the rat towards the operator. The placebo group received an intravenous injection of normal saline while the morphine group and opiorphin group received an intravenous injection of morphine sulphate (10 mg/mL) at 1 mg/kg and opiorphin (0.2 mg/mL) at 2 mg/kg formulated in a solution of 100 mM PBS (55%) and 0.01 N Acetic acid (45%) [2]. Tail flick test [18] was performed by immersing the tail of the rat in hot water maintained at 55 °C, prior to and 1 and 5 min after the injection of test drugs. Tail flick reaction time at each of the time-points was recorded. Naloxone HCl (0.4 mg/mL) at 1 mg/kg was injected sub-cutaneously after the third tail flick observation. Another tail flick test was performed 5 min after the naloxone injection. The cut off time for tail flick test was 10 s.

Hot plate test [12] was performed by placing rats on a hot plate at 50 °C. Response time for observed behavioural changes like paw licking, stomping, jumping and escaping from the hot plate was recorded prior to and 1 and 5 min after the injection of test drugs. Naloxone HCl at 1 mg/kg was injected sub- cutaneously after the third hot plate test observation. A subsequent hot plate test was performed 5 min after the naloxone injection. The cut off time for the hot plate test was 15 s.

Rats used for tail flick and hot plate tests were euthanized at end of the experiment using carbon dioxide.

EEG recording

EEG was recorded as described by Kongara et al. [16]. Briefly, rats ($n = 24$) were placed into an induction chamber and anaesthesia was induced with 2% halothane in oxygen. When the rat was unconscious, oro-tracheal intubation was performed with an 18-gauge cannula, which was connected to a T-piece breathing system. Anaesthesia was maintained with halothane in oxygen. The precision vaporizer (Fluothane; MedSource Ltd., Ashburton, NZ) was adjusted to maintain the end-tidal halothane tension (Et_{Hal}) between 1.2 and 1.25%. None of the rats showed any movement responses at this minimal plane of anaesthesia (see review by Murrell and Johnson for details on minimal anaesthesia model used for recording the EEG) Ventilation was controlled using an intermittent positive pressure ventilator (V valve ventilator; Vetronics, Bioanalytical Systems Inc., West LaFayette, IN, USA) and the end-tidal carbon dioxide concentration (Et_{CO2}) was maintained between 4.7 and 6.0 kPa. Airway gases were sampled continuously from the end of the endotracheal tube connected to the breathing circuit, using an anaesthetic gas analyzer (Hewlet Packard M1025B, Hewlet Packard, Hamburg, Germany). Rats' rectal temperature was monitored using a digital thermometer, and maintained between 37.0 and 38.5 °C with a circulating warm water blanket heating device.

Anaesthetised rats' head was secured in a stereotaxic frame to prevent any movement of the head during EEG recording. EEG was recorded using three subcutaneous 27-gauge stainless-steel needle electrodes (Medelec, Radiometer, Auckland, New Zealand). The three electrode montage comprised of an inverting electrode over the zygomatic process of the left frontal bone, non-inverting electrode over the left mastoid process and ground electrode caudal to the occipital process. Electrode cables were connected to a custom built break-out box that was plugged into a physiological signal amplifier (Iso-Dam Signal Amplifiers; World Precision Instruments, Sarasota, FL, USA). The signals were amplified with a gain of 1000× and a band pass of 0.1–100 Hz. EEG was recorded on a Powerlab 4/20 data acquisition system (Powerlab/4sp; AD Instruments Ltd., Sydney, Australia), which digitized the signal at a rate of 1.0 kHz.

EEG recording was started as soon as the rat was stabilized under anaesthesia and a 5 min baseline was recorded. The timeline for EEG recording and treatments is given in Fig. 1. At the end of the 5 min baseline, test drugs were injected. The placebo group ($n = 8$) received an intravenous injection of normal saline, while morphine (n = 8) and opiorphin (n = 8) groups received an intravenous injection of the respective drugs at 1 and 2 mg/kg. Five minutes after test drug administration and EEG recording, noxious stimuli (electrical or thermal) were applied randomly with a 10 min interval between each type of stimulus. Electrical stimulus (50 V at 50 Hz for 2 s; Valverde et al., [19]) was applied via two needle electrodes inserted to the lateral aspect of the tail base, using a Grass Stimulator (S48 K square pulse stimulator, Astro-Med Inc., Grass instrument division, Auckland, New Zealand), and thermal stimulus was applied by immersing the tail in a 55 °C hot water bath for 5 s [15].

EEG was sampled during and 5 min immediately after each type of stimulus. Naloxane HCl (1 mg/kg) was injected IV at the end of 5 min sampling after the second stimulus. Application of noxious stimuli and the EEG sampling pattern was the same as described above, after naloxane administration. Rats were euthanized at the end of the EEG recording with a halothane overdose while they were under anaesthesia.

Raw EEG data were inspected visually off-line and any out-of-range data resulting from movement artefact during noxious stimulation were excluded from analysis (Fig. 2). Data were multiplied using a Welch window and fast Fourier transformation applied to each epoch, generating sequential power spectra with one-hertz frequency bins [15, 16]. The F50, F95 and Ptot were calculated for consecutive non-overlapping one-second epochs, using purpose-built software (Spectral Analyser; Craig Johnson, Massey University, Palmerston North, NZ, 2002).

Statistical analyses

Differences in EEG variables (F50, F95 and Ptot) as well as tail flick and hot plate time, between treatment groups as well as time-points, were tested using generalised linear mixed model analysis (Littell et al. [20]) in SAS® 9.4 (SAS

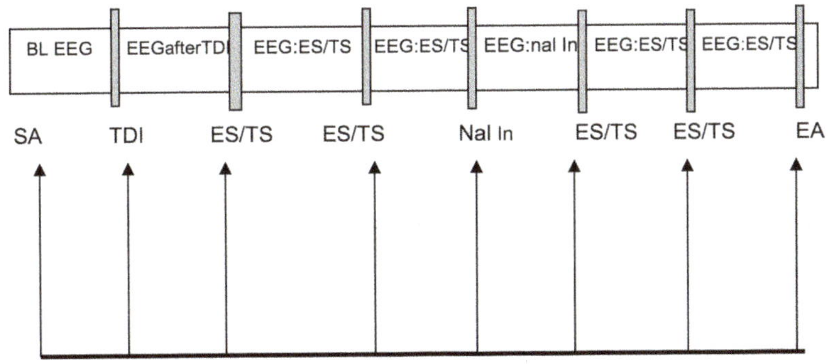

Fig. 1 Diagram of the EEG recording pattern at different time points in rats under minimal halothane anaesthesia. SA = stabilisation of anaesthesia; BL EEG = baseline EEG; TDI = test drug injection; EEG: ES/TS = EEG recording during and after electrical or thermal stimulation ES/TS = electrical or thermal stimulation; Nal In = naloxone injection; EEG: nal In = EEG recorded after naloxone injection; EA = end of anaesthesia

Institute Inc. Cary, NC, USA). The model in *proc. mixed* procedure included the fixed effects of group, time and their interaction, and random effects of animals. The covariance error structure for repeated measures over time-points, within animals in each group was determined using Akaike's information criterion. A first-order autoregressive model was found to be the most appropriate error structure. There were significant ($P < 0.05$) between-group differences in the baseline values of all variables and hence, baseline values were included as covariates in the model. The distribution of data for different variables were tested for normality using Shapiro-Wilk, Kolmogorov-Smirnov and Anderson-Darling tests using *proc. univariate* procedure in SAS® 9.4. The residuals of data for EEG variables were found to be non-normally distributed and hence, EEG variables were normalised by Blom's transformation employing *proc. rank* procedure in SAS® 9.4. The option of statement, NORMAL = BLOM, was used and this estimated the normal scores corresponding to the observations as per [21]. Least square means (LSM) and standard errors (SE) in original scale were used to plot graphs. Data are reported in mean ± standard errors.

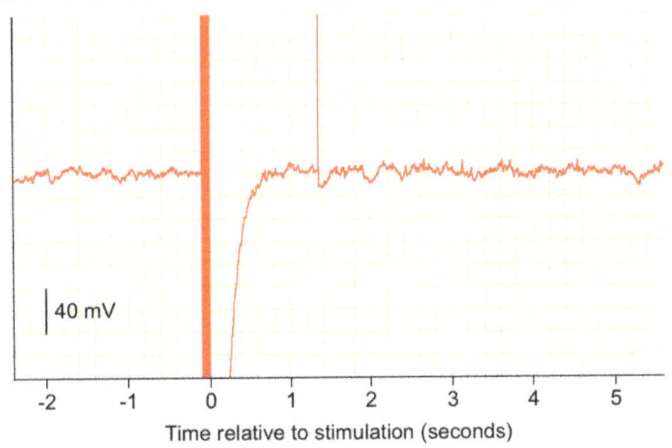

Fig. 2 Example of raw electroencephalogram of anaesthetized rat: before and after electrical stimulation. *Note the large movement artefact during electrical stimulation

Results

Tail flick test

Results from the tail flick test are shown in Fig. 3. There was a significant ($P < 0.05$) increase in the tail flick latencies at 5 min (5.32 s ± 0.17) after an injection of opiorphin as compared to the baseline (4.27 s ± 0.17) and this effect was blocked by an injection of naloxone (4.15 s ± 0.17). It took about 5 min for opiorphin to have its effect in the tail flick test as the tail flick latency at 1 min after the injection of opiorphin (4.56 s ± 0.17) was not significantly ($P > 0.05$) different from the baseline value. The effect of morphine on tail flick test was significant ($P < 0.05$) at 1 min after its administration (5.49 s ± 0.28) and was persistent till 5 min (5.71 s ± 0.28), after which naloxone blocked its effect (4.15 s ± 0.17).

In case of the saline group, the tail flick latencies at both time-points were non-significantly ($P > 0.05$) different from baseline reading. Comparison between groups, within a time-point, was also made. The tail flick latency at one-minute time-point in morphine group rats (5.49 s ± 0.28) was significantly ($P < 0.05$) higher than that in opiorphin group rats (4.56 s ± 0.17). Both morphine (5.71 s ± 0.28) and opiorphin (5.32 s ± 0.17) groups had significantly ($P < 0.05$) higher tail flick latencies at 5 min time-point, compared to saline group rats (4.49 secd±0.19).

Hot plate test

Figure 4 shows the results of the hot plate test. The hot plate test did not demonstrate the analgesic effects of opiorphin. There was a significant ($P < 0.05$) reduction in time spent on the hot plate in rats injected with either

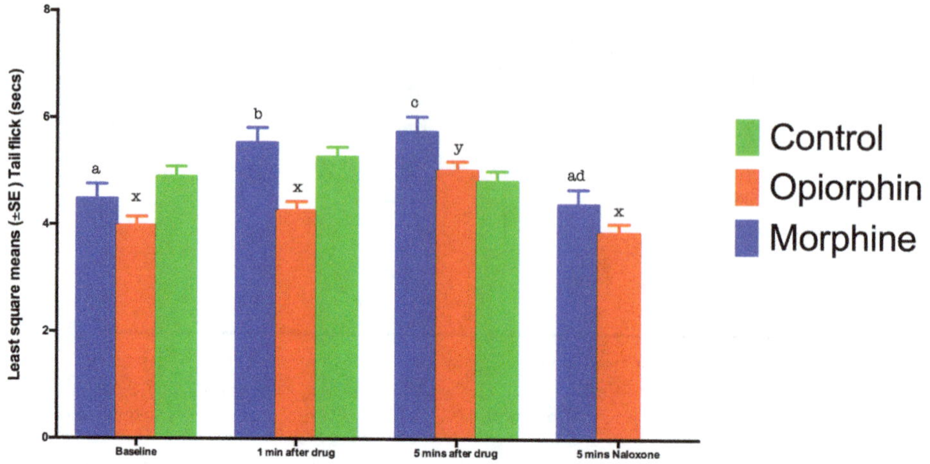

Fig. 3 Least square means for the tail immersion time (sec) at different time points. There was a significant increase in tail flick times at one and 5 min after an IV injection of morphine and 5 min after an injection of opiorphin. There was a significant decrease in tail flick times after an IV injection of naloxone. The control group did not receive an injection of naloxone. Note 1: Mean values with an asterisk over the error bars differed significantly ($p < 0.05$) from their respective baseline values. Note 2: Mean values with at least one common letter over the error bars, within the each time-point, did not differ significantly ($p > 0.05$). Note 3: Baseline = tail flick latency before the drug administration; 1 min after drug = tail flick latency 1 min after an i.v. injection of normal saline, opiorphin or morphine; 5 mins after drug = tail flick latency 5 min after an i.v. injection of normal saline, opiorphin or morphin; 5 mins Naloxone = tail flick latency 5 min after a s.c. injection of Naloxone

opiorphin or normal saline both at 1 and 5 min after injection, compared to the baseline observations. This effect was persistent after the injection of naloxone. The morphine group rats displayed typical analgesic effect. There was a significant ($P < 0.05$) increase in time spent on the hot plate at 5 after the injection of morphine. This effect was blocked by an injection of naloxone.

EEG responses

The median frequency (F50) significantly ($P < 0.05$) increased after thermal and electrical stimulation of rats injected with normal saline as compared to the baseline readings (Fig. 5). Rats in the opiorphin and morphine groups did not show any significant ($P > 0.05$) increase in F50 compared to the baseline values. There was a

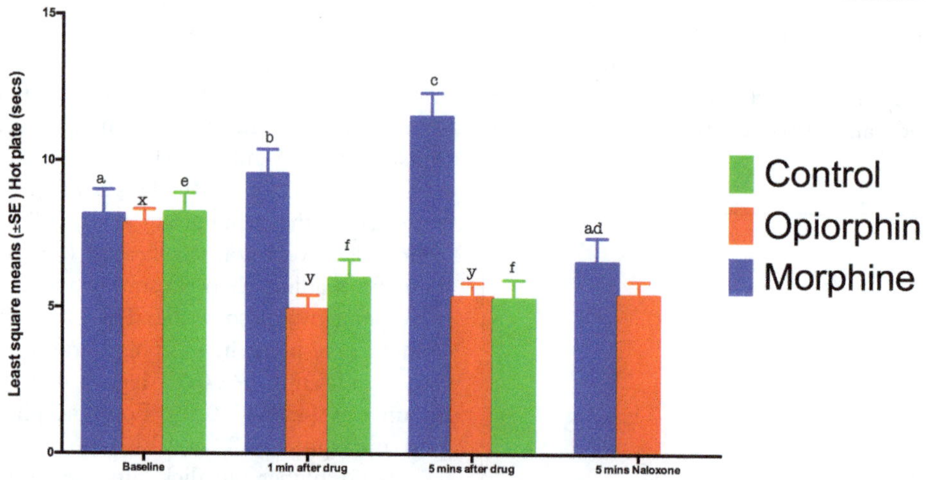

Fig. 4 Least square means for the time spent by rats on the hot plate before and after intravenous administration of normal saline, Opiorphin and morphine. There was a significant increase in time spent by rats after an injection of morphine, while there was a significant decrease in time spent by rats after an injection of either opiorphin or normal saline. Superscripts represent significant differences. Note 1: Mean values with an asterisk over the error bars differed significantly ($p < 0.05$) from their respective baseline values. Note 2: Mean values with at least one common letter over the error bars, within the each time-point, did not differ significantly ($p > 0.05$). Note 3: Baseline = hot plate latency before the drug administration; 1 min after drug = hot plate latency 1 min after an i.v. injection of normal saline, opiorphin or morphine; 5 mins after drug = hot plate latency 5 min after an i.v. injection of normal saline, opiorphin or morphin; 5 mins Naloxone = hot plate latency 5 min after a s.c. injection of Naloxone

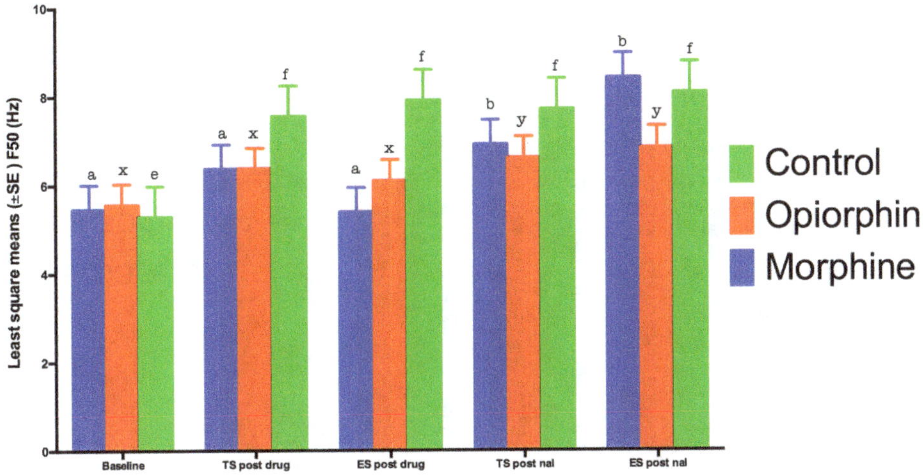

Fig. 5 Least square means for the median frequency (F50) during thermal (TS) and electrical stimulus (ES) in rats injected with normal saline (green bars), opiorphin (red bars) and morphine (blue bars). There was a significant increase in F50 in the normal saline injected rats both during the electrical and thermal stimulus. The morphine and opiorphin effect was blocked by naloxone as there was a significant increase in F50 after administration of naloxone during the electrical stimulus. Superscripts represent significant differences. Note 1: Mean values with an asterisk over the error bars differed significantly ($p < 0.05$) from their respective baseline values. Note 2: Mean values with at least one common letter over the error bars, within the each time-point, did not differ significantly ($p > 0.05$). Note 3: Baseline = F50 before the drug administration; TS post drug = F50 after an i.v. injection of normal saline, opiorphion or morphine during thermal nociceptive stimulus; ES post drug = F50 after an i.v. injection of normal saline, opiorphin or morphine during electrical nociceptive stimulus; TS post nal = F50 after a s.c. injection of naloxone

significant ($P < 0.05$) increase in F50 during the thermal and electrical stimuli after the injection of naloxone in both morphine and opiorphin groups. The morphine group rats, during the electrical stimulus after naloxone injection, had significantly ($P < 0.05$) higher F50 values as compared to opiorphin group. The saline group had significantly ($P < 0.05$) higher F50 compared to morphine and opiorphin groups during the electrical stimulation.

There was no significant ($P > 0.05$) difference in the spectral edge frequency (F95), compared to baseline values, following thermal and electrical stimuli in both morphine and opiorphin groups (Fig. 6). The saline group displayed significant ($P < 0.05$) increase in F95, compared to the baseline values during the electrical stimulus. The spectral edge frequency (F95) following both electrical and thermal stimuli, post- naloxone injection, significantly ($P < 0.05$) increased as compared to the baseline readings in the morphine group (Fig. 6). This increase was non-significant ($P > 0.05$) in case of opiorphin group.

The total power (Ptot), compared to baseline readings, did not show any significant ($P > 0.05$) difference during both electrical and thermal stimuli after the injection of morphine or opiorphin (Fig. 7). However, after the injection of naloxone, the Ptot during electrical stimulus significantly ($P < 0.05$) decreased in morphine rats. The rats injected with morphine had significantly ($P < 0.05$) higher Ptot values during electrical stimulus as compared to the control rats.

Discussion

The objective of this study was to compare the changes in EEG indices of nociception in response to noxious stimuli with the tail flick and hot plate latencies of rats administered opiorphin or morphine. A significant increase in F50 and F95 has been demonstrated to be the EEG responses indicating nociception after noxious stimulation of animals [16]. Studies have also demonstrated that these EEG indicators were similar to baseline during noxious stimulation after the administration of analgesic drugs. Changes in total power of the EEG may indicate a different aspect of nociception, and more related to degree of arousal during anaesthesia in animals [15]. F50 and F95 values similar to baseline after administration of either morphine or opiorphin suggests that both drugs could produce anti-nociception in response to noxious stimuli. Rats of saline group had a significant increase in F50 and F95 values compared to baseline during both electrical and thermal stimulation indicating nociception.

Following naloxone injection, F50 values in both opiorphin and morphine groups increased significantly during noxious stimulation. It is likely that naloxone displaced morphine or endogenous enkephalins from the opioid receptors and caused nociception due to noxious stimulation. Thus, opiorphin as expected functions to increase the half-life of endogenous opioids. When compared to morphine group, F50 of opiorphin group rats after an injection of naloxone

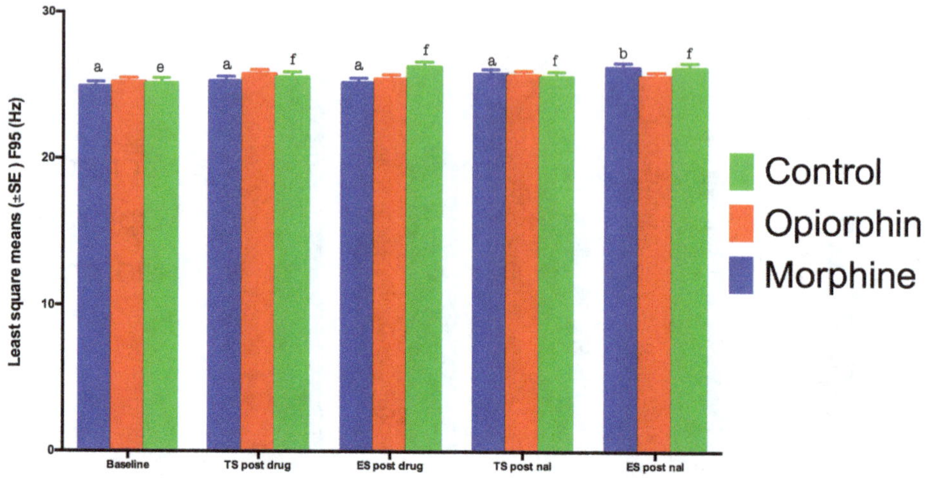

Fig. 6 Least square means for the spectral edge frequency (F95) during thermal (TS) and electrical stimulus (ES) in rats injected with normal saline (green bars), opiorphin (red bars) and morphine (blue bars). There was a significant increase in F95 in normal saline rats. There was a significant increase in F95 post naloxone injection in morphine administered rats, both during electrical and thermal stimulus. There was no such difference observed in opiorphin group rats. Superscripts represent significant differences. Note 1: Mean values with an asterisk over the error bars differed significantly ($p < 0.05$) from their respective baseline values. Note 2: Mean values with at least one common letter over the error bars, within the each time-point, did not differ significantly ($p > 0.05$). Note 3: Baseline = F95 before the drug administration; TS post drug = F95 after an i.v. injection of normal saline, opiorphion or morphine during thermal nociceptive stimulus; ES post drug = F95 after an i.v. injection of normal saline, opiorphin or morphine during electrical nociceptive stimulus; TS post nal = F95 after a s.c. injection of naloxone

during the electrical stimulus was significantly lower. The displacement of opioids by naloxone from its receptors in case of opiorphin rats was less as compared to morphine group. This could be due to continuous availability of endogenous opioids in the opiorphin administered rats that displaced naloxone from the opioid receptors. The fact that there was no significant difference in F95 after displacement of endogenous opioids in opiorphin injected rats reestablishes that naloxone may not completely block the opiorphin effect. A higher dose or continuous infusion of naloxone might be required to reverse the opiorphin

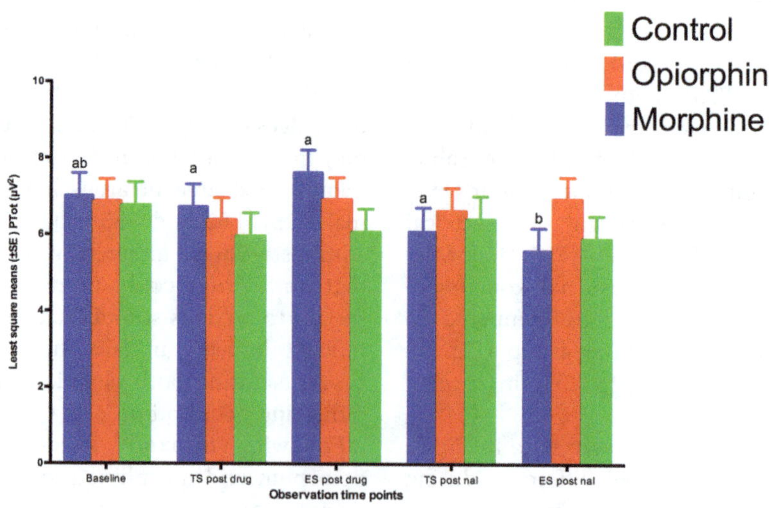

Fig. 7 Least square means for the total power (Ptot) during thermal (TS) and electrical stimulus (ES) in rats injected with normal saline (green bars), opiorphin (red bars) and morphine (blue bars). There was no significant difference in Ptot compared to baselines in any of the three groups. The Ptot in morphine group rats significantly decreased after an injection of naloxone. Superscripts represent significant differences. Note 1: Mean values with at least one common letter over the error bars, within the each time-point, did not differ significantly ($p > 0.05$). Note 2: Baseline = Ptot before the drug administration; TS post drug = Ptot after an i.v. injection of normal saline, opiorphion or morphine during thermal nociceptive stimulus; ES post drug = Ptot after an i.v. injection of normal saline, opiorphin or morphine during electrical nociceptive stimulus; TS post nal = Ptot after a s.c. injection of naloxone

effects. A continuous infusion of naloxone has been recommended to reverse the effects of the long acting potent opioid agonists [22]. The morphine group was injected only one IV bolus dose of morphine. A low dose continuous IV infusion of morphine may mimic the effects of continuous production of endogenous opioids, which was not followed in this current study.

Opiorphin caused a significant increase in tail flick latency of rats of the present study. This finding corroborates with the previously published studies in rats [2, 5]. The neurologic (reflexive) mechanisms that the tail flick test measures have been demonstrated to be spinally mediated responses to noxious stimuli [23]. This indicates the spinal analgesic effect of opiorphin in our study rats.

In this study the hot plate test was used to evaluate the supra-spinal analgesia of opiorphin, which did not show any analgesic effect of opiorphin. Wisner et al. [3] used mechanical nociceptive stimulus for assessing supraspinal analgesia after administration of opiorphin and morphine to rats, and found a significant increase in time spent on the pin areas (indicating analgesia) in both the opiorphin and morphine rats. The morphine injected rats spent higher time on the pin areas than opiorphin injected rats. Rougeot et al. [2] used formalin test as chemical induced peripheral inflammatory pain model and found significant reduction in paw flinches and body tremors after IV administration of opiorphin at 2 mg/kg. In case of morphine, a similar effect was seen, but the numbers of paw tremors was less, compared to opiorphin. Both these studies found morphine to have similar or better analgesic effect as compared to opiorphin. Opiorphin inhibits the activity of **enkephalinase enzymes**, further increasing the half-life of **endogenous opioids peptides**. The release of endogenous opioids depends on the type and intensity of the nociceptive stimulus. The endogenous opioids may not completely activate the opioids receptors. Thus, opiorphin may not exert a similar level of analgesia as compared to morphine. The present report was the only study that used hot plate test for assessing the supra-spinal effects of opiorphin. The lack of effect of opiorphin at supraspinal level (as assessed in the hot plate test) could also be due to the reduced permeability of the blood brain barrier to the peptides [24] or a lower dose of opiorphin. Bocsik et al. [25] demonstrated that only 3% of total IV dose of opiorphin crosses the blood brain barrier as compared to 26 to 40% of IV dose of morphine. The peptides can easily cross the blood spinal cord barrier due to reduction in pericytes as compared to the blood brain barrier [26]. Thus, the blood spinal cord barrier is more permeable as compared to the blood brain barrier and that could be the reason why opiorphin exhibited significant analgesic effect in the tail flick test, but not in the hot plate test.

In this study, three methods have been used to test the efficacy of opiorphin in rats. The hot plate and the EEG results contradicted each other in opiorphin group rats. This could be due to the nature of these two tests. The EEG measures the electrical activity of the cerebral cortex. It can indirectly reflect the activity of the lower centres of the brain (e.g. brain stem areas like thalamus, PAG, RVM etc.) that have diffuse connections with the spinal nociceptive pathways. These brain stem structures have a potential regulatory influence on cortical neuronal activity especially during periods of unconsciousness and anaesthesia [27, 28]. In the current study, the EEG has been recorded in anaesthetized rats. It is likely that the anti-nociceptive effect of the opiorphin demonstrated in EEG responses, might be due to its potent effect on spinal nociceptive mechanisms that has been reflected indirectly through diffuse connections with the cortical neurons. It is also possible that opiorphin might have a weak anti-nociceptive effect at supra spinal level due to its low permeability to blood brain barrier. The EEG could represent the combined effect of opiorphin at both spinal and supra spinal levels inhibiting changes in F50 and F95. Other objective (experimental) methods such as measuring the changes in electromyographic reflex thresholds [29] and expression of the neural marker of nociception, *c-fos* [30, 31] would further delineate the neural basis of the antinociceptive effects of opiorphin. In this study, only one dose of opiorphin (2 mg/kg) was tested based on the dose response curves previously reported [2, 3]. A dose response curve of opiorphin using the hot plate test should be conducted for further evaluation of supraspinal analgesia due to opiorphin administration. The hot plate test is a behavioural test in conscious subjects. The behavioural endpoints in rats associated with the hot plate test are complex and difficult to interpret which adds variability to the outcome of the test, as can learning. EEG is a more sensitive test as compared to the hot plate test.

One important factor that may influence the thermal test latencies in this study is the sex of the study rats. Previous studies have demonstrated the differences in pain perception between male and female rats and mice in a formalin induced pain model [32, 33]. Intact females showed significantly more nociceptive responses than intact males. In contrast, the influence of sex difference on hot plate latencies has been reported to be non-significant in rats [12]. In female rats, the stage of oestrous cycle may also affect the behavioural responses to nociceptive pressure stimuli [34], and the hot plate latencies [35]. When the rats were tested during the oestrus phase of the cycle a significant reduction in latencies was detected. In mice, the influence of stage of oestrous cycle on responses to formalin induced nociception was reported to be non-significant [32]. Based on the variable findings of the previous studies in rats and mice it appears that the influence of the sex and stage of the oestrous cycle on pain responses is dependent on the type of noxious stimulation and animal. It is likely that the thermal latencies reported in the female rats of the present study might differ in male rats but the significance of the difference is unknown.

Conclusion

There are several dual enkephalinase inhibitors currently under clinical trials show promising results in their preclinical studies [1]; especially orally administered P37 [36] which has potential to replace opioid pain management protocols in diabetic neuropathy.

Further research is required to enable to use opiorphin for clinical pain management. There is a need to conduct a proper pharmacokinetic study to know the half-life, distribution and elimination of opiorphin in the target species. The rapid breakdown of opiorphin peptide could be a hindrance in testing its analgesic efficacy. A different drug delivery approach may be required to make it a viable candidate for a new class of analgesic drugs.

Abbreviations

AP-N: Amino-peptidase N; EEG: Electroencephalogram; F50: Median Frequency; F95: Spectral edge frequency; IV: Intravenous; NEP: Endopeptidase; PBS: Phosphate buffer saline; Ptot: Total power; SC: Subcutaneous

Acknowledgments

We acknowledge Aimee Hamlin and Margaret Brown, staff of Small Animal Production Unit, Massey University, for routine care and husbandry of rats used in these studies. Prof Patrick Morel for translating manuscripts written in French to English.

Funding

The studies were funded by Massey University Research Funds.

Authors' contributions

PS designed the study, prepared the animal ethics and funding applications, conducted the study and participated in manuscript preparation and revision. KK helped in animal ethics, preparation and revision of the manuscript and conducted and designed the EEG studies. NW helped in acquisition of data in the hot plate and tail flick studies. CJ participated in animal ethics, study design, manuscript review and EEG studies. DH peptide synthesis and participated in study design and funding application. RD helped in statistical analysis. PC helped in designing and conducting the studies as well as in manuscript revisions. All the authors reviewed and accepted the final manuscript. All authors read and approved the final manuscript.

Competing interests

The authors declare that they have no competing interests.

Author details

[1]Massey University, Institute of Veterinary, Animal and Biomedical Sciences, Palmerston North, New Zealand. [2]Massey University, Institute of Fundamental Sciences, Palmerston North, New Zealand.

References

1. Roques BP, Fournié-Zaluski M-C, Wurm M. Inhibiting the breakdown of endogenous opioids and cannabinoids to alleviate pain. Nat Rev Drug Discov. 2012;11:292–310.
2. Rougeot C, Robert F, Menz L, Bisson J-F, Messaoudi M. Systemically active human opiorphin is a potent yet non-addictive analgesic without drug tolerance effects. J Physiol Pharmacol. 2010;61:483–90.
3. Wisner A, Dufour E, Messaoudi M, Nejdi A, Marcel A, Ungeheuer M-N, et al. Human Opiorphin, a natural antinociceptive modulator of opioid-dependent pathways. Proc Natl Acad Sci U S A. 2006;103:17979–84. pnas.org
4. Pinto M, Rougeot C, Gracia L, Rosa M, García A, Arsequell G, et al. Proposed bioactive conformations of opiorphin, an endogenous dual APN/NEP inhibitor. ACS Med Chem Lett. 2012;3:20–4.
5. Popik P, Kamysz E, Kreczko J, Wróbel M. Human opiorphin: the lack of physiological dependence, tolerance to antinociceptive effects and abuse liability in laboratory mice. Behav Brain Res. 2010;213:88–93.
6. Rougeot C, Messaoudi M. Identification of human opiorphin, a natural antinociceptive modulator of opioid-dependent pathways. Med Sci (Paris). 2007;23:37–9. EDK
7. Dufour E, Villard-Saussine S, Mellon V, Leandri R, Jouannet P, Ungeheuer MN, et al. Opiorphin secretion pattern in healthy volunteers: gender difference and organ specificity. Biochem Anal Biochem. 2013;2:1000136.
8. Bogeas A, Dufour E, Bisson J-F, Messaoudi M, Rougeot C. Structure-activity relationship study and function-based peptidomimetic design of human opiorphin with improved bioavailability property and unaltered analgesic activity. Biochem Pharmacol. 2013;2:2167–0501.
9. Mennini N, Mura P, Nativi C, Richichi B, Di Cesare Mannelli L, Ghelardini C. Injectable liposomal formulations of opiorphin as a new therapeutic strategy in pain management. Future Sci OA. 2015;1(3):FSO2. https://doi.org/10.4155/fso.14.3.
10. Benyhe Z, Toth G, Wollemann M, Borsodi A, Helyes Z, Rougeot C, et al. Effects of synthetic analogues of human opiorphin on rat brain opioid receptors. J Physiol Pharmacol. 2014;65:525–30.
11. Tian X-Z, Chen J, Xiong W, He T, Chen Q. Effects and underlying mechanisms of human opiorphin on colonic motility and nociception in mice. Peptides. 2009;30:1348–54.
12. Gunn A, Bobeck EN, Weber C, Morgan MM. The influence of non-nociceptive factors on hot-plate latency in rats. J Pain. 2011;12:222–7.
13. Ong RM, Morris JP, O'Dwyer JK, Barnett JL, Hemsworth PH, Clarke IJ. Behavioural and EEG changes in sheep in response to painful acute electrical stimuli. Aust Vet J. 1997;75:189–93.
14. Chen AC, Dworkin SF, Haug J, Gehrig J. Topographic brain measures of human pain and pain responsivity. Pain. 1989;37:129–41.
15. Murrell JC, Johnson CB. Neurophysiological techniques to assess pain in animals. J Vet Pharmacol Ther. 2006;29:325–35. Blackwell Publishing Ltd
16. Kongara K, McIlhone A, Kells N, Johnson C. Electroencephalographic evaluation of decapitation of the anaesthetized rat. Lab Anim. 2014;48:15–9. SAGE Publications
17. Fu S, Tar MT, Melman A, Davies KP. Opiorphin is a master regulator of the hypoxic response in corporal smooth muscle cells. FASEB J. 2014;28:3633–44.
18. Parle M, Yadav M. Laboratory models for screening analgesics. Int Res J Pharm. 2013;4:15–9.
19. Valverde, A., Dyson, D.H., McDonnell, W.N., 1989. Epidural morphine reduces halothane MAC in the dog. Can. J. Anaesth. 36, 629–632.
20. Littell, R.C., Henry, P.R., Ammerman, C.B., 1998. Statistical analysis of repeated measures data using SAS procedures. J. Anim. Sci. 76, 1216–1231.
21. Ludwig O. Blom, Gunnar: statistical estimates and transformed beta-variables. Wiley/New York, Almquist und Wiksell/Stockholm 1958. Biom J. 1961;3:285.
22. van Dorp ELA, Yassen A, Dahan A. Naloxone treatment in opioid addiction: the risks and benefits. Expert Opin Drug Saf. 2007;6:125–32.
23. Sora I, Takahashi N, Funada M, Ujike H, Revay RS, Donovan DM, et al. Opiate receptor knockout mice define mu receptor roles in endogenous nociceptive responses and morphine-induced analgesia. Proc Natl Acad Sci U S A. 1997;94:1544–9. National Acad Sciences
24. Banks WA. Peptides and the blood-brain barrier. Peptides. 2015;72:16–9.
25. Bocsik A, Darula Z, Tóth G, Deli MA, Wollemann M. Transfer of opiorphin through a blood-brain barrier culture model. Arch Med Res. 2015;46:502–6.

26. Winkler EA, Sengillo JD, Bell RD, Wang J, Zlokovic BV. Blood-spinal cord barrier pericyte reductions contribute to increased capillary permeability. J Cereb Blood Flow Metab. 2012;32:1841–52. SAGE Publications
27. Antognini JF, Atherley R, Carstens E. Isoflurane action in spinal cord indirectly depresses cortical activity associated with electrical stimulation of the reticular formation. Anesth Analg. 2003;96:999–1003. tableofcontents
28. Antognini JF, Wang XW, Carstens E. Isoflurane action in the spinal cord blunts electroencephalographic and thalamic-reticular formation responses to noxious stimulation in goats. Anesthesiology. 2000;92:559–66.
29. Benoist J-M, Keime F, Montagne J, Noble F, Fournié-Zaluski M-C, Roques BP, et al. Depressant effect on a C-fibre reflex in the rat, of RB101, a dual inhibitor of enkephalin-degrading enzymes. Eur J Pharmacol. 2002;445:201–10.
30. Harris JA. Using c-fos as a neural marker of pain. Brain Res Bull. 1998;45:1–8.
31. Le Guen S, Noble F, Fournié-Zaluski M-C, Roques BP, Besson J-M, Buritova J. RB101(S), a dual inhibitor of enkephalinases does not induce antinociceptive tolerance, or cross-tolerance with morphine: a c-Fos study at the spinal level. Eur J Pharmacol. 2002;441:141–50.
32. Kim SJ, Calejesan AA, Li P, Wei F, Zhuo M. Sex differences in late behavioral response to subcutaneous formalin injection in mice. Brain Res. 1999; 829:185–9.
33. Gaumond I, Arsenault P, Marchand S. The role of sex hormones on formalin-induced nociceptive responses. Brain Res. 2002;958:139–45.
34. Kayser V, Berkley KJ, Keita H, Gautron M, Guilbaud G. Estrous and sex variations in vocalization thresholds to hindpaw and tail pressure stimulation in the rat. Brain Res. 1996;742:352–4.
35. Stoffel EC, Ulibarri CM, Craft RM. Gonadal steroid hormone modulation of nociception, morphine antinociception and reproductive indices in male and female rats. Pain. 2003;103:285–302.
36. Tesfaye S. PL37: a new hope in the treatment of painful diabetic neuropathy? Pain Management. 2016;6:129–32. Future Medicine Ltd London, UK

20

Atypical central retinal artery occlusion as the first presentation of POEMS syndrome

Panitha Jindahra[1], Charungthai Dejthevaporn[1], Pimjai Niparuck[1], Jariya Waisayarat[2], Piyaphon Cheecharoen[3], Thanatporn Threetong[4], Purit Petpiroon[4], Tharikarn Sujirakul[4], Anuchit Poonyathalang[4] and Kavin Vanikieti[4*]

Abstract

Background: POEMS syndrome is a plasma cell disorder, which clinically manifests from paraneoplastic syndrome: polyneuropathy, organomegaly, endocrinopathy, monoclonal plasma cell disorder, and skin changes. The most common ocular manifestation is optic disc swelling, whereas other ocular manifestations; cystoid macular edema, serous macular detachment, venous sinus thrombosis, infiltrative orbitopathy, uveitis, neovascularization of the disc, peripapillary choroidal neovascularization and optic disc drusen, had also been reported.

Case presentation: A 52-year-old Thai man presented with 5-day sudden painless visual loss in the left eye. Ocular examination revealed visual acuity of 20/20 and no light perception in the right and left eye, respectively. Right fundoscopic examination was significant for hyperemic generalized optic disc swelling. Left fundoscopic examination revealed opaque and edematous entire retina giving the appearance of central retinal artery occlusion (CRAO) along with pallid "chalky white" optic disc swelling. Fluorescein angiography showed profound leakage of bilateral optic nerve heads and arteriolar filling defect in macular area along with leakage of small retinal arterioles in the left eye. Indocyanine green angiography demonstrated choroidal filling defect in the left eye only. Neuroimaging showed enhancement and luminal narrowing of left internal carotid artery, early subacute watershed infarctions in the left cerebral hemisphere and pachymeningeal enhancement. Cerebrospinal fluid analysis revealed high protein level with normal opening pressure. Intravenous methylprednisolone was initially started without any benefit. After extensive investigations, diagnosis of "POEMS syndrome" was made based on polyneuropathy, elevated lambda light chain level, elevated plasma vascular endothelial growth factor (VEGF), hepatomegaly, spinal sclerotic bone lesions, and thrombocytosis. Furthermore, sural nerve biopsy demonstrated neuropathy and positive VEGF staining. He was treated with eight cycles of bortezomib, cyclophosphamide and dexamethasone (BorCyDex). Polyneuropathy and thrombocytosis had remarkably improved after 2nd cycle, whereas, visual impairment had shown no recovery. Hepatomegaly was significantly reduced after the completion of BorCyDex. Our case eventually received autologous hematopoietic stem cell transplantation with high dose melphalan.

Conclusions: To our knowledge, we illustrated the first patient given CRAO as the first presentation and ocular finding ever reported in POEMS syndrome. Both cerebral and ocular infarctions were presumably the result of VEGF-induced cranial vasculopathy as evidenced by neuroimaging.

Keywords: POEMS syndrome, Central retinal artery occlusion, Anterior ischemic optic neuropathy, Visual loss

* Correspondence: vanikieti.kavin@gmail.com
[4]Department of Ophthalmology, Faculty of Medicine Ramathibodi Hospital, Mahidol University, 270 Rama VI Road, Bangkok 10400, Thailand
Full list of author information is available at the end of the article

Background

POEMS syndrome is a plasma cell disorder, which clinically manifests from paraneoplastic syndrome: polyneuropathy, organomegaly, endocrinopathy, monoclonal plasma cell disorder, and skin changes [1]. The most common ocular manifestation is optic disc swelling, whereas other ocular manifestations; cystoid macular edema (CME), serous macular detachment, venous sinus thrombosis, infiltrative orbitopathy, uveitis, neovascularization of the disc (NVD), peripapillary choroidal neovascularization and optic disc drusen, had also been reported [2–12]. To our knowledge, central retinal artery occlusion has never been reported in POEMS syndrome. We herein describe the first reported patient with POEMS syndrome who initially presented with atypical central retinal artery occlusion.

Case presentations

A 52-year-old Thai man presented with sudden painless visual loss in his left eye upon awakening 5 days prior to presentation. He had no visual complaints regarding his right eye. He reported no fever, jaw claudication, general malaise, anorexia, hearing of a whooshing sound, or new-onset headache. His ocular history was significant for bilateral hyperopia. His medical history was notable for 18.5-kg body weight loss in the past 2 years. He was not taking any medications and was a nonsmoker.

Ocular examination revealed visual acuity of 20/20 and no light perception in the right eye and left eye, respectively. The presence of a grade 4+ relative afferent pupillary defect of the left eye was noted. The intraocular pressure was 15 mmHg bilaterally. Slit-lamp examination showed a mild cortical cataract without signs of ocular inflammation bilaterally. Fundoscopic examination of the left eye showed that the entire retina was opaque and edematous, particularly in the posterior pole, and pallid "chalky white" generalized optic disc swelling was noted (Fig. 1b). Neither emboli nor cotton-wool spots were detected. Fundoscopic examination of the right eye was significant only for hyperemic generalized optic disc swelling; no hemorrhage, cotton-wool spots, or exudates were present (Fig. 1a).

A color vision test (Lanthony desaturated 15-hue test) of the right eye was unremarkable. The Humphrey 24-2 automated static perimetry program of the right eye showed blind spot enlargement. The average retinal nerve fiber layer thickness of the optic nerve head measured by

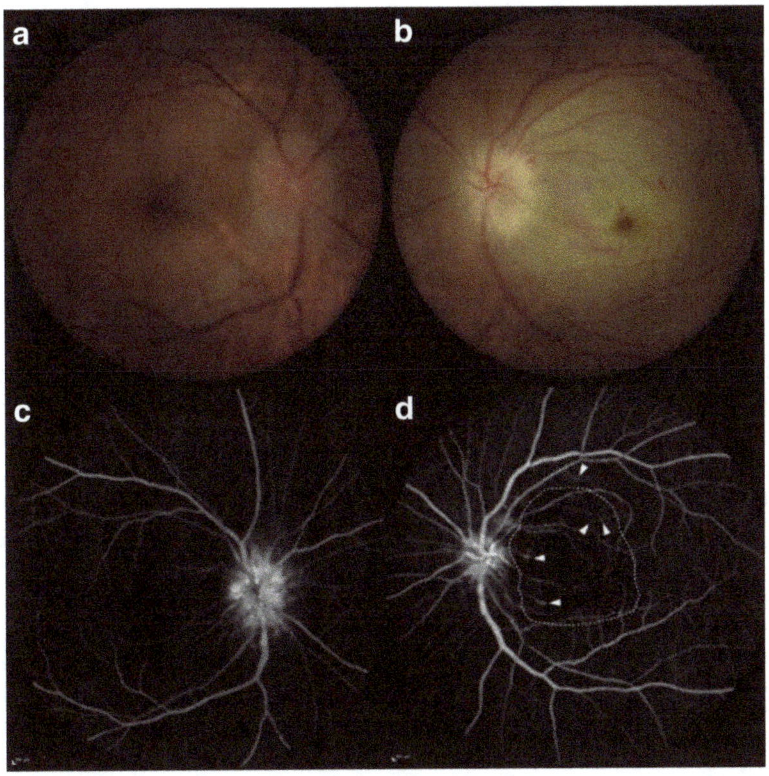

Fig. 1 Fundus photograph and fundus fluorescein angiography. **a** Hyperemic and generalized optic disc swelling is observed in the right eye. **b** An opaque and edematous retina in the posterior pole along with pallid "chalky white" generalized optic disc swelling is demonstrated in the left eye. **c** Fundus fluorescein angiography showing profound leakage of the optic nerve head in the right eye. **d** Leakage of the optic nerve head, filling defects in multiple arterioles predominantly in the macular area (*area within the dashed lines*), and leakage of small retinal arterioles (*arrowheads*) are observed in the left eye

spectral-domain optical coherence tomography (Cirrus HD-OCT, software version 6.0.0.599; Carl Zeiss Meditec, Inc., Dublin, CA, USA) was 554 and 187 μm in the right and left eye, respectively. Fundus fluorescein angiography (FFA) revealed profound leakage of the bilateral optic nerve heads, and filling defects were observed in multiple arterioles, predominantly in the macular area of the left eye, along with leakage of small retinal arterioles in the left eye (Fig. 1c, d). No filling defect or retinal vessel leakage was noted in the right eye. Indocyanine green angiography (ICG) demonstrated a choroidal filling defect in the left eye only. Partial occlusion of both retinal and choroidal circulation in the left eye was suspected. An electroretinogram (ERG) was evaluated according to the International Society for Clinical Electrophysiology of Vision standard (MonColor; Metrovision, Perenchies, France). A full-field ERG of the left eye showed a significant reduction of both the a-wave and b-wave amplitude, along with a decreased b:a ratio with a normal implicit time in the photopic and maximal combined responses, confirming both retinal and choroidal circulation in the left eye was affected. An ERG of the right eye was normal. Both sides of the superficial temporal artery were pulsatile and painless. The patient's blood pressure was 130/80 mmHg. A provisional diagnosis of atypical central retinal artery occlusion (CRAO) with anterior ischemic optic neuropathy (AION) in the left eye in conjunction with generalized right optic disc swelling was made. Treatment was started with intravenous methylprednisolone at 1 g once daily for 5 days.

A complete blood count showed 5.7×10^9/L white blood cells with 76% neutrophils; the platelet count was 595×10^9/L, and the hemoglobin level was 17.3 g/dL. The erythrocyte sedimentation rate was 9 mm/h, and the C-reactive protein level was 1.14 mg/L. The results of a comprehensive vasculitis panel, including measurement of antinuclear antibody, cytoplasmic antineutrophil cytoplasmic antibodies, perinuclear antineutrophil cytoplasmic antibodies, and anti-double-stranded DNA, were within normal limits. The results of the serum Venereal Disease Research Laboratory (VDRL) test, *Treponema pallidum* hemagglutination (TPHA) test, and anti-human immunodeficiency virus antibody test were negative. A metabolic panel, including liver function tests, the fasting blood sugar level, and a lipid profile, was unremarkable. Antiphospholipid antibodies were negative. The results of a coagulation panel were within normal limits.

Magnetic resonance imaging (MRI) of the brain with gadolinium injection revealed early subacute left anterior cerebral artery/middle cerebral artery watershed infarction, early subacute left middle cerebral artery/posterior cerebral artery watershed infarction, and marked pachymeningeal thickening with enhancement of the bilateral cerebral convexities (Fig. 2d). Diffusion weighted imaging (DWI) of the brain showed restricted diffusion involving gray-white matter of the left parietal lobe and centrum semiovale. Moreover, enhancement and luminal narrowing of the petrous and supraclinoid left internal carotid artery (ICA) were observed (Fig. 2a–c). The bilateral optic nerves showed a normal size and signal intensity. Magnetic resonance angiography (MRA) revealed luminal narrowing from the distal cervical left ICA extending to the supraclinoid left ICA. The patient was treated with aspirin. Echocardiography and electrocardiography showed normal results.

A lumbar puncture was then performed, and 6 mL of clear cerebrospinal fluid (CSF) was obtained with an opening pressure of 19 cmH_2O. CSF analysis revealed a significantly high protein level (234.6 mg/dL), normal glucose concentration (61 mg/dL), and white cell count of 4 cells/mm^3 (100% mononuclear cells). The VDRL test, TPHA test, polymerase chain reaction (PCR), and cultures for microorganisms were all negative in the CSF.

No clinical improvement was demonstrated during the 5-day course of methylprednisolone, and patient developed numbness in both feet.

Serum protein electrophoresis revealed no hypergammaglobulinemia, whereas, an IgGλ monoclonal gammopathy was detected by serum immunofixation electrophoresis (Fig. 3a). In addition, computed tomography (CT) of the whole spine showed multiple mixed lytic osteosclerotic bone lesions involving the T8 and L1 bodies (Fig. 3b), bilateral 8th ribs, right ilium, and right sacrum.

A more comprehensive systemic examination showed a symmetrical decrease in the motor power of the bilateral extensor hallucis longus and a symmetrical decrease in sensation (including proprioception, vibration, pain, and temperature) of both feet. The Achilles and patellar reflexes were absent bilaterally. A nerve conduction study also revealed sensory and motor demyelinating polyneuropathy. The Romberg sign was positive and steppage gait was noted. Moreover, hepatomegaly was observed on a CT scan of the whole abdomen, and localized hypertrichosis associated with hyperpigmentation involving the dorsal aspect of both feet was noted (Fig. 3c).

A diagnosis of POEMS syndrome was made. The levels of hormones, plasma interleukin-6, and plasma vascular endothelial growth factor (VEGF) were measured and PCR for human herpesvirus type 8 in serum was performed to support this diagnosis. The interleukin-6 level was < 1.5 pg/mL (reference range, 0–7 pg/mL), and the plasma VEGF level was 1828 pg/mL (reference range, 0–860 pg/mL). PCR for human herpesvirus type 8 in serum was negative. The levels of hormones, including testosterone, free T3, free T4, thyroid-stimulating hormone, and cortisol, were normal.

A bone marrow biopsy demonstrated normocellular bone marrow; adequate red cells, white cells, and platelets; and scattered plasma cells. CD138 immunohistochemistry showed only 5% plasma cells.

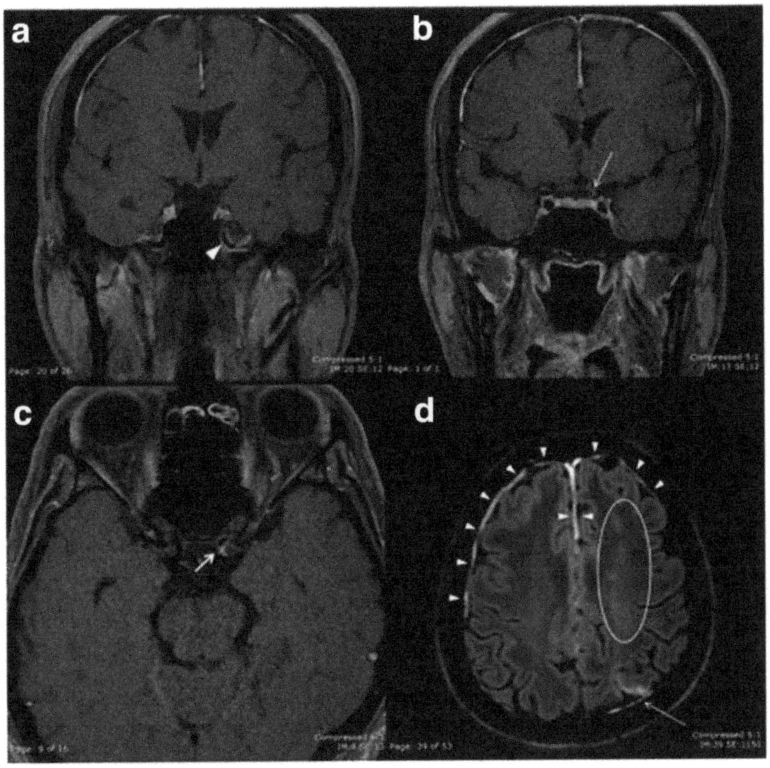

Fig. 2 Magnetic resonance imaging of the brain with gadolinium injection. **a**, **b** Coronal T1-weighted images with gadolinium injection showing enhancement and luminal narrowing of the petrous (*arrowhead*) and supraclinoid (*arrow*) left internal carotid artery. **c** Axial T1-weighted image with gadolinium injection showing enhancement and luminal narrowing of the supraclinoid (*arrow*) left internal carotid artery. **d** Axial fluid attenuation inversion recovery (FLAIR) image with gadolinium injection showing early subacute left anterior cerebral artery/middle cerebral artery watershed infarction (*area within the circle*), early subacute left middle cerebral artery/posterior cerebral artery watershed infarction (*arrow*), and marked pachymeningeal thickening with enhancement of the bilateral cerebral convexities (*arrowheads*)

Sural nerve biopsy was also undertaken and demonstrated neuropathy through slightly decreased myelinated fibers density (Fig. 3d). Mild to moderately increased small vessels in epineurium led to the diagnosis of POEMS syndrome, which confirmed by a positive VEGF (Fig. 3e). There was no evidence of vasculitis or amyloidosis. The patient was treated with eight cycles of bortezomib, cyclophosphamide, and dexamethasone (BorCyDex). After the 2nd cycle of BorCyDex, the polyneuropathy had remarkably improved and the platelet count returned to normal; however, the visual loss in the left eye was still present. Disease assessment was performed after the 4th and 8th cycles of BorCyDex. CSF was obtained and showed high protein levels (200 and 150 mg/dL after the 4th and 8th cycle of treatment, respectively). Hepatomegaly was significantly reduced based on CT. After eight cycles of BorCyDex, the patient finally underwent autologous hematopoietic stem cell transplantation with high-dose melphalan.

Discussion and conclusions

Our patient was diagnosed with POEMS syndrome based on demyelinating polyneuropathy, lambda light chain-restricted monoclonal plasma cell proliferative disorder, sclerotic bone lesions, plasma VEGF elevation, hepatomegaly, hypertrichosis associated with hyperpigmentation, thrombocytosis, and bilateral optic disc swelling [1].

To our knowledge, this is the first reported patient with POEMS syndrome to exhibit CRAO as the first presentation. Optic disc swelling is the most common ocular finding and occurs in 52.0 to 67.5% of affected patients [2, 3].

Other ocular manifestations reported in the literature include cystoid macular edema [4–6], serous macular detachment [7, 8], venous sinus thrombosis [9], infiltrative orbitopathy [10], uveitis [11], neovascularization of the disc [10], peripapillary choroidal neovascularization, and optic disc drusen [12].

Our patient was considered to have atypical CRAO given the demonstration of small retinal arteriole leakage on FFA, association with AION, and contralateral generalized optic disc swelling.

Our hypothesis regarding the mechanism causing leakage of small retinal arterioles on FFA in the present case is microvascular hyperpermeability induced by an increased plasma VEGF level. VEGF is thought to be the major contributor to various manifestations of POEMS syndrome, including ocular findings [1, 2, 6, 13].

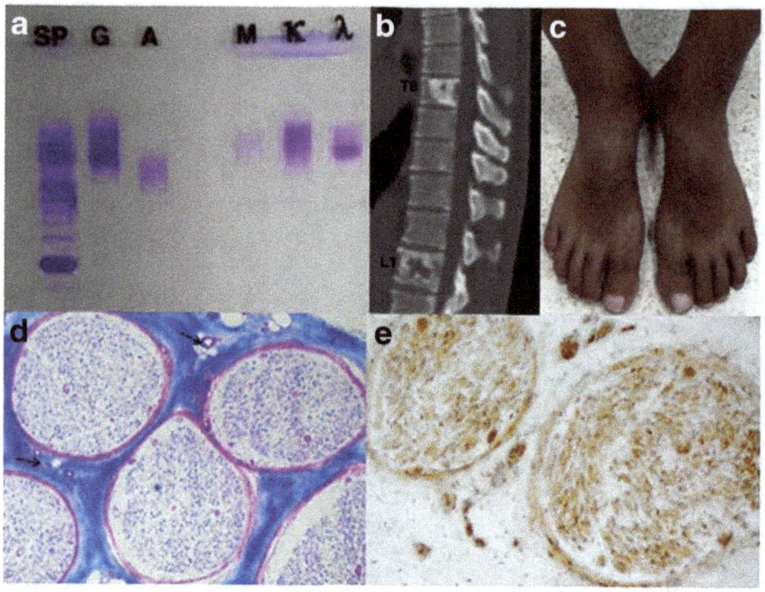

Fig. 3 Serum immunofixation electrophoresis, computed tomography of the spine, external appearance of both feet, and sural nerve biopsy. **a** Serum immunofixation electrophoresis showing an IgGλ monoclonal gammopathy. **b** Computed tomography of the spine with contrast showing multiple mixed lytic osteosclerotic bone lesions involving the T8 and L1 bodies. **c** Localized hypertrichosis associated with hyperpigmentation involving the dorsal aspect of both feet. Sural nerve biopsy showing neuropathy through slightly decreased myelinated fibers density with mild to moderate increase of small vessels in epineurium (arrows) (**d**: Luxol Fast Blue staining, 100×) and positive VEGF staining (**e**: VEGF staining, 200×)

The association with AION was the second atypical characteristic of CRAO in this case. The typical pallid "chalky white" generalized optic disc swelling led us to highly suspect paraoptic short posterior ciliary artery involvement. Inability to perceive light was caused by acute ischemia of not only the retina but also the optic nerve, which is supplied by the choroidal circulation. This was confirmed by a full-field ERG, which showed a significant reduction in both the a-wave and b-wave amplitude. Moreover, indocyanine green angiography of the left eye revealed a choroidal filling defect, consistent with short posterior ciliary artery occlusion. Ophthalmic artery occlusion was the most likely explanation for the ischemia of both the retina and optic nerve. This was supported by the findings of luminal narrowing of the left ICA on MRI and MRA.

The last atypical characteristic of CRAO was the generalized optic disc swelling in the right eye. Given the well-preserved visual function of the right eye despite the appearance of marked swelling of the optic disc, arteritic AION of the right eye was less of a concern. Considering the normal CSF opening pressure, the cause of the optic disc swelling in the right eye was probably microvascular hyperpermeability induced by the increased plasma VEGF level. This speculation is consistent with many previous reports [1, 2, 6, 13]. However, the pathophysiology of optic disc swelling remains unclear.

Cerebral infarctions in patients with POEMS syndrome have been previously described [14–18]. The area of infarction varies and may include the end arteries, watershed areas, and cervical and proximal intracranial vasculature [14]. Potential etiologies remain inconclusive. Dupont et al. [14] reported that an elevated platelet count and evidence of plasma cell proliferation on bone marrow biopsy lead to an increased risk of ischemic stroke. These findings are consistent with the present case.

In our patient, vasculopathy of the left ICA based on MRI and MRA could explain both the cerebral infarctions and the CRAO associated with AION. Moreover, hyperviscosity secondary to thrombocytosis was thought to be the synergic risk factor that led to the arterial thrombosis events.

Arterial walls enhancement has rarely been reported. Fu et al. [18] described a patient with POEMS syndrome who developed multiple acute watershed infarctions of the left cerebral hemisphere associated with enhancement and luminal narrowing of the ipsilateral ICA. These findings were similar to those in our patient. Moreover, generalized cranial pachymeningeal involvement was observed in our patient. This is consistent with a previous study reported by Briani et al. [19], who described nine patients with POEMS syndrome who showed pachymeningeal thickening with intense enhancement. Furthermore, two of nine patients showed hyperplasia of meningothelial cells, neovascularization, noninflammatory obstructive vessel remodeling, and strong coexpression of VEGF and VEGF receptor on meningeal biopsy. These findings suggest that VEGF might be a major contributor in the pathogenesis of pachymeningeal involvement in POEMS syndrome. We speculate that the possible cause of arterial wall enhancement might be similar to that of VEGF-induced pachymeningeal enhancement. However, we did not perform a biopsy of any affected vasculature or meninges.

With respect to the vasculopathy of the left ICA based on MRI and MRA and leakage of the bilateral optic nerve heads and small retinal arterioles in the left eye on FFA, our patient demonstrated involvement of all sizes of affected arterial vessels ranging from the distal cervical ICA to small retinal arterioles. Elevation of the plasma VEGF level is proposed to be the major contributor to these abnormalities.

Sural nerve biopsy is recommended at baseline if clinically indicated [1]. Symmetrical decrease in sensation of both feet was exhibited in our patient. This was supported by a nerve conduction study, which revealed sensory demyelinating polyneuropathy. Similarly, a reduction in the myelinated fiber population was revealed pathologically. In addition, VEGF overexpression and VEGF-related proliferation of endothelial cells as evidenced by the biopsy supported the diagnosis of POEMS syndrome [1].

In conclusion, we have herein reported the first patient with CRAO as the initial presentation and ocular finding of POEMS syndrome. The mechanism of occlusion remains unclear due to its rarity. Further studies are needed to determine the definite pathophysiology.

Abbreviations

AION: Anterior ischemic optic neuropathy; BorCyDex: Bortezomib, cyclophosphamide, and dexamethasone; CME: Cystoid macular edema; CRAO: Central retinal artery occlusion; CSF: Cerebrospinal fluid; CT: Computed tomography; ERG: Electroretinogram; FFA: Fundus fluorescein angiography; ICA: Internal carotid artery; ICG: Indocyanine green angiography; MRA: Magnetic resonance angiography; MRI: Magnetic resonance imaging; NVD: Neovascularization of the disc; PCR: Polymerase chain reaction; TPHA: *Treponema pallidum* hemagglutination; VDRL: Venereal disease research laboratory; VEGF: Vascular endothelial growth factor

Acknowledgements

We thank Angela Morben, DVM, ELS, from Edanz Group (www.edanzediting.com/ac), for editing a draft of this manuscript.

Authors' contributions

Study conception: PJ, KV, AP, and TT. Study design: KV, AP, and TT. Data acquisition: PJ and KV. Data analysis: KV, CD, PJ, PN, JW, PC, PP, and TS. Data interpretation: KV, CD, PJ, PN, JW, PC, PP, and TS. Drafting of the paper: KV, AP, CD, PJ, PN, JW, PC, PP, TT, and TS. Critical revision of the paper: KV. Final approval for submission: KV, AP, CD, PJ, PN, JW, PC, PP, TT, and TS.

Competing interests

The authors do not have any competing interests in the publication of this case report.

Author details

[1]Department of Medicine, Faculty of Medicine Ramathibodi Hospital, Mahidol University, 270 Rama VI Road, Bangkok 10400, Thailand.
[2]Department of Pathology, Faculty of Medicine Ramathibodi Hospital, Mahidol University, 270 Rama VI Road, Bangkok 10400, Thailand.
[3]Department of Radiology, Faculty of Medicine Ramathibodi Hospital, Mahidol University, 270 Rama VI Road, Bangkok 10400, Thailand.
[4]Department of Ophthalmology, Faculty of Medicine Ramathibodi Hospital, Mahidol University, 270 Rama VI Road, Bangkok 10400, Thailand.

References

1. Dispenzieri A. POEMS syndrome: update on diagnosis, risk-stratification, and management. Am J Hematol. 2015;90:951–62.
2. Kaushik M, Pulido JS, Abreu R, Amselem L, Dispenzieri A. Ocular findings in patients with polyneuropathy, organomegaly, endocrinopathy, monoclonal gammopathy, and skin changes syndrome. Ophthalmology. 2011;118:778–82.
3. Zhang X, Cai QQ, Huang XF, Cao XX, Cai H, Zhou DB, Dai RP, Li J. Ocular manifestations and treatment outcomes in Chinese patients with poems syndrome. Retina. 2017;37:1784–91.
4. Imai H, Kusuhara S, Nakanishi Y, Escaño MF, Yamamoto H, Tsukahara Y, Negi A. A case of POEMS syndrome with cystoid macular edema. Am J Ophthalmol. 2005;139:563–6.
5. Prost MG, Gilhuis HJ, Brouwer RE, Gawda P. Local treatment with triamcinolone acetonide and bevacizumab for ocular symptoms in a patient with POEMS syndrome. Case Rep Ophthalmol. 2014;5:416–22.
6. Chong DY, Comer GM, Trobe JD. Optic disc edema, cystoid macular edema, and elevated vascular endothelial growth factor in a patient with POEMS syndrome. J Neuroophthalmol. 2007;27:180–3.
7. Ecsedy M, Schneider M, Nemes J, Nemeth J, Recsan Z. Optical coherence tomography features of POEMS syndrome and Castleman disease-associated papillopathy. Ocul Immunol Inflamm. 2014;22:454–60.
8. Kimura S, Morizane Y, Hosogi M, Hosokawa M, Shiode Y, Kawata T, Kondo E, Shiraga F. POEMS syndrome in a 20-year-old patient diagnosed following a complaint of reduced visual acuity. Acta Med Okayama. 2014;68:379–83.
9. Witoonpanich R, Phankhian S, Jootar S, Poonyathalang A, Worapongpaiboon S, Phudhichareonrat S, Chanplakorn N. POEMS syndrome with venous sinus thrombosis and visual failure: a case report. J Med Assoc Thail. 2005;88:690–4.
10. Bourdette DN, Rosenberg NL. Infiltrative orbitopathy, optic disk edema, and POEMS. Neurology. 1984;34:532–3.
11. Arnold PD, Kinyoun JL, Guzak SV. Poems syndrome: an unusual cause of neovascularization. Retina. 1999;19:166–8.
12. Diduszyn JM, Quillen DA, Cantore WA, Gardner TW. Optic disk drusen, peripapillary choroidal neovascularization, and POEMS syndrome. Am J Ophthalmol. 2002 Feb 28;133(2):275–6.
13. Rahimy E, Sarraf D. Paraneoplastic and non-paraneoplastic retinopathy and optic neuropathy: evaluation and management. Surv Ophthalmol. 2013 Oct 31;58(5):430–58.
14. Dupont SA, Dispenzieri A, Mauermann ML, Rabinstein AA, Brown RD. Cerebral infarction in POEMS syndrome incidence, risk factors, and imaging characteristics. Neurology. 2009;73:1308–12.
15. Kang K, Chu K, Kim DE, Jeong SW, Lee JW, Roh JK. POEMS syndrome associated with ischemic stroke. Arch Neurol. 2003;60:745–9.
16. Erro ME, Lacruz F, Aymerich N, Ayuso T, Soriano G, Gállego J, Villanueva JA. Acute carotid obliteration: a new vascular manifestation in POEMS syndrome. Eur J Neurol. 2003;10:383–4.
17. Garcia T, Dafer R, Hocker S, Schneck M, Barton K, Biller J. Recurrent strokes in two patients with POEMS syndrome and Castleman's disease. J Stroke Cerebrovasc Dis. 2007;16:278–84.
18. Fu FW, Rao J, Zheng YY, Wang HL, Yang JG, Zheng GQ. Ischemic stroke in patients with POEMS syndrome: a case report and comprehensive analysis of literature. Oncotarget. 2017;8:89406.
19. Briani C, Fedrigo M, Manara R, Castellani C, Zambello R, Citton V, Campagnolo M, Dalla Torre C, Lucchetta M, Orvieto E, Rotilio A. Pachymeningeal involvement in POEMS syndrome: MRI and histopathological study. J Neurol Neurosurg Psychiatry. 2012;83:33–7.

21

Hopkins syndrome following the first episode of bronchial asthma associated with enterovirus D68

Fumie Hayashi[1], Shintaro Hayashi[1], Dai Matsuse[1], Ryo Yamasaki[1], Keiji Yonekura[2] and Jun-ichi Kira[1*]

Abstract

Background: Hopkins syndrome (HS) is a rare disorder presenting with acute flaccid paralysis of the limbs following an asthma attack. Neurologists encounter a diagnostic challenge if patients without a history of bronchial asthma develop neurologic features mimicking HS following acute respiratory distress. We report a case of HS occurring after a first episode of bronchial asthma associated with enterovirus D68 infection.

Case presentation: A 5-year-old girl developed acute respiratory distress. On the fourth hospital day, both her legs became paralyzed except for slight muscle contraction in the right lower limb. Tendon reflexes in the lower limbs were diminished and there was a positive Babinski sign on the right. Sensation was normal in all modalities, and there was no uro-rectal disturbance. Spinal magnetic resonance imaging identified T2-hyperintense lesions with spinal cord edema, mainly involving the bilateral T11 to L1 anterior horns, with left side dominance extending to the left posterior horn. The neurological and neuro-radiological findings of our case were suggestive of HS; however, she had no history of bronchial asthma. An acetylcholine inhalation challenge eventually proved the presence of reversible airway hyper-responsiveness, allowing us to diagnose HS. We identified enterovirus D68 in the patient's intratracheal aspirates using a sensitive polymerase chain reaction assay. Intravenous immunoglobulin administrations at 2 g/kg^2 for 5 consecutive days were repeated every month up to four times. After these treatments, the muscle strength of her right lower limb slightly improved while her left lower leg remained completely paralyzed.

Conclusion: This case emphasizes the importance of provocation tests to reveal the presence of airway hyper-responsiveness when a child shows neurological signs mimicking HS following acute respiratory distress. Furthermore, the present case suggests a possible link between HS and acute flaccid paralysis following lower respiratory tract infection by enterovirus D68.

Keywords: Hopkins syndrome, Bronchial hyper-reactivity, Intravenous immunoglobulin, Enterovirus D68, First asthma attack

Background

Hopkins syndrome (HS) is a poliomyelitis-like illness that occurs acutely after an asthmatic attack. It was first reported in 1974 [1], and so far only about 40 cases have been reported. HS mostly affects children, typically occurs within several days to a few weeks following an acute asthmatic attack, and presents as flaccid paralysis of one or more extremities. Due to its rarity, the pathogenesis and effective therapy of HS remains to be elucidated. We report a case of HS occurring after a first episode of bronchial asthma (BA), associated with enterovirus D68 infection, in which the presence of airway hyper-responsiveness was confirmed by provocation tests.

* Correspondence: kira@neuro.med.kyushu-u.ac.jp
[1]Department of Neurology, Neurological Institute, Graduate School of Medical Sciences, Kyushu University, 3-1-1 Maidashi, Higashi-ku, Fukuoka 812-8582, Japan
Full list of author information is available at the end of the article

Case presentation

A healthy 5-year-old girl developed acute respiratory distress and became unconscious. On arrival at the Emergency Room, venous blood gas analysis showed type II respiratory failure and respiratory acidosis (pH 7.011, partial pressure of O_2 93.7 mmHg, partial pressure of CO_2 112.0 mmHg, serum bicarbonate concentration

27.0 mmol/l, base excess − 7.3 on room air). She was mechanically ventilated under midazolam sedation. Initially, anaphylactic shock of unknown origin was suspected. Epinephrine (0.03 mg/kg) was administered subcutaneously, leading to partial improvement in tidal volume. Serum immunoglobulin E (IgE) concentration was elevated (166 IU/ml, normal < 70 IU/ml for her age), and specific IgE to house dust mites was strongly positive (*Dermatophagoides pteronyssinus* 91.8 UA/ml; *Dermatophagoides farinae* > 100 UA/ml).

Although the patient had no history of BA, a first asthma attack was suspected, and methylprednisolone (2 mg/kg/day) and ampicillin/sulbactam (100 mg/kg/day) were given. Serologic tests for infection on the 2nd day after the onset of respiratory distress, including echovirus, enterovirus, coxsackievirus, poliovirus, herpes simplex virus, and *Mycoplasma* were negative. On the 4th day after symptom onset, she was weaned off mechanical ventilation and extubated. At this time, when her level of consciousness improved, her legs showed no paralysis. However, a few hours later when she woke from sleep, both her legs were paralyzed except for weak motor activity in the right anterior tibialis muscle. Patellar and Achilles tendon reflexes were diminished; there were no pathologic reflexes. Cerebrospinal fluid (CSF) analysis on the 21st day after symptom onset showed 7 cells/μl (100% mononuclear cells), elevated protein concentration (120 mg/dl, normal 15–40 mg/dl), and normal myelin basic protein concentration. Virus isolation culture did not detect any viruses in the CSF. Spinal magnetic resonance imaging (MRI) on the 21st day after symptom onset identified T2-hyperintense lesions with spinal cord edema, mainly involving the anterior horns bilaterally from T11 to L1, with left side dominance extending to the left posterior horn (Fig. 1). On the 23rd day after the onset, HS was suspected and intravenous immunoglobulin (IVIg) (400 mg/kg/day for 5 days) followed by intravenous methylprednisolone (30 mg/kg/day for 3 days) were administered, but there was no improvement over the next 3 weeks.

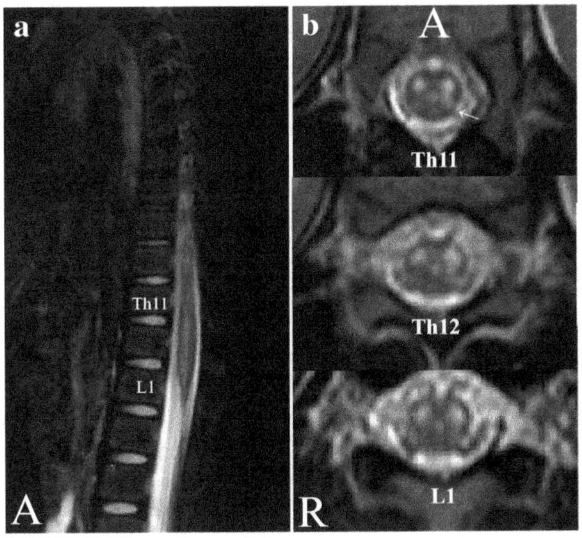

Fig. 1 **a** Sagittal T2-weighted magnetic resonance image showing a hyperintense lesion and spinal cord edema continuously from the T11 to L1 spinal levels; **b** axial T2-weighted images at T11, T12 and L1 show hyperintense lesions in both anterior horns, worse on the left, with left posterior horn involvement (arrow). Key: R, right; A, anterior

On the 47th day after symptom onset, she was transferred to our institution. She was alert and orientated, and her cranial nerves were intact. She had diffuse muscle atrophy in the left lower limb, with diminished tone but no fasciculation. Marked muscle weakness was evident in iliopsoas (Medical Research Council [MRC] scale grade right/left 0/0), the thigh adductors (0/0) and abductors (0/0), gluteus maximus (0/0), quadriceps femoris (0/0), biceps femoris (0/0), anterior tibialis (3/0), gastrocnemius (3/0), and dorsi- (3/0) and plantar-flexors of the toes (3/0). Tendon reflexes in the lower limbs were diminished. The Babinski sign was positive on the right. Sensation was normal in all modalities, and there was no uro-rectal disturbance. Complete blood count, including eosinophil count, blood biochemistry, coagulation status, and the concentrations of D-dimer, proteins S and C and lupus anticoagulant were normal. Serum myeloperoxidase and proteinase-3 anti-neutrophil cytoplasmic antibodies were negative, and autoantibodies against aquaporin-4 and phospholipid-bound β2–glycoprotein I were absent. Enterovirus D68 was detected in endotracheal aspirates (obtained on the 2nd day after symptom onset), but not in the CSF (obtained on the 21st day after onset), using a consensus-degenerate hybrid oligonucleotide primer polymerase chain reaction (PCR) method with direct sequencing,. Nerve conduction studies identified decreased compound muscle action potential amplitudes in the left tibial nerve (0.04 mV, normal > 2.9 mV). There was no evidence of arteriovenous malformation or arteriovenous fistula on spinal MR angiography. With parental permission, an acetylcholine (ACh) bronchial stimulation test was undertaken by a pulmonologist, which showed that inhalation of 5000 μg/ml ACh provoked wheezing and a rapid reduction in forced expiratory volume from 0.86 l/min to 0.50 l/min and a flow-volume loop typical of peripheral airway obstruction, both of which were reversed by 1.0 mg inhaled salbutamol. These findings were diagnostic of BA, and consequently HS.

Intravenous immunoglobulin 0.4 g/kg was administered for five consecutive days a month for 4 months, based on previous case reports showing its efficacy in HS [2, 3]. After treatment, power in the right anterior tibialis, dorsi- and plantar-flexors of the toes and gastrocnemius muscles improved to MRC grade 4, but power remained MRC grade 0 throughout the left lower limb. Spinal MRI undertaken on the 103rd day after symptom onset showed atrophy of the left anterior horn. She was transferred to another hospital for rehabilitation.

Discussion and conclusion

In this patient, airway hypersensitivity provoked by ACh inhalation and reversed by a β-adrenoreceptor agonist together with atopy to *Dermatophagoides* suggests that her episode of acute respiratory distress was the first manifestation of BA [4]. Consequently, we judge her diagnosis to be HS following a first episode of BA associated with enterovirus D68 infection. Besides flaccid paraparesis due to lumbar anterior horn cell involvement, the patient had right pyramidal tract signs and left posterior horn involvement on MRI. Involvement of the pyramidal tracts and posterior horns have also been reported in HS [5, 6].

Although the pathogenesis of HS is not understood, infectious and immune mechanisms are thought to be responsible [2, 5, 7, 8]. We identified enterovirus D68 in our patient's intratracheal aspirates using a sensitive assay, even though serum anti-enterovirus antibodies were negative. Intriguingly, a series of cases of acute flaccid paralysis was reported after an outbreak of lower respiratory tract infection by enterovirus D68 in the USA in 2014 [9, 10]. In a nationwide survey undertaken in Japan in 2015, three out of 205 individuals diagnosed with enterovirus D68 infection exhibited flaccid paralysis (one of whom was our patient) (https://www.niid.go.jp/niid/en/iasr-vol37-e/6283-inx432-e.html). Both our and the former cases [9, 10] are similar in that they showed severe paralysis and longitudinally extending spinal cord lesions of the central grey matter with predominant anterior horn involvement. However, the current case also had posterior horn involvement and no brainstem lesions, which distinguishes it from the cases with enterovirus D68 infection-related flaccid paralysis [9, 10]. Unfortunately, provocation tests to reveal the presence of airway hyper-responsiveness were not performed in any of the former cases with enterovirus D68 infection-related flaccid paralysis. Negative findings for enterovirus D68 in our patient's CSF do not support direct CNS invasion by the virus, but enterovirus D68 infection in the context of BA causing acute respiratory distress appears to have been the trigger for HS. The effectiveness of repeated IVIg in this case supports an immune-mediated mechanism for the pathogenesis of her flaccid myelitis, although the natural progression of the disease course is also a plausible explanation for her limited amelioration.

Alternatively, it is possible that the patient developed acute flaccid paralysis in the context of enterovirus D68 respiratory infection, which became particularly severe because she had asthma. Even in this case, we consider that IVIg administration is reasonable for treating acute flaccid paralysis caused by EVD68. IVIg contains neutralizing antibodies to EVD68 [11, 12] and has been shown to be effective in experimental animal infection by EVD68 [13] and in a patient with acute flaccid myelitis associated with EVD 68 infection [14]. Thus, the diagnosis of asthma is not pre-requisite for deciding the indication of immunotherapy in the present, and similar, cases.

Given that a number of viruses can cause respiratory illness, to perform PCR targeting for enterovirus D68 in all patients with solely respiratory symptoms might not be acceptable to all clinicians. However, to detect enterovirus D68 prior to full development of paralysis is of great significance to avoid devastating sequelae, as seen in our patient and previously reported children with enterovirus D68 infection-related flaccid paralysis [9, 10]. Therefore, evaluating the presence of enterovirus D68 and strain differences [14] in both the CSF and intratracheal aspirates from patients with respiratory illness followed by paralysis is warranted in future to clarify any pathogenic roles. Additionally, development of more sensitive assays to detect enterovirus D68 in CSF may further illuminate the involvement of enterovirus D68 in HS.

Abbreviations

ACh: Acetylcholine; BA: Bronchial asthma; CSF: Cerebrospinal fluid; HS: Hopkins syndrome; IgE: Immunoglobulin E; IVIg: Intravenous immunoglobulin; MRC: Medical Research Council; MRI: Magnetic resonance imaging; PCR: Primer polymerase chain reaction

Acknowledgements

The authors thank Edanz Group Japan for the English language review.

Authors' contributions

FH analyzed the data and drafted the manuscript; KY acquired clinical data and drafted the manuscript; SH, DM and RY conceptualized and revised the manuscript; JK drafted and revised the manuscript critically, and gave final approval of the version to be published. All authors read and approved the final manuscript.

Competing interests

The authors declare that they have no competing interests.

Author details

[1]Department of Neurology, Neurological Institute, Graduate School of Medical Sciences, Kyushu University, 3-1-1 Maidashi, Higashi-ku, Fukuoka 812-8582, Japan. [2]Department of Pediatrics, Kure Medical center, Hiroshima, Japan.

References

1. Hopkins IJ. Poliomyelitis-like illness associated with asthma in childhood. Lancet. 1974;1:760.
2. Cantarín-Extremera V, González-Gutiérrez-Solana L, Ramírez-Orellana M, López-Marín L, Duat-Rodríguez A, Ruíz-Falcó-Rojas ML. Immune-mediated mechanisms in the pathogenesis of Hopkins syndrome. Pediatr Neurol. 2012;47:373–4. https://doi.org/10.1016/j.pediatrneurol.2012.08.006
3. Cohen HA, Ashkenasi A, Ring H, Weiss R, Wolach B, Paret G, Barzilai A. Poliomyelitis-like syndrome following asthmatic attack (Hopkins' syndrome) –recovery associated with i.v. gamma globulin treatment. Infection. 1998;26: 247–9. http://www.ncbi.nlm.nih.gov/pubmed/9717685
4. Arakawa H, Hamasaki Y, Kohno Y, Ebisawa M. Allergology international Japanese guidelines for childhood asthma 2017. Allergol Int. 2017;66:190–204. https://doi.org/10.1016/j.alit.2016.11.003
5. Yeung SCM, Antonio G, Ip KS. Flaccid paralysis of the limbs after an asthmatic attack. Pediatr Neurol. 2010;42:133–6. https://doi.org/10.1016/j.pediatrneurol.2009.09.013
6. Piero P, Longo MR, Scalia F, Polosa R, Kira JI, Falsaperla R. Recurrent Hopkin's syndrome: a case report and review of the literature. J Neurol Sci. 2010;297: 89–91. https://doi.org/10.1016/j.jns.2010.07.005
7. Mizuno Y. Poliomyelitis-like illness after acute asthma (Hopkins syndrome)- a histological study of biopsied muscle in a case. Brain and Development. 1995;17:126–9.
8. Manson JI. Immunological abnormalities in the syndrome of poliomyelitis-like illness associated with acute bronchial asthma (Hopkins' syndrome). Arch Dis Child. 1980;55:26–32.
9. Greninger AL, Naccache SN, Messacar K, Clayton A, Yu G, Somasekar S, Federman S, Stryke D, Anderson C, Yagi S, Messenger S, Wadford D, Xia D, Watt JP, Van Haren K, Dominguez SR, Glaser C, Aldrovandi G, Chiu CY. A novel outbreak enterovirus D68 strain associated with acute flaccid myelitis cases in the USA (2012-14): a retrospective cohort study. Lancet Infect Dis. 2015;15:671–82. https://doi.org/10.1016/S1473-3099(15)70093-9
10. Messacar K, Schreiner TL, Maloney JA, Wallace A, Ludke J, Oberste MS, Nix WA, Robinson CC, Glodé MP, Abzug MJ, Dominguez SR. A cluster of acute flaccid paralysis and cranial nerve dysfunction temporally associated with an outbreak of enterovirus D68 in children in Colorado, USA. Lancet. 2015;385: 1662–71.
11. Arora R, Kaplan M, Nelson M. Enterovirus-specific IgG in intravenous immunoglobulin preparations. J Clin Virol. 2015;106:172–5. https://doi.org/10.1016/S1473-3099(18)30094-X
12. Zhang Y, Moore DD, Nix WA, Oberste MS, Weldon WC. Neutralization of enterovirus D68 isolated from the 2014 US outbreak by commercial intravenous immune globulin products. J Clin Virol. 2015;69:172–5. https://doi.org/10.1016/j.jcv.2015.06.086
13. Hixon AM, Clarke P, Tyler KL. Evaluating treatment efficacy in a mouse model of enterovirus D68-associated paralytic myelitis. J Infect Dis. 2017;216: 1245–53.
14. Esposito S, Chidini G, Cinnante C, Napolitano L, Giannini A, Terranova L. Acute flaccid myelitis associated with enterovirus-D68 infection in an otherwise healthy child. Virol J. 2017;14:1–5. https://doi.org/10.1186/s12985-016-0678-0

22

A heterozygous deletion (2791_2805 del) in exon 18 of the filamin C gene causing filamin C-related myofibrillar myopathies in a Chinese family

Jing Miao[1†], Fei-fei Su[1†], Xue-mei Liu[1], Xiao-jing Wei[1], Yun Yuan[2] and Xue-fan Yu[3*]

Abstract

Background: Filamin C-related myofibrillar myopathies (MFM) are progressive skeletal myopathies with an autosomal dominant inheritance pattern. The conditions are caused by mutations of the filamin C gene (*FLNC*) located in the chromosome 7q32-q35 region. Genetic variations in the *FLNC* gene result in various clinical phenotypes.

Case presentation: We describe a 43-year-old woman who suffered filamin C-related MFM, with symptoms first presenting in the proximal muscles of the lower limbs and eventually spreading to the upper limbs and distal muscles. The patient's serum level of creatine kinase was mildly increased. Mildy myopathic changes in the electromyographic exam and moderate lipomatous alterations in lower limb MRI were found. Histopathological examination revealed increased muscle fiber size variability, disturbances in oxidative enzyme activity, and the presence of abnormal protein aggregates and vacuoles in some muscle fibers. Ultrastructural analysis showed inclusions composed of thin filaments and interspersed granular densities. DNA sequencing analysis detected a novel 15-nucleotide deletion (c.2791_2805del, p.931_935del) in the *FLNC* gene. The patient's father, sister, brother, three paternal aunts, one paternal uncle, and the uncle's son also had slowly progressive muscle weakness, and thus, we detected an autosomal dominant inheritance pattern of the disorder.

Conclusions: A novel heterogeneous 15-nucleotide deletion (c.2791_2805del, p.931_935del) in the Ig-like domain 7 of the *FLNC* gene was found to cause filamin C-related MFM. This deletion in the *FLNC* gene causes protein aggregation, abnormalities in muscle structure, and impairment in muscle fiber function, which leads to muscle weakness.

Keywords: Deletion, Filamin C gene, Dominant, Myofibrillar myopathy, Case report

Background

Filamin C-related myofibrillar myopathies (MFM) caused by mutations in the filamin C gene (*FLNC*) are autosomal dominant inherited and characterized by progressive myopathies that eventually result in wheelchair dependence. The *FLNC* gene is located in the 7q32-q35 chromosome band and includes 48 coding exons. To date, a continually increasing number of mutations in the *FLNC* gene have been reported in various populations worldwide. Among these mutations, codon 2710 is a mutational hotspot [1]. Mutations in different functional domains of filamins can cause various clinical phenotypes [2, 3]. Most patients with mutations in FLNC-Ig-like domains 7, 22, and 24 present with weakness in limb-girdle muscles, cardiomyopathy, and typical protein aggregation [1, 2, 4, 5], while those with mutations in the actin-binding domains or Ig-like domain 15 mostly present with weakness in the distal muscles and no cardiomyopathy or typical pathology [6, 7]. Here, we report a Chinese family suffering from filamin-C-related MFM caused by a novel 15-bp deletion in exon 18 of the *FLNC* gene.

* Correspondence: dr_yuxuefan@126.com
†Jing Miao and Fei-fei Su contributed equally to this work.
[3]Department of Neurology and Neuroscience Center First Affiliated Hospital of Jilin University, Changchun, 130021 Jilin, People's Republic of China

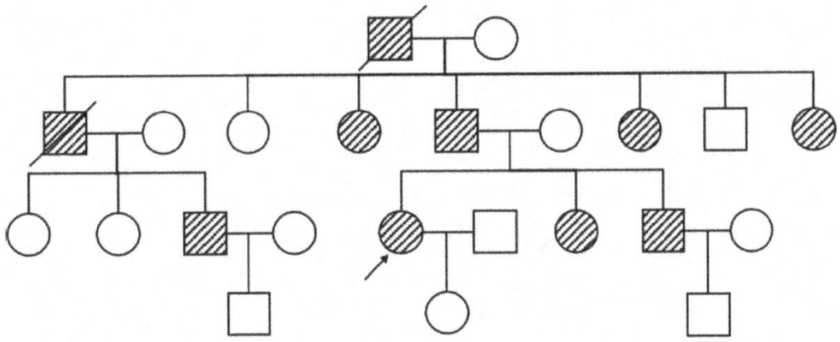

Fig. 1 Pedigree of the patient's family. The affected members are indicated with shading. Squares and circles represent males and females, respectively. Arrow indicates the case of the report

Case presentation

A 43-year-old woman suffered progressively worsening proximal muscle weakness for 10 years resulting in difficulties with fast walking, climbing stairs, and rising from a chair. She had experienced normal growth and development. She reported lumbar back pain. Now, the symptom of proximal lower limb weakness had spread to her arms, causing her difficulty in washing clothes. Her father, sister, brother, three paternal aunts, one paternal uncle, and the uncle's son also had slowly progressive proximal muscle weakness, but not as severe as hers. The pedigree of her family revealed an autosomal dominant inheritance pattern (Fig. 1). Muscle weakness was detected in the biceps and triceps muscles (MRC4+/5), wrist flexor extensor muscles (MRC 4/5), iliopsoas muscles (MRC 3/5), and quadriceps muscles (MRC 4−/5). Her distal arm strength was 4. She had a waddling gait and muscle atrophy in the quadriceps and distal lower legs. In her most recent examination, she could not walk on her toes. Deep tendon reflexes were absent. Gower's sign was present. No cranial nerve dysfunction or sensory disturbance was noted. Her serum level of creatine kinase was 2-fold higher than the upper normal value. An electromyogram revealed mild myogenic changes. Echocardiography and electrocardiogram evaluations did not detect any cardiac abnormalities. Fatty degeneration was detected in a few lower limb muscles by magnetic resonance imaging (MRI), including the vastus intermedius, vastus lateralis, semimembranosus, adductor magnus and the long head of the biceps femoris muscles. The rectus femoris was slightly involved. No abnormalities were detected in the gracilis, sartorius, or semitendinosus muscles. At the distal leg level, the soleus, gastrocnemius medialis, and gastrocnemius lateralis showed degeneration with fatty infiltration (Fig. 2). After the patient provided written consent, a skeletal muscle biopsy was taken from the tibial anterior muscle, precooled with isopentane, and frozen in liquid nitrogen. Frozen sections of 8 μm were prepared and histopathological examination showed increased fiber size variability with atrophic and hypertrophic fibers. Muscle fiber necrosis and phagocytosis were observed. There was a mild increase in connective tissue. Non-rimmed vacuoles were commonly present. Some fibers showed structural changes with abnormal material deposits after staining with hematoxylin-eosin (HE), modified Gomori's trichrome (MGT) (Fig. 3a and b). Oxidative enzyme activities were reduced focally in some fibers, occasionally resulting in core-like lesions after staining with succinate dehydrogenase (SDH), NADH-tetrazolium

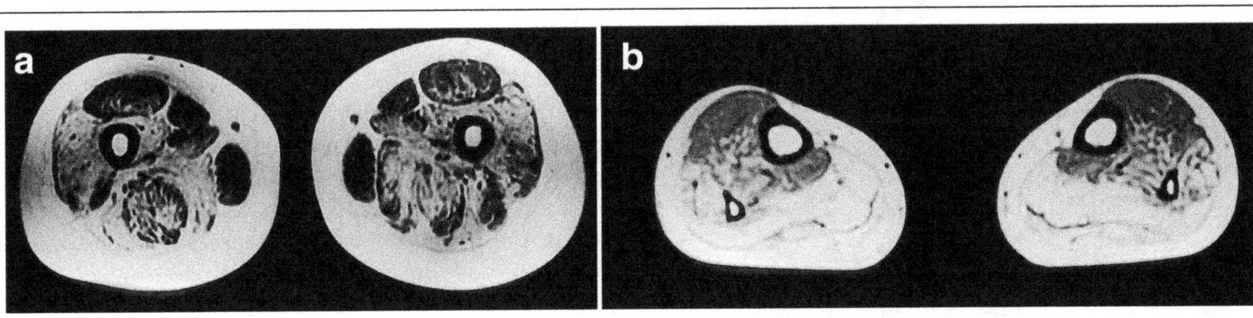

Fig. 2 Image and transverse T1-weighted muscle MR image from the patient. MR images demonstrated a typical pattern of muscle involvement (hyperintensities reflect lipomatous alterations). On the thigh level **a** the vastus intermedius, vastus lateralis, semimembranosus, adductor magnus and long head of the biceps femoris muscles showed moderate lipomatous alterations. On the lower leg level **b** the soleus, gastrocnemius medialis, and gastrocnemius lateralis muscles show pronounced fatty changes

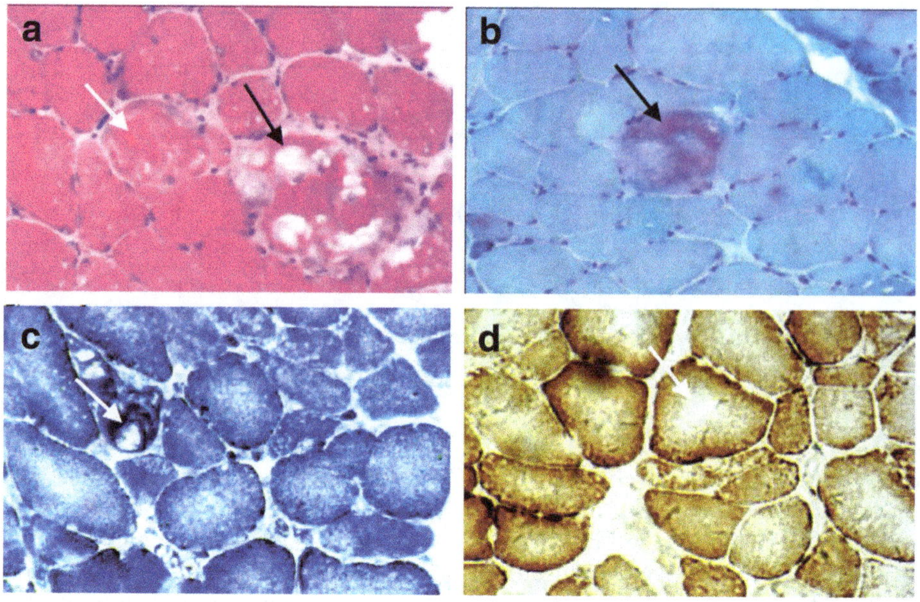

Fig. 3 Histopathological examination of the skeletal muscles. **a** HE staining showed muscle fibers of variable sizes, vacuoles (black arrow), and abnormal material deposits (white arrow). **b** MGT staining showed abnormal material deposits in a muscle fiber (black arrow).**c** NADH-TR and (**d**) COX staining showed reduced oxidative enzyme activities in some fibers, like core-like lesions (white arrow)

reductase (NADH-TR), and cytochrome c oxidase (COX) (Fig. 3c and d). Electron microscopy showed myofibrillar deposits of thin filaments interspersed with dense granular material between myofibrils, frequently in spheroid shape. These structures were surrounded by radially arranged thin filaments (Fig. 4). Next generation sequencing identified a 15-nucleotide deletion (c.2791_2805del, p.931_935del) in the immunoglobulin (Ig)-like domain 7 of the *FLNC* gene (Fig. 5). Genetic testing revealed that this deletion had been passed to the patient from her father and carried by her other symptomatic relatives. The patient and her relatives were administered 10 mg per day coenzyme Q10 and some vitamins for about 1 year, but their symptoms were not relieved.

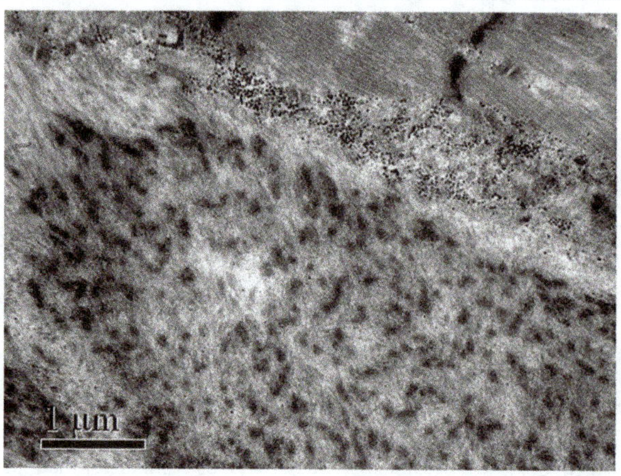

Fig. 4 Ultrastructural examination of the skeletal muscle fibers showed deposits of dense granular material and thin filaments

Discussions and conclusions

In the current case, a novel 15-bp deletion in the *FLNC* gene showed an autosomal dominant inheritance pattern and caused muscle weakness in all limbs, a mildly elevated serum level of creatine kinase, slight myogenic changes on EMG, variations in muscle fiber size, and the presence of abnormal protein aggregates and vacuoles in some muscle fibers. These phenotypic manifestations were also observed in the previously identified *FLNC* gene mutation-mediated MFM cases [1, 2, 4, 5].

The *FLNC* gene is located in the 7q32-q35 chromosome band and contains 48 coding exons. In general, three different domains harbored in the filamin-C protein may have different filaminS C-related myopathy phenotypes: N-terminal acting-binding domain and the frameshift deletion c.5161delG mutation in the rod domain involved with distal muscle weakness [6, 8], 24 Ig-like repeat domains, and a C-terminal dimerization domain associated with limb-girdle proximal muscle weakness [1]. In 2016, a 15-bp (c.2786_2800del) mutation in the Ig-like domain 7 of the *FLNC* gene was reported to cause limb-girdle muscular dystrophy (LGMD) [9], whereas the novel 15-bp (c.2791_2805del) mutation in the same domain in our case obviously caused the clinical phenotypes of filamin C–related MFM and displayed a typical autosomal dominant inheritance pattern. The two deletions in the same domain are very likely to

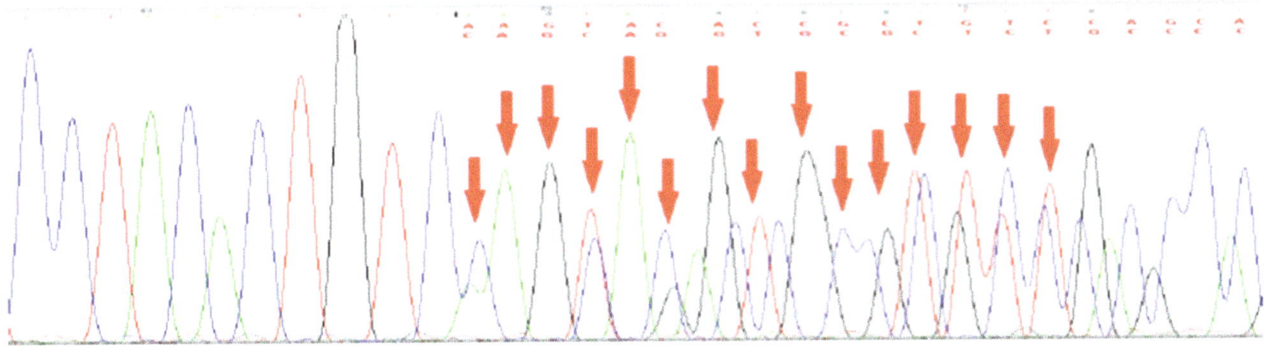

Fig. 5 DNA sequencing analysis showed an internal 15-nucleotide deletion in exon 18 of the *FLNC* gene (red arrows)

result in protein aggregation in muscle fibers, causing similar clinical phenotypes [4, 5, 10]. The variation in fiber size and the presence of necrosis and fatty degeneration in muscle tissues in our case, which were also observed in cases harboring different mutations in the same Ig-like domain [4, 5], indicate that mutations in the Ig-like domain 7 of the *FLNC* gene lead to structural changes in skeletal muscles. The presence of phagocytosis, non-rimmed vacuoles, and abnormal material deposits in the muscles in our case, which is in agreement with the observations in other Ig-like domain 7 mutation-mediated filamin C–related MFM cases [4, 5] and in cultured cells transfected with expression vectors for the *FLNC* gene with a mutation in Ig-like domain 7 [10], indicates that the 15-bp deletion in the Ig-like domain 7 of the *FLNC* gene in our case may lead to protein misfolding, trigger aggregation of the mutant filamin C protein, and decrease the efficiency of both the ubiquitin–proteasome system and autophagy system to degrade protein aggregates [10–13]. These events ultimately result in disruption of myofibrils [10, 14] and muscle weakness.

In conclusion, a novel 15-nucleotide deletion (c.2791_2805del, p.931_935del) in the Ig-like domain 7 of the *FLNC* gene was found to cause filamin C–related MFM. This deletion in the *FLNC* gene causes protein aggregation, abnormalities in muscle structure, and impairment in muscle fiber function, which leads to muscle weakness.

Abbreviations

COX: Cytochrome c oxidase (COX; HE: Hematoxylin-eosin; LGMD: Limb-girdle muscular dystrophy; MFM: Myofibrillar myopathies; MGT: Modified Gomori-trichrome; MRI: Magnetic resonance imaging;; NADH-TR: NADH-tetrazolium reductase; PAS: Periodic acid-schiff; SDH: Succinate dehydrogenase

Acknowledgements

The authors thank Medjaden Bioscience Limited for proofreading the manuscript.

Funding

This work was supported by the National Natural Science Foundation of China (No, 81601088), Natural Science Foundation of Jilin Province (No, 20160520164JH) and the 7th Youth Foundation of the First Hospital of Jilin University (No, JDYY72016028).

Authors' contributions

JM drafted the manuscript and figures; FS designed and analyzed the study; XL and XW analyzed and interpreted histological data; YY analyzed and interpreted the electron microscopy imaging; XY revised the manuscript and gave the final approval of the version to be published. All authors read and approved the contents of the case report.

Authors' information

All of authors are from the Department of Neurology and the Neuroscience Center of the First Affiliated Hospital of Jilin University.

Competing interests

The authors declare that they have no competing interests.

Author details

[1]Department of Neurology and Neuroscience Center, First Affiliated Hospital of Jilin University, Changchun, 130021 Jilin, People's Republic of China. [2]Department of Neurology, Peking University First Hospital, #8 Xishiku St, Xicheng District, Beijing 100034, China. [3]Department of Neurology and Neuroscience Center First Affiliated Hospital of Jilin University, Changchun, 130021 Jilin, People's Republic of China.

References

1. Vorgerd M, van der Ven PF, Bruchertseifer V, Löwe T, Kley RA, Schröder R, et al. A mutation in the dimerization domain of filamin c causes a novel type of autosomal dominant myofibrillar myopathy. Am J Hum Genet. 2005;77:297–304.
2. Tasca G, Odgerel Z, Monforte M, Aurino S, Clarke NF, Waddell LB, et al. Novel FLNC mutation in a patient with myofibrillar myopathy in combination with late-onset cerebellar ataxia. Muscle Nerve. 2012;46: 275–82.
3. Avila-Smirnow D, Gueneau L, Batonnet-Pichon S, Delort F, Bécane HM, Claeys K, et al. Cardiac arrhythmia and late-onset muscle weakness caused by a myofibrillar myopathy with unusual histopathological features due to a novel missense mutation in FLNC. Rev Neurol (Paris). 2016;172:594–606.
4. Luan X, Hong D, Zhang W, Wang Z, Yuan Y. A novel heterozygous deletion-insertion mutation (2695-2712 del/GTTTGT ins) in exon 18 of the filamin C gene causes filaminopathy in a large Chinese family. Neuromuscul Disord. 2010;20:390–6.
5. Shatunov A, Olivé M, Odgerel Z, Stadelmann-Nessler C, Irlbacher K, van Landeghem F, et al. In-frame deletion in the seventh immunoglobulin-like repeat of filamin C in a family with myofibrillar myopathy. Eur J Hum Genet. 2009;17:656–63.
6. Duff RM, Tay V, Hackman P, Ravenscroft G, McLean C, Kennedy P, et al.

Mutations in the N-terminal actin-binding domain of filamin C cause a distal myopathy. Am J Hum Genet. 2011;88:729–40.

7. Guergueltcheva V, Peeters K, Baets J, Ceuterick-de Groote C, Martin JJ, Suls A, et al. Distal myopathy with upper limb predominance caused by filamin C haploinsufficiency. Neurology. 2011;77:2105–14.
8. Rossi D, Palmio J, Evilä A, Galli L, Barone V, Caldwell TA, et al. A novel FLNC frameshift and an OBSCN variant in a family with distal muscular dystrophy. PLoS One. 2017;12:e0186642.
9. Evilä A, Arumilli M, Udd B, Hackman P. Targeted next-generation sequencing assay for detection of mutations in primary myopathies. Neuromuscul Disord. 2016;26:7–15.
10. Kley RA, Serdaroglu-Oflazer P, Leber Y, Odgerel Z, van der Ven PF, Olivé M, et al. Pathophysiology of protein aggregation and extended phenotyping in filaminopathy. Brain. 2012;135:2642–60.
11. Kley RA, van der Ven PF, Olivé M, Höhfeld J, Goldfarb LG, Fürst DO, et al. Impairment of protein degradation in myofibrillar myopathy caused by FLNC/filamin C mutations. Autophagy. 2013;9:422–3.
12. Chevessier F, Schuld J, Orfanos Z, Plank AC, Wolf L, Maerkens A, et al. Myofibrillar instability exacerbated by acute exercise in filaminopathy. Hum Mol Genet. 2015;24:7207–20.
13. Fürst DO, Goldfarb LG, Kley RA, Vorgerd M, Olivé M, van der Ven PF. Filamin C-related myopathies: pathology and mechanisms. Acta Neuropathol. 2013; 125:33–46.
14. Löwe T, Kley RA, van der Ven PF, Himmel M, Huebner A, Vorgerd M, et al. The pathomechanism of filaminopathy: altered biochemical properties explain the cellular phenotype of a protein aggregation myopathy. Hum Mol Genet. 2007;16:1351–8.

23

Myalgia caused by chronic myositis associated with plasmacytosis

Taku Hatano[1*], Masashi Takanashi[1,2], Hitoshi Tsuchihashi[3], Shin-Ichi Ueno[1], Arisa Hayashida[1], Yutaka Tsukune[4], Kazuaki Kanai[1], Yasushi Shimo[1,5] and Nobutaka Hattori[1]

Abstract

Background: Cutaneous and systemic plasmacytosis are skin disorders characterized by cutaneous polyclonal plasma cell infiltration accompanied by polyclonal hypergammaglobulinemia. Cutaneous plasmacytosis involvement is limited to the skin, mainly on the face and trunk, while systemic plasmacytosis also involves 2 or more organ systems. However, there have been no reports of inflammatory myositis due to plasmacytosis. Here, we report a patient with plasmacytosis who developed myalgia and easy fatigability due to inflammatory myositis.

Case presentation: A 54-year-old man with cutaneous plasmacytosis on the face, chest, and back complained of a history of atypical facial and lower leg pain and easy fatigability since the age of 45 years. Muscle-strength tests revealed bilateral trivial gastrocnemius weakness with myalgia. The results of routine blood analysis, including creatine kinase and thyroid function, were normal, but levels of several inflammation markers and autoantibodies were elevated. Additionally, lower leg magnetic resonance imaging and gastrocnemius muscle biopsy revealed inflammatory myositis mimicking polymyositis. His plasmacytosis, myalgia, and lower leg weakness were ameliorated by prednisolone.

Conclusion: The patient was diagnosed with inflammatory myositis due to plasmacytosis. Given that plasmacytosis has previously been reported to disrupt the immune status, myositis in this patient might have been associated with abnormal autoimmune inflammation. Neurologists and physicians should thus be aware that plasmacytosis might be associated with inflammatory myositis accompanied by myalgia.

Keywords: Plasmacytosis, Chronic myositis, Myalgia, Autoimmune disease, Lymphoproliferative disease

Background

Cutaneous and systemic plasmacytosis are skin disorders characterized by cutaneous polyclonal plasma cell infiltration accompanied by polyclonal hypergammaglobulinemia [1]. Although plasmacytosis is a rare condition, its prevalence in the Japanese population is relatively high [2–7]. Shimizu et al. reviewed 26 previously published cases with this disease, and found that all but two patients were Japanese [2]. But the precise prevalence of the disease in Japan, and other countries, remains unclear. Plasmacytosis has 2 different clinical phenotypes: cutaneous plasmacytosis, which is limited to the skin and characterized by reddish-brown plaques, mainly on the face and trunk; and systemic plasmacytosis, which involves 2 or more organ systems [1]. However, the association between systemic plasmacytosis and muscle involvement has not been reported. Here, we describe a patient with cutaneous plasmacytosis who complained of myalgia followed by the emergence of blown plaques on his face and trunk. Although serum studies failed to detect any elevation of creatinine kinase, magnetic resonance imaging (MRI) revealed abnormalities of the lower leg muscles. Histological analysis of a leg muscle biopsy revealed inflammatory myositis.

* Correspondence: thatano@juntendo.ac.jp
[1]Department of Neurology, Juntendo University Graduate School of Medicine, 2-1-1 Hongo, Bunkyo-ku, Tokyo 113-8421, Japan
Full list of author information is available at the end of the article

Case presentation

A 54-year-old man with cutaneous plasmacytosis of the face, chest, and back consulted the neurology service at our hospital with complaints of tingling pain in his face, tenderness in the bilateral lower legs, and easy fatigability. He had developed red-brown plaques on his face and trunk at age 45 years, and consulted his local hospital at age 47. Skin biopsy was performed at that time and histological examination revealed characteristic findings of cutaneous plasmacytosis. At about the same time as he was diagnosed with skin plasmacytosis, the patient also complained of myalgia with easy fatigability and was diagnosed with fibromyalgia. His other medical history was remarkable for hypertension, angina pectoris, left mastoiditis, lumbar stenosis, and osteoarthritis of bilateral knees. Nine years after the onset of myalgia, the patient consulted our neurological service and was admitted to our department to identify the cause of facial and lower leg pain.

On admission, the patient had red-brown plaques on his face and trunk (Fig. 1a). He complained of myalgia in his bilateral vastus lateralis muscles, hip adductors, and gastrocnemius, which worsened with pressure. Muscle strength tests revealed bilateral trivial weakness of the gastrocnemius with normal muscular tone. The results of general and neurological examinations and routine blood analysis, including creatine kinase 95 U/L (normal range 57–240) and thyroid function, were all normal. Serum antibodies specific to syphilis, neurotrophic viruses, human immunodeficiency virus, and thyroid and autoimmune diseases, including interleukin-6 (IL-6), IgG4, antinuclear, anti-Sm, anti-mitochondria M2, anti-SS-A/SS-B, anti-Jo-1, anti-Scl-70, anti-acetylcholine receptor, myeloperoxidase-, and proteinase 3-anti-neutrophil cytoplasmic antibodies were all normal. Rheumatoid factor and anti-cardiolipin antibodies were positive, but anti-citrullinated protein antibody and lupus anticoagulant were negative. Serum levels of soluble IL-2 receptor 873 U/mL (normal range 145–519), IgG 1914 mg/dL (normal range 870–1700) and IgA 619 mg/dL (normal range 110–410) were all elevated. However, both Bence Jones protein and M protein were negative. We performed a repeat skin biopsy to confirm the diagnosis of plasmacytosis. The biopsy specimen (Fig. 1c, d) showed prominent

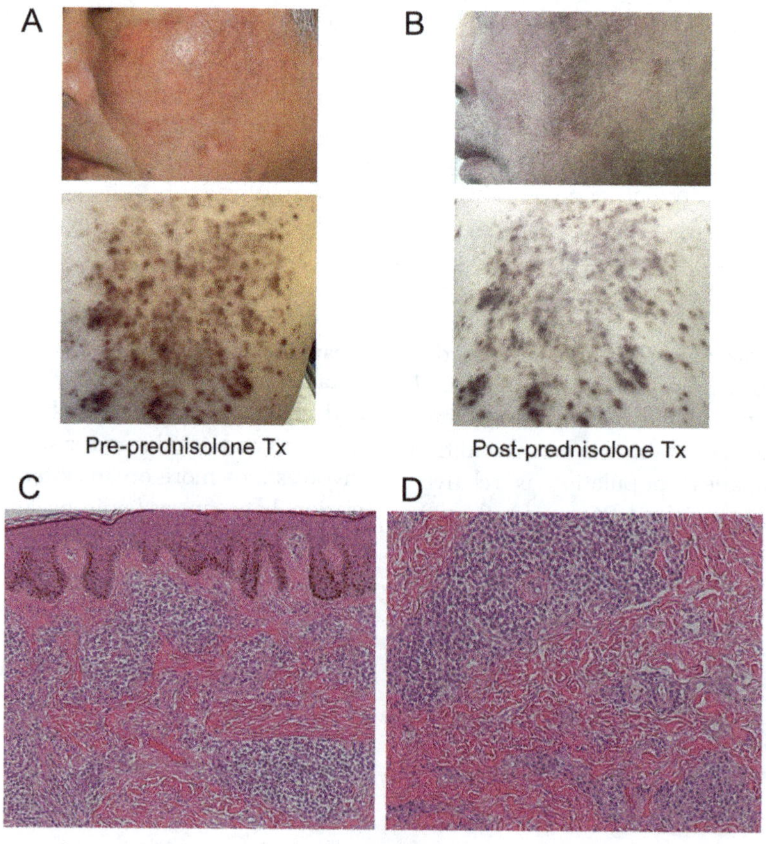

Fig. 1 Cutaneous plasmacytosis in the patient. The patient presented with red-brown plaques on his face and trunk (**a**) which were ameliorated by prednisolone therapy. Although the pigmentation of facial lesions remained, redness and swelling improved to some extent (**b**). Histological examination revealed characteristic findings of cutaneous plasmacytosis (**c**, **d**). There was no abnormality in either the stratum corneum or epidermis, but plasma cells infiltrated the dermis. Tx, treatment

dermal perivascular proliferation of mature plasma cells, with a normal gamma chain kappa/lambda ratio, and a MIB-1-labeling index of less than 5%. In the specimen, CD79a expression was positive but CD56, cyclin D1, and Epstein Barr virus-encoded RNA were negative. There was no evidence of immunoglobulin heavy-chain gene rearrangements. Therefore, these findings were compatible with cutaneous plasmacytosis, not multiple myeloma. The findings of a nerve conduction study were all normal, but gastrocnemius needle electromyography revealed positive sharp waves, repetitive discharge, and polyphasic motor unit potentials. However, there was no evidence of early recruitment. These findings suggested denervation, but myogenic changes were inconclusive. T1- and T2-weighted MRI of the lower legs revealed abnormal high intensity in several muscles, including bilateral adductors, quadriceps, semimembranosus, and gastrocnemius muscles. Short tau inversion recovery imaging also showed abnormal intensity of the bilateral quadriceps and gastrocnemius muscles (Fig. 2a–c). These findings indicated myositis with chronic inflammation, and we therefore performed a biopsy of the right gastrocnemius muscle. Morphological analysis of the muscle specimen showed fiber size variability, scattered necrotic and regenerated fibers, and lymphocyte infiltration predominantly in the endomysium rather than the perimysium or the vessels (Fig. 2d), but no perifascicular atrophy or rimmed vacuoles. CD8+ toxic T cells surrounded the non-necrotic fibers and major histocompatibility complex (MHC) class 1 antigen expression was ubiquitous (Fig. 2e, f). There were almost no B cells, CD4+ cells, macrophages, or membrane attack complexes around the small vessels. A few plasmacytes were visible in the endomysium (Fig. 2g), and they stained negative for IgG4. These pathological features were compatible with European Neuromuscular Center classification criteria of polymyositis [8].

The patient's muscle pain was unaffected by acetaminophen and pregabalin, but his myalgia and cutaneous plasmacytosis on his face and back were ameliorated by prednisolone (20 mg/day) (Fig. 1b).

Discussion and conclusion

Plasmacytosis can be either localized, as in plasma-cell type giant lymph node hyperplasia, or systemic [1]. The current patient showed multiple reddish-brown skin lesions, typical of cutaneous plasmacytosis, scattered over his face and back. Serum and dermal pathological analyses revealed elevated levels of IgG and IgA, without Bence Jones or M protein, and proliferation of mature plasma cells in the dermis. These findings suggested plasmacyotosis rather than multiple myeloma. The abnormally high intensity of muscles in T1- and T2-weighted MRI indicated chronic myositis with fatty degeneration. The needle electromyography failed to provide conclusive evidence for myogenic changes, although the results might be influenced by the neurogenic changes from lumbar stenosis. Plasmacytosis occasionally proliferates systemically, similar to the skin. However, although several previous reports have described the involvement of superficial lymph nodes, liver, spleen and lung [1, 5, 6], there have been no reports of an association between proliferating plasma cells and myopathy. Muscle biopsy in the current case showed proliferation of lymphocytes, but not plasma cells, suggesting that the myositis in this case might have been related to chronic inflammation, rather than to the invasion of plasma cells into the muscles.

The proliferation of lymphocytes in the muscle suggested that the inflammation might be related to an autoimmune response. Pathological investigation indicated that the myositis could be a compatible finding of polymyositis. Inflammatory myopathies, such as polymyositis, dermatomyositis, and inclusion body myositis, are known to be associated with autoimmune disorders. Plasma cells are antibody-producing, terminally differentiated quiescent B cells [9], and abnormal plasma cells might thus perturb the immune system. Indeed, autoimmune disorders and lymphoproliferative diseases, including Castleman's disease, chronic lymphocytic leukemia, and lymphoma, share a bidirectional relationship [10]. Dermatomyositis and polymyositis are occasionally associated with lymphoma development [10]. Additionally, Kiniwa et al. reported a patient with autoimmune hemolytic anemia due to cutaneous plasmacytosis [7]. Notably, serum examinations in the present case failed to reveal any abnormalities of myositis-associated biomarkers, including IL-6, anti-nuclear antibodies, or anti-Jo1 antibodies; however, he had abnormally high serum levels of soluble IL-2 receptor, rheumatoid factor, and anti-cardiolipin antibody, suggesting an immunological perturbation. In this context, we concluded that his myositis might have been caused by an immunological abnormality related to plasmacytosis. This was supported by the fact that his skin lesions and myalgia were ameliorated by prednisolone, but not by non-steroidal anti-inflammatory drugs. Skin lesions in most patients with plasmacytosis are resistant to several therapies, but the current case suggests that immunomodulation using steroids and cyclophosphamide might be an effective option [3], and that inflammation might play an important role in the pathogenesis of skin lesions in patients with plasmacytosis.

We should consider some of the shortcomings of our case assessment. The patient's myositis could be considered an idiopathic inflammatory myositis, including polymyositis, dermatomyositis, and inclusion body

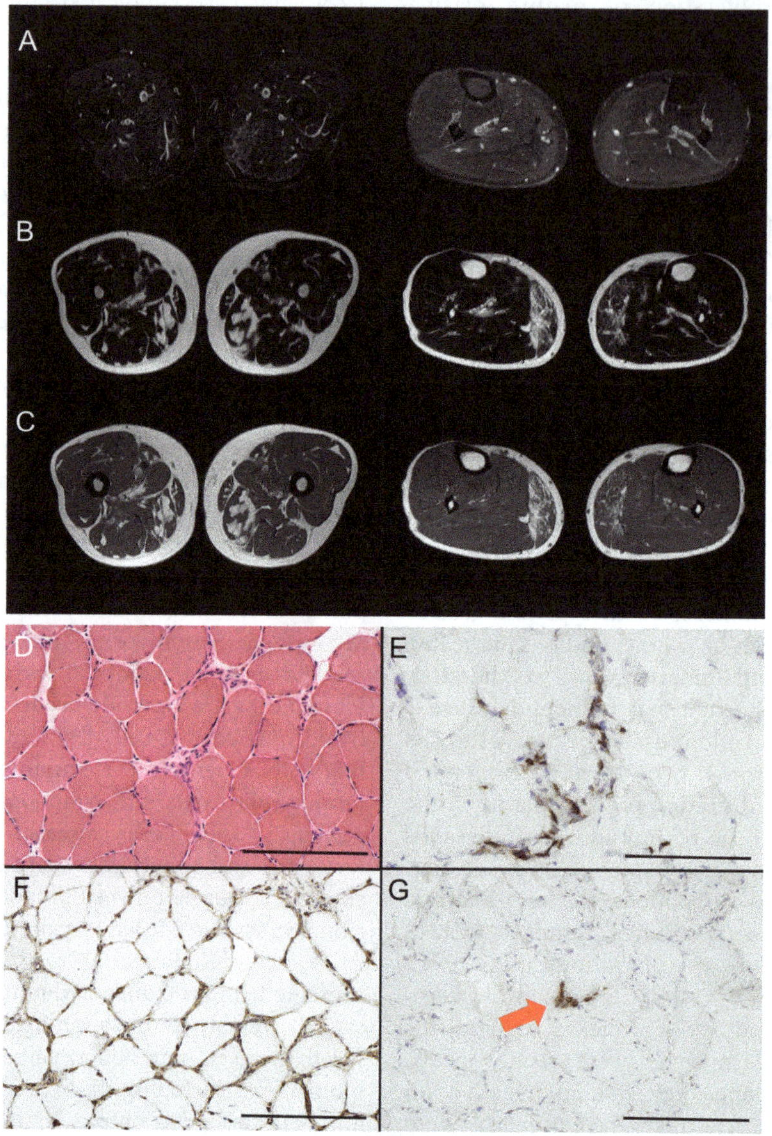

Fig. 2 MRI and histological findings of myositis in the patient. Short tau inversion recovery (**a**), T2-weighted (**b**), and T1-weighted (**c**) MRI revealed inflammation of several muscles in the bilateral lower legs. **d–g** Gastrocnemius muscle pathology. Inflammatory cells invaded the endomysium (**d**, hematoxylin and eosin, bar 200 μm). Lymphocytes surrounding non-necrotic fibers were CD8+ cytotoxic T cells (**e**, CD8 immunostaining, bar 100 μm). Non-necrotic fibers showed ubiquitous MHC-class 1 antigen expression (F, MHC-class 1 immunostaining, bar 500 μm). A few plasmacytes were seen in the endomysium (**g**, red arrow, CD138 immunostaining, bar 200 μm)

myositis, incidentally combined with plasmacytosis. Prednisolone and immunomodulation therapy also have an effect on idiopathic inflammatory myositis. Additionally, the patient was not examined for the presence of several autoimmune inflammatory myositis-associated antibodies, except for anti-Jo1 antibody. However, his myositis showed atypical findings of idiopathic inflammatory myositis, such as very slow progression without rimmed vacuole, no elevation of creatine kinase, and no characteristic skin lesions in dermatomyositis. Therefore, we believe that the myositis was associated with plasmacyotosis.

To the best of our knowledge, this is the first report of a patient with inflammatory myositis mimicking polymyositis and plasmacytosis. Physicians and neurologists should be aware of the co-existence of plasmacytosis and inflammatory myositis.

Abbreviations

Ig: Immunoglobulin; IL-2: Interleukin-2; IL-6: Interleukin-6; MHC: Major histocompatibility complex; MRI: Magnetic resonance imaging; Tx, treatment

Acknowledgements

The authors thank Mrs. Akiko Sumii for technical assistance.

Funding
This study was supported by a Strategic Research Foundation Grant-in-Aid for Private Universities, and Grants-in-Aid for Scientific Research on Priority Areas (to TH, 25461290).

Authors' contributions
Study concept and design: TH. Acquisition of data: TH, MT, HT, SU, AH, and YT. Analysis and interpretation of data: TH, MT, HT, and KK. Drafting of the manuscript: TH. Critical revision of the manuscript for important intellectual content: MT, HT, SU, AH, YT, KK, YS and NH. Study supervision: YS and NH. All authors read and approved the final manuscript.

Competing interests
M. Takanashi, H Tsuchihashi, SI. Ueno, A. Hayashida, Y Tsukune, K. Kanai, Y. Shimo, and N Hattori report no conflict of interests.
T. Hatano is an associate editor/member of the editorial board for BMC Neurology.

Author details
[1]Department of Neurology, Juntendo University Graduate School of Medicine, 2-1-1 Hongo, Bunkyo-ku, Tokyo 113-8421, Japan. [2]Department of Neurology, Juntendo Koshigaya Hospital, 560 Fukuroyama, Koshigayashi, Saitama 343-0032, Japan. [3]Department of Dermatology, Juntendo University Graduate School of Medicine, 2-1-1 Hongo, Bunkyo-ku, Tokyo 113-8421, Japan. [4]Department of Internal Medicine, Division of Hematology, Juntendo University Graduate School of Medicine, 2-1-1 Hongo, Bunkyo-ku, Tokyo 113-8421, Japan. [5]Department of Research and Therapeutics for Movement Disorders, Juntendo University Graduate School of Medicine, 2-1-1 Hongo, Bunkyo-ku, Tokyo 113-8421, Japan.

References

1. Watanabe S, Ohara K, Kukita A, Shigeo M. Systemic plasmacytosis. A syndrome of peculiar multiple skin eruptions, generalized lymphadenopathy, and polyclonal hypergammaglobulinemia. Arch Dermatol. 1986;122:1314–20.
2. Shimizu S, Tanaka M, Shimizu H, Han-yaku H. Is cutaneous plasmacytosis a distinct clinical entity? J Am Acad Dermatol. 1997;36:876–80.
3. Carey WP, Rico MJ, Nierodzik ML, Sidhu G. Systemic plasmacytosis with cutaneous manifestations in a white man: successful therapy with cyclophosphamide/prednisone. J Am Acad Dermatol. 1998;38:629–31.
4. Leonard AL, Meehan SA, Ramsey D, Brown L, Sen F. Cutaneous and systemic plasmacytosis. J Am Acad Dermatol. 2007;56:S38–40.
5. Honda R, Cerroni L, Tanikawa A, Ebihara T, Amagai M, Ishiko A. Cutaneous plasmacytosis: report of 6 cases with or without systemic involvement. J Am Acad Dermatol. 2013;2013:978–85.
6. Chantachaeng W, Chularojanamontri L. Cutaneous plasmacytosis: a case report and review of pulmonary findings. Dermatol Reports. 2011;3:e39.
7. Kiniwa Y, Matoba H, Hamano H, Sendo Y, Okuyama R. Cutaneous plasmacytosis associated with autoimmune hemolytic anemia. J Dermatol. 2016;43:343–5.
8. Hoogendijk JE, Amato AA, Lecky BR, Choy EH, Lundberg IE, Rose MR, Vencovsky J, de Visser M, Hughes RA. 119th ENMC international workshop: trial design in adult idiopathic inflammatory myopathies, with the exception of inclusion body myositis, 10-12 October 2003, Naarden, The Netherlands. Neuromuscul Disord. 2004;14:337–45.
9. Nutt SL, Hodgkin PD, Tarlinton DM, Corcoran LM. The generation of antibody-secreting plasma cells. Nat Rev Immunol. 2015;15:160–71.
10. Stubgen JP. Inflammatory myopathies and lymphoma. J Neurol Sci. 2016; 369:377–89.

24

Miller Fisher syndrome, Bickerstaff brainstem encephalitis and Guillain-Barré syndrome overlap with persistent non-demyelinating conduction blocks

Angela Puma[1,2*], Jeanne Benoit[1], Sabrina Sacconi[1,3] and Antonino Uncini[4]

Abstract

Background: Miller Fisher syndrome (MFS) and Bickerstaff's Brainstem Encephalitis (BBE) share some clinical features and a common immunological profile characterized by anti-GQ1b antibodies. Some MFS patients overlap with Guillain-Barré syndrome (GBS) or BBE. We report a patient with MFS, BBE, and axonal GBS overlap in whom serial electrophysiological studies showed persistent motor conduction blocks (CBs).

Case presentation: A 61-year-old man acutely developed ophtalmoparesis, ataxia and areflexia suggesting MFS. Paresthesias, severe weakness, and drowsiness rapidly developed indicating an overlap with BBE and GBS. Preceding infection with *Mycoplasma Pneumoniae* and anti-GQ1b antibodies were detected. On day 4, nerve conduction study showed reduced or non-recordable compound muscle action potentials (CMAPs) and sensory nerve action potentials (SNAPs) without demyelinating features, indicating the electrodiagnosis of acute motor and sensory axonal neuropathy and suggesting a poor prognosis. Intravenous immunoglobulins (IVIg) were given but clinical status worsened to ophthalmoplegia, tetraplegia and coma needing mechanical ventilation. A second IVIg course was given and the patient was weaned off ventilation on day 41 and transferred to rehabilitation on day 57 with partial resolution of the ophthalmoplegia and limited recovery of muscle strength. Electrophysiology showed, after 10 weeks, greatly improved distal CMAP amplitudes suggesting the resolution of distal CBs while CBs in intermediate and proximal nerve segments emerged. CBs unusually persisted for four to 6 months without development of abnormal temporal dispersion. A third IVIg course was started on day 179 and the resolution of CBs mirrored the clinical improvement.

Conclusions: GQ1b gangliosides are expressed in the nodal region of oculomotor nerves, muscle spindle afferents, peripheral nerves and possibly in the brainstem reticular formation. Anti-GQ1b antibodies may explain the complex symptomatology and the overlap between MFS, BBE, and GBS.
CBs that persisted and recovered without the development of temporal dispersion suggest that weakness was due to a sustained, antibody-mediated, attack at the nodal region inducing a non-demyelinating conduction failure as expression of an acute onset, long lasting, nodopathy. Serial electrophysiological studies allowed not only to understand the underlying pathophysiology and formulate a more correct prognosis but also to guide the treatment.

Keywords: Guillain-Barré syndrome, Miller Fisher syndrome, Bickerstaff brainstem encephalitis, Anti-GQ1b antibody, Nodopathy, Persistent motor conduction block

* Correspondence: puma.ar@chu-nice.fr
[1]Peripheral Nervous System, Muscle & ALS Department, University of Nice and Côte d'Azur (UCA), Nice, France
[2]UMR7370 CNRS, LP2M, Faculté de Médecine, University Côte d'Azur, Nice, France
Full list of author information is available at the end of the article

Background

In the 1950s, Miller Fisher Syndrome (MFS) and Bickerstaff brain encephalitis (BBE) were independently described [1, 2]. Both disorders were related a preceding infection, showed ophthalmoplegia and ataxia, and presented a spontaneous recovery in most cases. MFS patients were areflexic, in keeping with a peripheral nerve etiology, whereas BBE was characterized by altered consciousness and hyperreflexia in some patients, supporting a central pathology. Interestingly, both Fisher and Bickerstaff recognized in the diseases they described similarities with Guillain–Barré syndrome (GBS) [1, 2].

In the early 1990s, the discovery of anti-GQ1b IgG antibodies in MFS and BBE provided evidence that both disorders were part of the same disease spectrum, later referred to as anti-GQ1b antibody syndrome [3–5]. MFS patients who develop limb weakness overlapping with Guillain Barré syndrome (GBS), or drowsiness overlapping with BBE [6, 7] also support a common immunological profile and clinical spectrum.

We report a patient who developed, after a *Mycoplasma Pneumoniae* infection, an overlap of MFS, BBE and axonal GBS with GQ1b IgG antibodies and showing, at serial conduction studies, persistent motor conduction blocks (CB).

Case presentation

A 61-year-old man acutely developed diplopia and balance disorders. 24 h after onset, he was admitted in the hospital due to ascending paresthesias and an emerging tetraparesis. On day 4 after onset, examination showed a drowsy patient with ophthalmoparesis, areflexia and severe tetraparesis. Plantar responses were flexor. The cerebrospinal fluid study was normal. IgM to *Mycoplasma Pneumoniae* and IgG anti-GQ1b (1:2560) were detected. IgG and IgM anti- GM1, -GD1a, -GD1b and -GM2 were absent. Two MRIs of the brain, one with gadolinium, were normal. The patient was treated with intravenous immunoglobulin (IVIg) (0,4 g/kg/day X 5 days) but worsened to complete ophthalmoplegia, tetraplegia and coma needing mechanical ventilation. Considering the severity of the condition a second IVIg course was started on day 24. A few days later he began to improve, with initial resolution of the drowsiness and bulbar symptoms, and partial resolution of the ophtalmoplegia. The patient was weaned off ventilation on day 41 and transferred to rehabilitation on day 57 with improved muscle strength (MCR scale: 2–3/5 in the lower and 2/5 in the upper limbs). After considering the results of the nerve conduction studies performed on days 72 and 128, we searched for antibodies to Neurofascin155, Contactin1 and Contactin associated protein1 that resulted negative. On the other hand, five months after the onset of symptoms, the anti GQ1b IgG rate remained elevated (1:2560).

A third IVIg course was started on day 179. On day 240, the patient had recovered muscle strength, except in the right upper limb (MCR scale: 3–4/5) and showed mild gait ataxia.

Nerve conduction studies

Four serial conduction studies were performed (Table 1, Fig. 1). On day 4 compound muscle action potentials (CMAPs) were not recordable or were very reduced in amplitudes with slightly prolonged distal motor latencies (DML) and normal motor conduction velocities (MCVs). Sensory nerve action potentials (SNAPs) showed reduced amplitudes in the right sural nerve and were not recordable in the five other nerves. On day 72, distal CMAPs, previously undetectable, were measured at 5.3 and 2.6 mV in the median nerves, and 1.1 mV in the left ulnar nerve. CMAP amplitude of the right ulnar nerve was increased by 512%. Partial CBs, defined as > 30% decrease of proximal CMAP amplitude without abnormal temporal dispersion of proximal CMAP (< 30% increased CMAP duration) [8], emerged in intermediate nerve segments of both median and ulnar nerves with decrements of proximal CMAP amplitudes ranging from 30.2 to 73% (Fig. 1). An additional partial CB was detectable in the right median nerve in the Erb's point-axilla segment (Fig. 1). MCVs were slow. SNAPs with reduced amplitude were recordable in 7/8 nerves. On day 128, distal CMAP amplitudes furtherly increased with however persistently low distal CMAP amplitudes for the common peroneal nerves. Partial CBs improved in the intermediate segments of left median and right ulnar nerves.

The last study on day 240 showed distal CMAP amplitudes in the normal range, except in the left peroneal nerve as well as the resolution of CBs in all nerves with the exception of the emergence of a partial CB in the intermediate segment of the left peroneal nerve, possibly revealed by the increased distal CMAP amplitude due to the resolution of a distal CB. MCV were still slow in some nerve segments. SNAPs amplitudes remained reduced reaching the normal range in only 1/8 nerves.

Discussion and conclusions

The patient we describe presented with signs suggesting MFS but rapidly developed impaired consciousness and tetraplegia indicating an overlap with BBE and GBS. IgG anti-GQ1b were detected and serology documented a recent *Mycoplasma Pneumoniae* infection. MFS overlapping with GBS or BBE has been reported respectively in 15 and 12% of cases but the triple overlap has rarely been described [6, 7]. Prior *Mycoplasma Pneumoniae* infection has been reported in GBS, MFS and also in BBE [9]. A common denominator to MFS, BBE and GBS is

Table 1 Nerve conduction studies

Nerve	cMAP (mV)	Proximal/Distal CMAP Amplitude (%)	Motor Latencies (ms)	Proximal/Distal CMAP Duration (%)'	CV (m/s)	SNAP (μV)
Right Median (ABP)						
Day 4						
Wrist	NR	NR	NR	NR	NR	NR
Elbow	NR	NR	NR	NR	NR	
Axilla	NR	NR	NR	NR	NR	
Erb's Point	NR		NR			
Day 72						
Wrist	5,3	69,8	3,79	73,7	31,8	2,1
Elbow	3,7	83,8	11,8	105,3	36,2	
Axilla	3,1	64,5	13,6	125,4	35,2	
Erb's Point	2		22,4			
Day 128						
Wrist	8,3	59	4	98,4	39,3	3,6
Elbow	4,9	93,9	11	92,3	43,8	
Axilla	4,6	54,3	12,6	120	44	
Erb's Point	2,5		17			
Day 240						
Wrist	8,5	91,8	3,92	100	43,2	7,5
Elbow	7,8	97,4	10,4	104	50	
Axilla	7,6	72,3	12,2	113,7	36,2	
Erb's Point	5,5		18			
Left Median (ABP)						
Day 4						
Wrist	NR	NR	NR	NR	NR	NR
Elbow	NR	NR	NR	NR	NR	
Axilla	NR	NR	NR	NR	NR	
Erb's Point	NR		NR			
Day 72						
Wrist	2,6	47,6	4,54	75,8	29,3	NR
Elbow	1,24	84,7	11,5	101,4	25,6	
Axilla	1,05		15,2			
Day 128						
Wrist	5	62	3,26	91,3	31,2	3,9
Elbow	3,1		11,6NR			
Day 240						
Wrist	6,2	83,8	3,26	92,1	36,6	7,2
Elbow	5,2	100	10,5	106,8	64,3	
Axilla	5,2	92,3	11,9	109,5	41,8	
Erb's Point	4,8		18			
Right Ulnar (ADM)						
Day 4						
Wrist	0,8	75	4,1	95,3	49	NR
Below Elbow	0,6	100	7,8	108	47	

Table 1 Nerve conduction studies *(Continued)*

Nerve	cMAP (mV)	Proximal/Distal CMAP Amplitude (%)	Motor Latencies (ms)	Proximal/Distal CMAP Duration (%)'	CV (m/s)	SNAP (μV)
Above Elbow	0,6	83,3	9,5	95,5	50	
Axilla	0,5		11,3			
Day 72						
Wrist	4,1	27,3	3,74	128	35,6	5,2
Below Elbow	1,12	71,4	10,9	117,8	38,2	
Above Elbow	0,8		13,5			
Day 128						
Wrist	5,7	45,6	2,3	92,2	40,1	5,4
Below Elbow	2,6	80,8	8,54	102,8	37,6	
Above Elbow	2,1		11,2			
Day 240						
Wrist	6,8	86,7	2,03	107,7	43,8	6,7
Below Elbow	5,9	81,3	7,63	107,1	39,3,	
Above Elbow	4,8	79,2	10,3	108,3	38,5	
Axilla	3,8		11,6			
Left Ulnar (ADM)						
Day 4						
Wrist	NR	NR	NR	NR	NR	NR
Below Elbow	NR	NR	NR	NR	NR	
Above Elbow	NR	NR	NR	NR	NR	
AXILLA	NR		NR			
Day 72						
Wrist	1,12	41,9	4,54	98,5	30,9	3,3
Below Elbow	0,47	65,9	11,5	97	32	
Above Elbow	0,31		15,2			
Day 128						
Wrist	3,1	42,2	2,75	83,5	32	3
Below Elbow	1,31	91,6	9,94	100	21,5	
Above Elbow	1,2		11,8			
Day 240						
Wrist	5,1	80,3	2,89	113,3	48,4	5,7
Below Elbow	4,1	80,5	8,06	111,8	34,7	
Above Elbow	3,3	69,7	10,8	107	47,1	
Right Peroneal (EDB)						
Day 4						
Ankle	0,9	22,2	5,9	125,2	56	NR
Below fibular head	0,2	50	11,5	83,5	46	
Above fibular head	0,1		13,5			
Day 72						
Ankle	0,75	49,3	8,13	104,4	25,3	2,1
Below fibular head	0,37	81	20,8	91,5	25	
Above fibular head	0,3		23			

Table 1 Nerve conduction studies *(Continued)*

Nerve	cMAP (mV)	Proximal/Distal CMAP Amplitude (%)	Motor Latencies (ms)	Proximal/Distal CMAP Duration (%)'	CV (m/s)	SNAP (μV)
Day 128						
Ankle	0,92	71,7	4,04	97	29,4	2,7
Below fibular head	0,66	87,9	14,6	95,3	36,1	
Above fibular head	0,58		16,4			
Day 240						
Ankle	3,3	78,7	3,9	94,2	33,3	11,6
Below fibular head	2,6	100	13,2	93,9	42,9	
Above fibular head	2,6		15,3			
Left Peroneal (EDB)						
Day 4						
Ankle	NR	NR	NR	NR	NR	NR
Below fibular head	NR	NR	NR	NR	NR	
Above fibular head	NR		NR			
Day 72						
Ankle	NR	NR	NR	NR	NR	2,6
Below fibular head	NR	NR	NR	NR	NR	
Above fibular head	NR		NR			
Day 128						
Ankle	0,24	91,6	6,35	94,6	29,8	4
Below fibular head	0,22	81,8	18,1	90	32,3	
Above fibular head	0,18		19,7			
Day 240						
Ankle	1,77	61	5,34	90	31,1	6,3
Below fibular head	1,08	100	15,3	104,7	34,2	
Above fibular head	1,08		17,2			
RighT sural						
Day 4						
Lateral malleolus						3
Day 72						
Lateral malleolus						3,2
Day 210						
Lateral malleolus						6,6
Left sural						
Day 4						
Lateral malleolus						NR
Day 72						
Lateral malleolus						3,3
Day 240						
Lateral malleolus						9

Control Values: median nerve: distal CMAP amplitude ≥5 mV, DML ≤ 4 ms, MCV ≥ 45 m/s; ulnar nerve: distal CMAP amplitude ≥6 mV, DML ≤ 3,5 ms, MCV ≥ 45 m/s; peroneal nerve: distal CMAP amplitude ≥3 mV, DML ≤ 5,5 ms, MCV ≥ 40 m/s; tibial nerve: distal CMAP amplitude ≥5 mV, DML ≤ 6 ms. Sensory Action Potential Amplitude: ≥ 10 μV for all nerves

Abbreviations: *APB* abductor pollicis brevis, *ADM* abductor digiti minimi, *EDB* extensor digitorum brevis, *AH* abductor hallucis, *CMAP* compound muscle action potential, *DML* distal motor latency, *CV* conduction velocity, *SNAP* sensory nerve action potential, *NR* not recordable the presence of anti-GQ1b antibody [6].GQ1b gangliosides are highly expressed in the nodal and paranodal regions of the oculomotor nerves, muscle spindle afferents, peripheral nerves and possibly in the brainstem reticular formation [10, 11]. The presence of anti-GQ1b antibodies may explain the complex symptomatology of the patient we report. The overlap among MFS, BBE, and GBS reemphasizes that these disorders are all part of a wide clinical spectrum [12]. The patient presented electrophysiologically with severely reduced or non-recordable CMAPs and SNAPs without demyelinating features indicating, at first test, the electrodiagnosis of acute motor and sensory axonal neuropathy with axonal degeneration and suggesting, in presence of tetraplegia, a poor prognosis. However, distal CMAPs greatly improved in 10 weeks suggesting the resolution of distal CBs whereas CBs in intermediate and proximal nerve segments emerged and unusually persisted for four to 7 months without the development of excessive temporal dispersion of CMAPs, which is considered one of the electrophysiological correlates of de-remyelination [13, 14]. These electrophysiological features and the fact that the resolution of CBs mirrored the clinical improvement suggest that weakness was due to a sustained, antibody-mediated attack at the nodal region inducing a non-demyelinating conduction failure [15–17]. CBs in axonal GBS predominate where the blood-nerve barrier is anatomically deficient, as in the nerve endings, nerve roots, and the common entrapment sites [15, 18]. We hypothesize that, in the patient we report, the improving of distal conduction blocks revealed already existing proximal conduction blocks that persisted for months [8]. Alternatively, the persistence of the autoimmune attack, supported by the high rate of IgG anti GQ1b 5 months after the onset of symptoms, might have caused the appearance of new CBs in more proximal sites.In this last case, other humoral factors present in our patient's serum probably intervened favoring the disruption of the blood-nerve barrier [19].

Currently, axonal GBS subtypes and MFS are thought to represent acute autoimmune nodopathies with a common pathogenic mechanism characterized by anti-gangliosides mediated dysfunction/disruption of the NAv channel clusters at the Ranvier node and by an electrophysiological continuum from conduction failure, reversible in few weeks, to axonal degeneration [20, 21]. Acute onset and long lasting CBs as in the patient we report, have been described in few patients with IgM antibodies against GM1, GD1a or GD1Q and variably categorized as acute variant

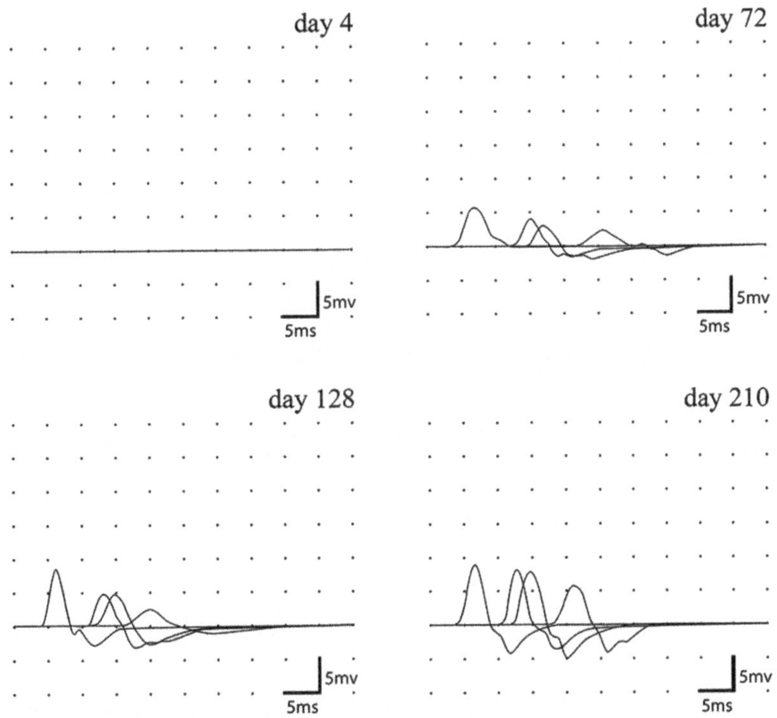

Fig. 1 Serial motor conduction recordings of the right median nerve. Superimposed compound muscle action potentials (CMAPs) recorded from the abductor pollicis brevis after median nerve stimulation at wrist, elbow, axilla and Erb's point. On day 4, distal CMAP was not recordable. On day 72, distal CMAP was 5,3 mV and partial CB was detectable in the elbow-wrist segment (proximal CMAP amplitude reduction = 30,2%; proximal CMAP area reduction = 51,3%) and in the Erb's point-axilla segment (proximal CMAP amplitude reduction = 35%; proximal CMAP area reduction = 30%). On day 128 distal CMAP amplitude was 8.3 mV but CBs persisted. The last recording on day 210 showed resolution of CBs. In all recordings there was no evidence of CMAP abnormal temporal dispersion

of multifocal motor neuropathies or chronic forms of acute motor conduction block neuropathies [22–24]. In neuropathies with anti-ganglioside antibodies it is not explained why most patients have an acute onset with conduction failure that may be promptly reversible or progress to axonal degeneration whereas few others are characterized by persistent CBs. In addition to the duration of the immune attack, intrinsic properties of anti-ganglioside antibodies, such as isotype, affinity and capability to activate complement may be implicated.

Notably, except in the first electrophysiological study, the patient showed slowing of nerve conduction that is commonly assumed to be a characteristic of a de-remyelinating process. However, inactivation of Nav channels by intravenous infusion of lidocaine or tetrodotoxin intoxication reduces conduction velocity, even reaching the "demyelinating" range, possibly by increasing the rise time of the action potential and the internodal conduction time [25, 26]. These findings may well explain the occurrence of slow conduction velocity in an autoimmune neuropathy targeting the excitable axolemma of the node of Ranvier as in the patient we describe [27].

In conclusion, in this patient with an unusual and severe clinical overlap of MFS, BBE, and GBS, serial electrophysiological studies allowed to understand the underlying pathophysiology as attributable to an acute onset, long lasting, nodopathy. Moreover, serial electrophysiology allowed by the second study to formulate a more correct prognosis and guided the treatment as the persistence of CBs encouraged us to carry out a third cycle of IVIg which possibly accelerated the clinical recovery and prevented further axonal degeneration.

Abbreviations

BBE: Bickerstaff Brainstem Encephalitis; CB: Conduction block; CMAP: Compound muscle action potential; DML: Distal motor latency; ENMG: Electroneuromyography; GBS: Guillain Barré syndrome; IgG: immunoglobulin G; IVIg: Intravenous immunoglobulin; MCR scale: Medical Research Council scale; MCV: Motor conduction velocity; MFS: Miller-Fischer syndrome; RCF: Reversible conduction failure; SNAP: Sensory nerve action potential

Acknowledgments

The authors thank Jerome Devaux and Emilien Delmont for antibody assay.

Funding

None of the authors have received any financial assistance for this manuscript.

Authors' contributions

AP and AU made the clinical and electrophysiological diagnosis. JB, AP and SS were involved in the direct management of the patient. AP, SS and AU reviewed the literature. JB and AP drafted the first manuscript and AU reviewed all manuscript versions. All authors read and approved the final manuscript.

Competing interests

The authors declare that they have no competing interests.

Author details

[1]Peripheral Nervous System, Muscle & ALS Department, University of Nice and Côte d'Azur (UCA), Nice, France. [2]UMR7370 CNRS, LP2M, Faculté de Médecine, University Côte d'Azur, Nice, France. [3]Université Côte d'Azur, Centre National de la Recherche Scientifique, Institut de Pharmacologie Moléculaire et Cellulaire, Valbonne, France. [4]Department of Neuroscience, Imaging and Clinical Sciences, University "G. d'Annunzio", Chieti-Pescara, Italy.

References

1. Fisher M. An unusual variant of acute idiopathic polyneuritis (syndrome of ophthalmoplegia, ataxia and areflexia). N Engl J Med. 1956;255:57–65.
2. Bickerstaff ER. Brain-stem encephalitis; further observations on a grave syndrome with benign prognosis. Br Med J. 1957;1:1384–7.
3. Chiba A, Kusunoki S, Shimizu T, Kanazawa I. Serum IgG antibody to ganglioside GQ1b is a possible marker of miller fisher syndrome. Ann Neurol. 1992;31:677–9.
4. Yuki N, Sato S, Tsuji S, Hozumi I, Miyatake T. An immunologic abnormality common to Bickerstaff's brain stem encephalitis and Fisher's syndrome. J Neurol Sci. 1993;118:83–7.
5. Odaka M, Yuki N, Hirata K. Anti-GQ1b IgG antibody syndrome: clinical and immunological range. J Neurol Neurosurg Psychiatry. 2001;70:50–5.
6. Sekiguchi Y, Mori M, Misawa S, Sawai S, Yuki N, Beppu M, et al. How often and when fisher syndrome is overlapped by Guillain-Barré syndrome or Bickerstaff brainstem encephalitis? Eur J Neurol. 2016;23:1058–63.
7. Pegg EJ, Chhetri SK, Lekwuwa UG, Majeed T. An overlapping case of miller fisher syndrome, Bickerstaff's encephalitis, and the ASMAN variant of Guillain-Barre syndrome. Case Rep Neurol Med. 2016;2016:1596850.
8. Uncini A, Ippoliti L, Shahrizaila N, Sekiguchi Y, Kuwabara S. Optimizing the electrodiagnostic accuracy in Guillain-Barré syndrome subtypes: criteria sets and sparse linear discriminant analysis. Clin Neurophysiol Off J Int Fed Clin Neurophysiol. 2017;128:1176–83.
9. Kuwahara M, Samukawa M, Ikeda T, Morikawa M, Ueno R, Hamada Y, et al. Characterization of the neurological diseases associated with mycoplasma pneumoniae infection and anti-glycolipid antibodies. J Neurol. 2017;264: 467–75.
10. Scherer SS. Molecular specializations at nodes and paranodes in peripheral nerve. Microsc Res Tech. 1996;34:452–61.
11. Shahrizaila N, Yuki N. Bickerstaff brainstem encephalitis and fisher syndrome: anti-GQ1b antibody syndrome. J Neurol Neurosurg Psychiatry. 2013;84:576–83.
12. Wakerley BR, Uncini A, Yuki N. GBS classification group, GBS classification group. Guillain-Barré and miller fisher syndromes--new diagnostic classification. Nat Rev Neurol. 2014;10:537–44.
13. Uncini A, Manzoli C, Notturno F, Capasso M. Pitfalls in electrodiagnosis of Guillain-Barré syndrome subtypes. J Neurol Neurosurg Psychiatry. 2010;81: 1157–63.
14. Uncini A, Kuwabara S. Electrodiagnostic criteria for Guillain-Barrè syndrome: a critical revision and the need for an update. Clin Neurophysiol Off J Int Fed Clin Neurophysiol. 2012;123:1487–95.
15. Kuwabara S, Yuki N, Koga M, Hattori T, Matsuura D, Miyake M, et al. IgG anti-GM1 antibody is associated with reversible conduction failure and axonal degeneration in Guillain-Barré syndrome. Ann Neurol. 1998;44:202–8.
16. Rajabally YA, Hassan-Smith G, Notturno F, Eames PJ, Hayton T, Capasso M, et al. Motor and sensory conduction failure in overlap of Guillain-Barré and miller fisher syndrome: two simultaneous cases. J Neurol Sci. 2011;303:35–8.
17. Umapathi T, Tan EY, Kokubun N, Verma K, Yuki N. Non-demyelinating, reversible conduction failure in fisher syndrome and related disorders. J Neurol Neurosurg Psychiatry. 2012;83:941–8.
18. Hong Y-H, Sung J-J, Oh M-Y, Moon H-J, Park K-S, Lee K-W. Axonal conduction block at intermediate nerve segments in pure motor Guillain-Barré syndrome. J Peripher Nerv Syst JPNS. 2011;16:37–46.

19. Saito K, Shimizu F, Koga M, Sano Y, Tasaki A, Abe M, et al. Blood-brain barrier destruction determines fisher/Bickerstaff clinical phenotypes: an in vitro study. J Neurol Neurosurg Psychiatry. 2013;84:756–65.
20. Uncini A, Susuki K, Yuki N. Nodo-paranodopathy: beyond the demyelinating and axonal classification in anti-ganglioside antibody-mediated neuropathies. Clin Neurophysiol Off J Int Fed Clin Neurophysiol. 2013;124: 1928–34.
21. Uncini A, Kuwabara S. Nodopathies of the peripheral nerve: an emerging concept. J Neurol Neurosurg Psychiatry. 2015;86:1186–95.
22. Lefaucheur J-P, Gregson NA, Gray I, von Raison F, Bertocchi M, Créange A. A variant of multifocal motor neuropathy with acute, generalised presentation and persistent conduction blocks. J Neurol Neurosurg Psychiatry. 2003;74: 1555–61.
23. Manganelli F, Pisciotta C, Iodice R, Calandro S, Dubbioso R, Ranieri A, et al. Case of acute motor conduction block neuropathy (AMCBN). Muscle Nerve. 2009;39:224–6.
24. Uncini A, Manzoli C, Capasso M. Acute motor conduction block neuropathy or acute multifocal motor neuropathy: an attempt at a nosological systematization. Muscle Nerve. 2010;41:283–5. author reply 285
25. Oda K, Araki K, Totoki T, Shibasaki H. Nerve conduction study of human tetrodotoxication. Neurology. 1989;39:743–5.
26. Yokota T, Saito Y, Miyatake T. Conduction slowing without conduction block of compound muscle and nerve action potentials due to sodium channel block. J Neurol Sci. 1994;124:220–4.
27. Uncini A, Vallat J-M. Autoimmune nodo-paranodopathies of peripheral nerve: the concept is gaining ground. J Neurol Neurosurg Psychiatry. 2018; 89:627–35.

25

Hashimoto's encephalitis associated with AMPAR2 antibodies

Mingqin Zhu[1], Xuefan Yu[1], Caiyun Liu[1], Chenchen Duan[1], Chunxiao Li[1], Jie Zhu[2] and Ying Zhang[1*]

Abstract

Background: Hashimoto's encephalitis (HE) is a rare neurological complication of Hashimoto's thyroiditis (HT), while limbic encephalitis (LE) is an autoimmune inflammatory disorder frequently associated with anti-neuronal antibodies. The glutamate receptor α-amino-3-hydroxy-5-methyl-4-isoxazole-propionic acid receptor (AMPAR) is important for synaptic transmission, memory, and learning. The etiology of HE remains unclear. We present a case of HE with antibodies to AMPAR2 both in the serum and cerebrospinal fluid.

Case presentation: The patient presented with progressive memory loss and subsequently went into a coma. Magnetic resonance imaging revealed temporal lobe and hippocampal lesions, while the electrocardiogram showed paroxysmal delta waves. Elevated serum levels of antibodies against thyroid globulin, thyroid peroxidase, and thyroid stimulating receptor were also noted. Ultrasonography showed enlargement of the thyroid gland. Therefore, the diagnosis was established as HE. Both the CSF and serum samples of the patient tested positive for antibodies to the cell-surface antigen AMPAR2. Intravenous injection of immunoglobulin followed by dexamethasone treatment resulted in recovery from the coma. Follow-up examination three months later showed some improvement of memory. To our knowledge, this is the first report on the detection of AMPAR2 antibodies in HE.

Conclusions: Our findings suggest that antibodies to AMPAR2 may be involved in the pathogenesis of HE. Elevated levels of thyroid antibodies possibly cause immune dysfunction, leading to the production of anti-AMPAR2 antibodies that are detrimental to the neurons. We believe that encephalitis patients with thyroid abnormalities should undergo screening for anti-neuronal antibodies, and early immune therapy may improve prognosis.

Keywords: Limbic encephalitis, Autoimmune thyroid disease, AMPAR, Hashimoto's thyroiditis, Hashimoto's encephalitis, Case report

Background

Hashimoto's thyroiditis (HT) is the most common type of autoimmune thyroid disease (AITD); it is characterized by the presence of high titers of anti-thyroid antibodies in the blood [1]. The neurological complication of HT, namely, Hashimoto's encephalitis (HE,) was first reported in the 1960's by Brain et al. [2]. The clinical presentations of HE are diverse, ranging from focal signs similar to those manifested in stroke-like events to those reflecting diffuse panencephalitis, such as altered cognition and psychosis [3, 4].

Limbic encephalitis (LE) is an autoimmune inflammatory disorder of the limbic system, involving the medial temporal lobe, amygdala, and cingulate gyri. Clinically, it is clinically manifested by short-term memory deficit, psychosis, and seizures [5]. Recent studies have suggested that the pathogenesis of LE is mediated by anti-neuronal antibodies, including antibodies to both intra-neuronal and cell-surface antigens. Intra-neuronal antigens are usually paraneoplastic, while cell-surface antigens are thought to be immune-mediated [5–7]. The glutamate receptor α-amino-3-hydroxy-5-methyl-4-isoxazole-propionic acid receptor (AMPAR) is a cell-surface ionotropic receptor that plays important roles in synaptic transmission, memory, and learning [8]. Anti-AMPAR encephalitis was first reported in 2009 in a cohort study of ten patients [9]. Exposure of neurons to the antibodies causes a significant decrease in the total amount of AMPAR cluster and synaptic locations of GluA1- and GluA2-containing AMPARs

* Correspondence: rose19700@sina.com
[1]Department of Neurology and Neuroscience Center, First Hospital of Jilin University, Xinmin Street No 71, Changchun 130000, China

[10], which demonstrates the pathogenic effect of anti-AMPAR antibodies.

Even to date, the pathogenesis of HE is largely unclear and widely debated. Several mechanisms, such as vasculitis, cerebral hypoperfusion and cerebral tissue specific autoimmunity, have been postulated thus far. In this paper, we present a case of HE with evidence of antibodies against AMPAR2 positive both in the serum and cerebrospinal fluid (CSF) [4].

Case presentation

A 54-year-old previously healthy woman was admitted to our hospital for progressive cognitive decline and memory loss since 5 days. The patient's symptoms started with the inability to remember the names and the functions of the condiments on the first day. The next day, the patient had difficulty in recollecting the names of her close relatives, in addition to dizziness and fatigue. At the time of admission, the patient was conscious, but confused. History taking revealed no fever, headache, or significant weight loss during the past three months, and no family history of auto-immune diseases. On further clinical examination, long-term and short-term memory, the ability of calculation, as well as temporal and spatial perception were found to be impaired. No other neurological signs were present, expect for a positive Chaddok sign on the left side.

The first magnetic resonance image (MRI) obtained at the local hospital showed normal findings. The second MRI repeated on the next day at our hospital revealed patchy lesions in the left temporal lobe and hippocampal area. The lesions showed high signal intensity on T1- and T2-weighted imaging and high signal intensity on the fluid-attenuated inversion recovery (FLAIR) sequence (Fig 1a-c). Electrocardiography (EEG) revealed paroxysmal delta waves in the left temporal lobe. Ultrasonographic examination showed enlargement of the thyroid gland (left thyroid lobe: 16 mm × 6 mm, and right thyroid lobe: 15 mm × 16 mm × 43 mm), with irregular echogenicity. However, ultrasonography examination of the abdominal organs, including the liver, kidney, pancreas and uterus, as well as other organs,

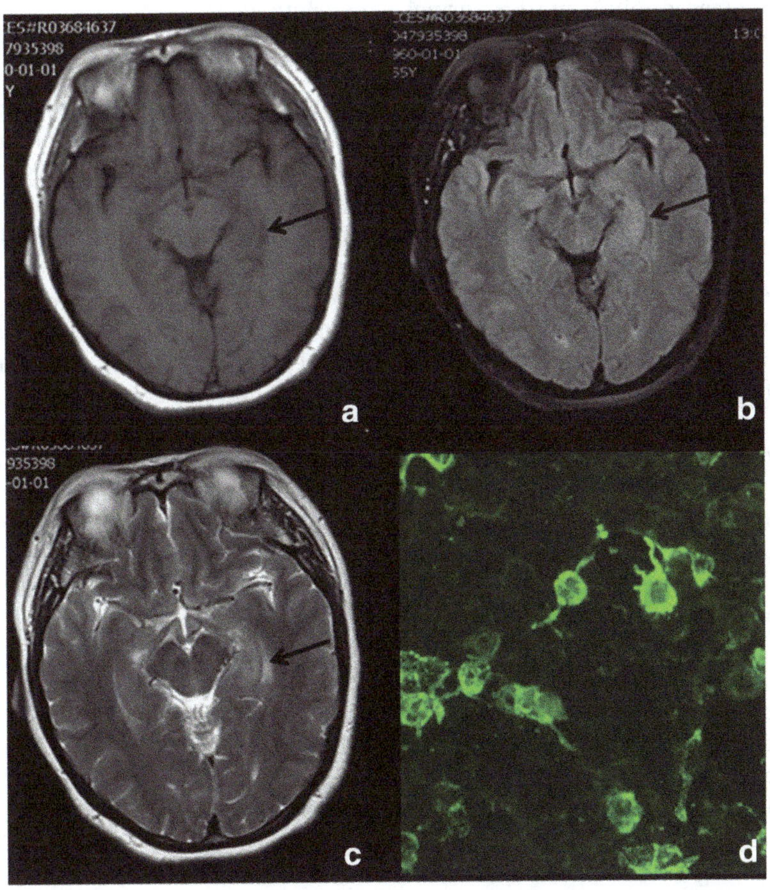

Fig. 1 a-d. Axonal magnetic resonance imaging (MRI) scans revealed patchy lesions in the left temporal lobe and hippocampus. The lesions were represented by areas of low signal intensity on T1-weighted imaging (**a**) and high signal intensity on T2-weighted imaging (**b**) sequence and high signal intensity on the fluid-attenuated inversion recovery (FLAIR) sequence (**c**). Anti-AMPAR2 antibodies in the serum of the patient was positive, as tested by CBA method (**d**)

such as mammary glands, did not reveal any abnormality. Pulmonary computed tomography (CT) scan was negative for neoplasia.

The findings of routine blood tests were normal, except for slightly low levels of sodium (133.9, normal range: 137–147 mmol/L) and chloride (97, normal range: 99–110 mmol/L). The screening assay for viral infection showed elevated levels of antibodies against herpes simplex virus I (HSV I) (8.023 S/CO, normal range: <1.00 S/CO), rubella virus (0.927 S/CO, normal range: <1.00 S/CO), and cytomegalovirus (CMV) (6.332 S/CO, normal range, normal range: <1.00 S/CO) in the serum but not in the CSF. The results of the lumbar puncture test showed increased intracranial pressure (230 mm H_2O; normal range: 70–180 mm H_2O). Routine analysis of the CSF showed increased concentration of protein (0.50 g/L, normal range 0.15–0.45 g/L) and elevated white blood cell count (63×10^6/L, normal range: $0–8 \times 10^6$/L), with 89% lymphocytes, 7% eosinophils, and 4% monocytes. The CSF was negative for oligoclonal bands. Further, the levels of the immunoglobulin (Ig) G were also found to be slightly increased (49.1 mg/L; normal range: 0–34.0 mg/L) in the CSF. The results of the autoimmune encephalitis test using cell-based assay (CBA) for antibodies against AMPAR2 were positive for both the serum and CSF (Fig 1d), but negative for other antibodies, including NMDA-R, CASPR2, AMPA1-R, and LGI1. Screening tests were also negative for paraneoplastic markers, including Hu, Yo, Ri, paraneoplastic Ma2 (PNMA2), CV2/collapsing response mediator 5 (CRMP5), and amphiphysin. Additionally, tests for tuberculosis were negative. Thyroid function-related tests showed slightly lower levels of thyroid stimulating hormones (TSH) (0.26 mIU/L; normal range: 0.27–4.2 mIU/L), while the serum levels of free T3 and T4 were within the normal range. Levels of the antibodies against the thyroid globulin (TG) (2006 IU/ml, normal range <115 IU/ml), thyroid peroxidase (TPO) (276.9 IU/ml, normal range <35 IU/ml), and thyroid stimulating receptor (TSHR) (13.6 IU/ml, normal range 0.3-1.75 IU/ml) were found to be elevated. Tests for antibodies against and antigen of hepatitis B and C virus were all negative. Antibody tests for human immunodeficiency virus (HIV) and syphilis were also negative, as were the screening tests for the tumor biomarkers. The results of routine urine analysis and tests for liver and kidney function were normal. The blood levels of lipids and glucose were also within the normal range. The erythrocyte sedimentation rate and levels of the C-reactive proteins were also within the normal range.

On the basis of the results of the preliminary physical examination and the laboratory tests conducted on the day of admission, viral encephalitis was suspected. Accordingly, the patient was treated with the anti-virus drug acyclovir. However, there was no significant relief in the patient's symptoms. Four days later, the patient's conditions worsened and the patient went into a coma; therefore, she was shifted to the intensive care unit. There, anti-AMPAR2 antibodies were detected in the serum and CSF, and accordingly, the patient was treated with intravenous injection of immunoglobulin (IVIG) for 3 days followed by dexamethasone. Once the IVIG treatment was initiated, the patient recovered from coma. Follow-up examination after 3 months showed that her memory function had improved to some extent, but not completely restored.

Discussion

In this paper, we presented a case of HE in which both serum and CSF were positive for antibodies to AMPAR2. HE is a rare neurological complication of HT, and approximately, one-third of HE cases occur in the euthyroid state of HT [11]. Although HE has been a known clinical entity since 50 years, its etiology is still not fully understood.

Our patient had progressive memory loss and eventually slipped into a coma. MRI scan showed lesions in the temporal lobe and hippocampus, while the EEG showed paroxysmal delta waves. Furthermore, the patient had elevated serum levels of antibodies to TG, TPO, and TSHR. In the light of these findings, the diagnosis was established as HE. High levels of anti-thyroid antibodies have been previously reported in the CSF of HE patients [12].

Moreover, anti-thyroid antibodies have been showed to bind to astrocytes [13], suggesting a direct pathogenic link between the two. However, the levels of anti-thyroid antibodies do not correlate with the severity of the clinical syndrome, and immunotherapy does not always reduce the levels of anti-thyroid antibodies despite reliving the clinical symptoms [14]; these findings suggest that there are more mechanisms, hitherto undiscovered, may be involved in the pathogenesis of HE. It has been suggested that anti-thyroid antibodies could serve as markers for autoimmune disease in the brain and anti-neuronal auto-antibodies may exist in HE. Oide et al. showed that serum of HE patients contained an anti-neuronal autoantibody that reacted with a 36-kDa antigenic protein from human cerebral cortex [15]. Moreover, the CSF of HE patients has been shown to test positive for other anti-neuronal auto-antibodies against enzymes expressed by neurons [16].

The antibodies to the cell surface antigen AMPAR2 were found positive both in the CSF and in the serum of this patient. To our knowledge, this is the first report on the detection of AMPAR2 antibodies in HE patients. Since the first report of AMPAR encephalitis in 2009, no more than 50 cases have been reported thus far [17]. One peculiar feature of this case is that the clinical presentation in this case is also consistent with the diagnosis of AMPAR2 LE. More than half of the cases of AMPAR encephalitis show evidence of coexistent tumor [17, 18]. Therefore, to rule out coexistent neoplasia, we performed ultrasonography of the abdominal organs and mammary glands in addition to pulmonary CT. However, no evidence of tumors was obtained in these scans. Moreover, screening for tumor markers and paraneoplastic auto-antibodies also did not yield any significant findings. Thus, caner was ruled out in this patient. In the light of our experience in this case, we speculate that the elevated levels of anti-thyroid antibodies may have caused immune dysfunction in the brain; this may have triggered the production of AMPAR2 antibodies, which, in turn, have a detrimental effect on neurons. It would be worthwhile to further investigate whether anti-thyroid antibodies have a causative relationship with the\production of AMPAR2 antibodies.

Vasculitis is another leading theory used to explain the etiology of HE. An autopsy study in a 77-year-old female patient showed infiltration of inflammatory CD3-positive T-lymphocytes in the brain stem, cerebellum, and cortex. In line with this hypothesis, increased concentrations of protein were found in the CSF of our patient, indicating the disruption of the blood brain barrier (BBB). Furthermore, increases were noted in the number of monocytes and eosinophils in our patient. Increase of the inflammatory cells in the CSF can produce inflammatory cytokines, which can cause damage to the neurons.

The patient's symptoms improved after initiation of IVIG treatment. Immunotherapy should be considered as the first-line-treatment for both HE and LE, and most of the patients show immediate response to the treatment, with reversal of the symptoms as well as MRI changes. However, the persistence of the neurologic deficits and eventual fatality may occur depending on the severity of the disease and complication of other organs. This patient's memory deficits did not completely recover despite administration of immunotherapy. Therefore, IVIG or glucocorticoid treatment alone or their combination is recommended as soon as the diagnosis is established.

Conclusions

Our findings in this case support the role of inflammatory autoimmunity in the pathogenesis of HE. Anti-thyroid antibodies may cause dysregulation of the immune cells in the brain, leading to the production of antibodies to AMPAR2, which in turn are detrimental to neurons. Our experience in this case also indicates that encephalitis patients with autoimmune thyroid disease should undergo screening for anti-neuronal antibodies and receive early immune therapy for a better prognosis.

Abbreviations

AMPAR: α-amino-3-hydroxy-5-methyl-4-isoxazole-propionic acid receptor; BBB: Blood–brain barrier; CMV: Cytomegalovirus; CSF: Cerebral spinal fluid; ESR: Erythrocyte sedimentation rate; HE: Hashimoto's encephalitis; HSV: Herpes simplex virus; HT: Hashimoto's thyroiditis; Ig: Immunoglobulin; IVIG: Intravenous injection of immunoglobulin; LE: Limbic encephalitis; MRI: Magnetic resonance imaging; TSH: Thyroid stimulating hormones

Acknowledgements

None.

Funding

There's no funding for this case report.

Authors' contributions

MZ drafted the manuscript; XY, CD and CXL collected the patient information; CYL performed the CBA test for this patient; JZ and YZ did manuscript editing and data interpretation. All authors read and approved the final manuscript.

Competing interests

The authors declare that they have no competing interests.

Author details

[1]Department of Neurology and Neuroscience Center, First Hospital of Jilin University, Xinmin Street No 71, Changchun 130000, China. [2]Division of Neurodegerneration, Department of Neurobiology, Care Sciences & Society, Karolinska Institutet, SE 14157, Huddinge, Stockholm, Sweden.

References

1. Leyhe T, Mussig K. Cognitive and affective dysfunctions in autoimmune thyroiditis. Brain Behav Immun. 2014;41:261–6.
2. Brain L, Jellinek EH, Ball K. Hashimoto's disease and encephalopathy. Lancet. 1966;2(7462):512–4.
3. Olmez I, Moses H, Sriram S, Kirshner H, Lagrange AH, Pawate S. Diagnostic and therapeutic aspects of Hashimoto's encephalopathy. J Neurol Sci. 2013; 331(1-2):67–71.
4. Tamagno G, Federspil G, Murialdo G. Clinical and diagnostic aspects of encephalopathy associated with autoimmune thyroid disease (or Hashimoto's encephalopathy). Intern Emerg Med. 2006;1(1):15–23.
5. Melzer N, Budde T, Stork O, Meuth SG. Limbic encephalitis: potential impact of adaptive autoimmune inflammation on neuronal circuits of the amygdala. Front Neurol. 2015;6:171.
6. Vincent A, Bien CG, Irani SR, Waters P. Autoantibodies associated with diseases of the CNS: new developments and future challenges. Lancet Neurol. 2011;10(8):759–72.
7. Lancaster E, Martinez-Hernandez E, Dalmau J. Encephalitis and antibodies to synaptic and neuronal cell surface proteins. Neurology. 2011;77(2):179–89.
8. Derkach VA, Oh MC, Guire ES, Soderling TR. Regulatory mechanisms of AMPA receptors in synaptic plasticity. Nat Rev Neurosci. 2007;8(2):101–13.

9. Lai M, Hughes EG, Peng X, Zhou L, Gleichman AJ, Shu H, Mata S, Kremens D, Vitaliani R, Geschwind MD, et al. AMPA receptor antibodies in limbic encephalitis alter synaptic receptor location. Ann Neurol. 2009;65(4):424–34.
10. Peng X, Hughes EG, Moscato EH, Parsons TD, Dalmau J, Balice-Gordon RJ. Cellular plasticity induced by anti-alpha-amino-3-hydroxy-5-methyl-4-isoxazolepropionic acid (AMPA) receptor encephalitis antibodies. Ann Neurol. 2015;77(3):381–98.
11. Chong JY, Rowland LP, Utiger RD. Hashimoto encephalopathy: syndrome or myth? Arch Neurol. 2003;60(2):164–71.
12. Ferracci F, Moretto G, Candeago RM, Cimini N, Conte F, Gentile M, Papa N, Carnevale A. Antithyroid antibodies in the CSF: their role in the pathogenesis of Hashimoto's encephalopathy. Neurology. 2003;60(4):712–4.
13. Blanchin S, Coffin C, Viader F, Ruf J, Carayon P, Potier F, Portier E, Comby E, Allouche S, Ollivier Y, et al. Anti-thyroperoxidase antibodies from patients with Hashimoto's encephalopathy bind to cerebellar astrocytes. J Neuroimmunol. 2007;192(1-2):13–20.
14. Kothbauer-Margreiter I, Sturzenegger M, Komor J, Baumgartner R, Hess CW. Encephalopathy associated with Hashimoto thyroiditis: diagnosis and treatment. J Neurol. 1996;243(8):585–93.
15. Oide T, Tokuda T, Yazaki M, Watarai M, Mitsuhashi S, Kaneko K, Hashimoto T, Ohara S, Ikeda S. Anti-neuronal autoantibody in Hashimoto's encephalopathy: neuropathological, immunohistochemical, and biochemical analysis of two patients. J Neurol Sci. 2004;217(1):7–12.
16. Gini B, Lovato L, Cianti R, Cecotti L, Marconi S, Anghileri E, Armini A, Moretto G, Bini L, Ferracci F, et al. Novel autoantigens recognized by CSF IgG from Hashimoto's encephalitis revealed by a proteomic approach. J Neuroimmunol. 2008;196(1-2):153–8.
17. Hoftberger R, van Sonderen A, Leypoldt F, Houghton D, Geschwind M, Gelfand J, Paredes M, Sabater L, Saiz A, Titulaer MJ, et al. Encephalitis and AMPA receptor antibodies: Novel findings in a case series of 22 patients. Neurology. 2015;84(24):2403–12.
18. Joubert B, Kerschen P, Zekeridou A, Desestret V, Rogemond V, Chaffois MO, Ducray F, Larrue V, Daubail B, Idbaih A, et al. Clinical spectrum of encephalitis associated with antibodies against the alpha-amino-3-hydroxy-5-methyl-4-isoxazolepropionic acid receptor: case series and review of the literature. JAMA Neurol. 2015;72(10):1163–9.

Kikuchi-Fujimoto disease (histiocytic necrotizing lymphadenitis) with atypical encephalitis and painful testitis

Hidenori Kido[1*†], Osamu Kano[2†], Asami Hamai[1], Hiroyuki Masuda[3], Yutaka Fuchinoue[3], Masaaki Nemoto[3], Chiaki Arai[4], Teppei Takeda[4], Fumihito Yamabe[5], Toshihiro Tai[5], Mizuki Kasahara[5], Kenichi Suzuki[6], Nobuyuki Shiraga[6], Sota Sadamoto[7], Megumi Wakayama[7], Yukitoshi Takahashi[8], Yasuo Iwasaki[2], Kazutoshi Shibuya[7] and Yoshihisa Urita[1]

Abstract

Background: Kikuchi-Fujimoto disease is a self-limited clinicopathologic entity that is increasingly recognized worldwide. Kikuchi-Fujimoto disease is characterized by cervical lymphadenopathy occurring in young adults. Neurologic involvement is rare, and testitis directly caused by Kikuchi-Fujimoto disease has not yet been reported.

Case presentation: A 19-year-old man was brought to our clinic with complaints of fever, headache, fatigue, and left lower quadrant pain that had persisted for 3 weeks. On physical examination, painful cervical lymphadenopathies were observed. Meningitis was suspected based on a cerebrospinal fluid examination, and left-sided orchitis was diagnosed based on findings from magnetic resonance imaging and ultrasonography. However, neither antibiotics nor antiviral drugs were effective in treating the patient's symptoms. On the 20th day of hospitalization, the patient experienced a loss of consciousness, and brain T2-weighted magnetic resonance imaging showed asymmetrical, high-signal intensities in both basal nuclei and the left temporal lobe. Encephalitis was suspected, and the patient was treated with intravenous prednisolone pulse therapy (1 g/day) for 3 days and intravenous immunoglobulin therapy for 5 days. A left cervical lymph node biopsy showed apoptotic necrosis in paracortical and cortical areas with an abundance of macrophages and large lymphoid cells, which had irregular nuclei suggestive of Kikuchi-Fujimoto disease; the pathological findings from a brain biopsy were the same as those of the cervical lymph node biopsy. The encephalitis and cervical lymphadenopathies followed a benign course, as did the testitis.

Conclusions: This is the first report of Kikuchi-Fujimoto disease involving painful testitis and pathologically proven asymmetrical brain regions. Kikuchi-Fujimoto disease should be included in the differential diagnosis when a patient presents with encephalitis, testitis, and fever of unknown origin.

Keywords: Encephalitis, Fever of unknown origin, Histiocytic necrotizing lymphadenitis, Kikuchi-Fujimoto disease, Testitis

* Correspondence: hidenori775@gmail.com
†Equal contributors
[1]Department of General Medicine and Emergency Care, Toho University School of Medicine, 6-11-1 Omorinishi Ota-ku, Tokyo 143-8541, Japan
Full list of author information is available at the end of the article

Background

Kikuchi-Fujimoto disease (KFD), or histiocytic necrotizing lymphadenitis, is known to be a benign disease that usually resolves spontaneously. It is a rare disease and was first reported in Japan in 1972 [1, 2]. KFD usually affects female patients under the age of 30 years and is characterized by regional lymphadenopathy with tenderness, predominantly in the cervical region, and is usually accompanied by mild fever and night sweats. It is of clinical importance because it is often misdiagnosed as tuberculosis, lymphoma, or systemic lupus erythematosus (SLE); therefore, the diagnosis should be confirmed by biopsy study. Diseases that generally accompany KFD are SLE, arthritis, mixed connective tissue disease, and similar conditions; however, comorbid testitis has not yet been reported. Neurological complications occur in about 11% of cases, as revealed by a review of 244 cases in which a minority of cases evolved to developing encephalitis [3]. Brain magnetic resonance imaging (MRI) includes symmetrical hyperintense T2-weighted and FLAIR (fluid-attenuated inversion recovery) signals in the temporal lobes, pons, and periaqueductal gray matter [4–7]. This is the first report of KFD occurring with testitis and pathologically proven asymmetrical brain regions.

Case presentation

A 19-year-old man presented to our hospital with complaints of fever (39.5 °C), headache, fatigue, night sweats, and lower abdominal pain, which had been present for about 1 month. For 20 days, he had used anti-flatulent medications before presenting to our hospital. He had no history of close contact with pets, he did not travel often, and similar complaints were not present in his social circle. According to the patient's physical examination on admission, his general health status was good; body temperature, pulse, and blood pressure were 37.2 °C, 102 beats/min, and 106/70 mmHg, respectively. He was alert, oriented, and cooperative. Mobile, painful lymphadenopathies were observed on both sides of the cervical region, of which the largest was 2 × 1.6 cm in size. Bilateral cervical lymphadenopathy was present and involved a posterior group of cervical lymph nodes. Cardiac, respiratory, and neurological examination revealed no abnormality; vegetation was not detected by transthoracic echocardiography. Laboratory investigations showed leukopenia (total leucocyte count: 3200 cells/mm^3). Cerebrospinal fluid (CSF) analyses were normal. No positive results that could explain the high body temperature were found during serological testing for Epstein Barr virus (EBV); cytomegalovirus (CMV); hepatitis A, B, and C; parvovirus; human herpesvirus; chlamydia trachomatis; mumps; human immunodeficiency virus; echo virus; coxsackie virus enterovirus; and measles spp. Results of tests for rheumatologic markers (ferritin, anti-nuclear antibody, anti-neutrophil cytoplasmic antibody, anti-cyclic citrullinated peptide antibodies, extractable nuclear antigen antibody panel, anti-double stranded DNA, and rheumatoid factor) were also negative. Results of tuberculosis polymerase chain reaction (PCR) and herpes simplex PCR were also negative in the CSF. Blood and CSF cultures showed no growth after incubation for 6 to 8 weeks. Brain T2-weighted and FLAIR MRI sequences showed a slightly hyperintense signal of about 4 mm in the left temporal lobe (Fig. 1), and antibiotics and acyclovir treatment were begun because we could not rule out encephalitis. However, the patient's body temperature could not be reduced by routine anti-inflammatory drugs and intravenous paracetamol. Thoracic and abdominal computed tomography (CT) and MRI scans revealed a testicular lesion having no contrast effect (Fig. 2); lymph nodes were predominantly located on the right side of the cervical region, with the largest measuring 2 cm in diameter. Thus, one of the lymph nodes located in the right cervical region was removed and sent to pathology for analysis. On the 4th

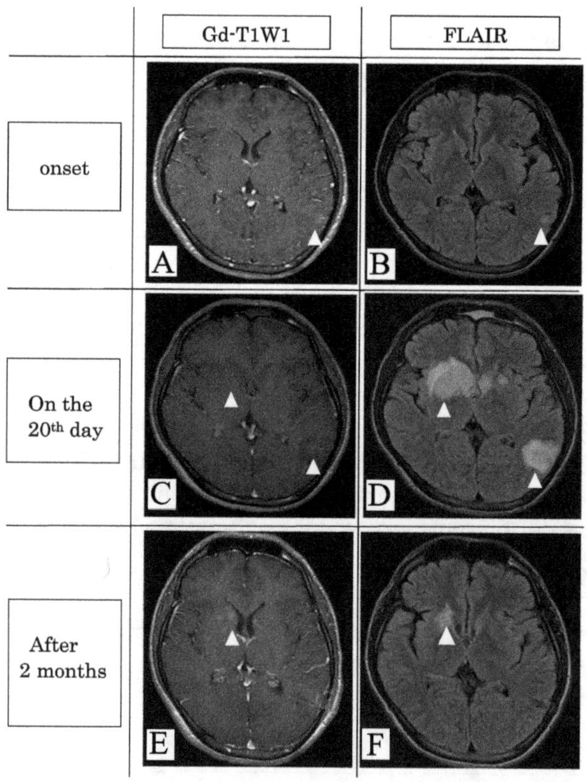

Fig. 1 Axial T1-weighted MRI with gadolinium contrast (**a**) and FLAIR-weighted MRI (**b**) show mild enhancement and a high-intensity area, respectively, in the left temporal lobe at onset (*arrow heads*). Following periods of acute exacerbation on the 20th day, axial T1-weighted MRI with gadolinium contrast (**c**) showed slightly larger enhancement, and FLAIR-weighted MRI (**d**) revealed an asymmetrical hyperintense signal in the left temporal lobe and both basal nuclei. After 2 months of hospitalization, the abnormal lesions became smaller (**e**, **f**)

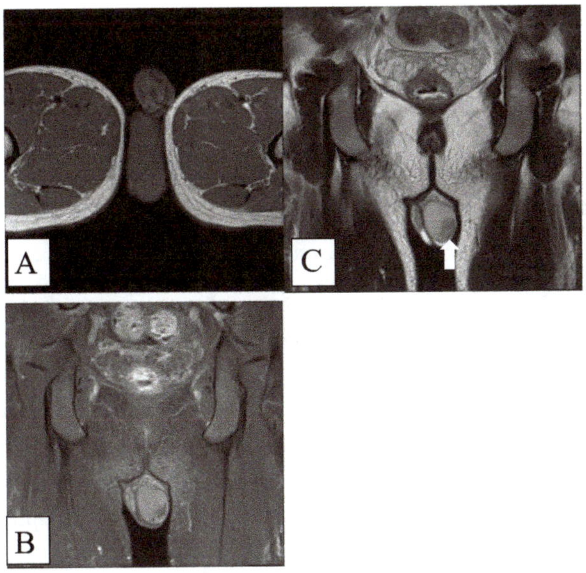

Fig. 2 a Axial T1-weighted magnetic resonance image shows that the lesion has an isointense signal. **b** After administration of gadolinium contrast, material internal enhancement is not observed. **c** Coronal T2-weighted magnetic resonance image shows that the lesion has low signal intensity (*arrow*)

day of hospitalization, an excision biopsy of the cervical lymph node was performed. Microscopic examination showed that the lymph nodes were expressed in paracortical and cortical areas of conspicuous apoptotic necrosis with an abundance of enlarged lymphocytes, which had prominent nucleoli in the absence of neutrophils and a proliferation of macrophages (Fig. 3). Results of tests using in situ hybridization to detect EBV with marked paracortical expansion due to a proliferation of immunoblasts were negative. On the 20th day of hospitalization, the patient's general status suddenly and temporarily worsened. The signal intensity on brain MRI had changed and showed an asymmetrical hyperintense signal in the wider larger left temporal lobe and both basal nuclei (Fig. 1) with slight Gd-enhancement. CSF protein levels and pleocytosis were increased (protein: 50 mg/dL; pleocytosis: 24 cells/μL), but CSF cultures were negative, and cytology showed no malignant findings. Anti-NMDA, CO, Tr, GAD65, Zic4, Titin, SOX1, Rec, Hu, Yo, Ri, Ma-2/Ta, Cv2, and Amp antibodies associated with auto-immune-mediated encephalomyelitis were all absent. Oligoclonal bands were also not detected in the CSF sample. Since acute disseminated encephalomyelitis (ADEM) was suspected, the patient was managed with intravenous prednisolone pulse treatment (1 g/day) for 3 days and intravenous immunoglobulin treatment for 5 days, and these therapies were repeated 3 times every 3 weeks. Electroencephalography showed no waves characteristic of epilepsy, but levetiracetam 1000 mg/day was begun. On the 34th day of hospitalization, MRI investigation of the brain revealed that the previous abnormalities were present and had not changed. Since the cervical lymph node biopsy before steroid therapy did not reveal lymphoma, a brain biopsy of the temporal lobe was performed. Steroids can obscure diffuse large B-cell lymphoma or intravascular lymphomatosis; however, no recurrence was experienced. The pathological results revealed many CD68+ macrophages and histiocytes, as in the cervical lymph node, suggestive of KFD (Fig. 4). The cervical lymphadenopathies disappeared after 2 months of hospitalization, and the previous abnormalities on MRI became smaller during follow-up. The testicular mass that showed a contrast effect on MRI and CT similarly was smaller (Fig. 1); therefore, we suspected that the testitis had been caused by KFD. His complaints of fever, headache, and fatigue gradually improved; he was discharged on the 90th day of hospitalization. He was followed for more than 3 months in our clinic and did not show any recurrence.

Discussion and Conclusions

KFD was first described in Japan in 1972 and has increasingly been recognized worldwide since 1982

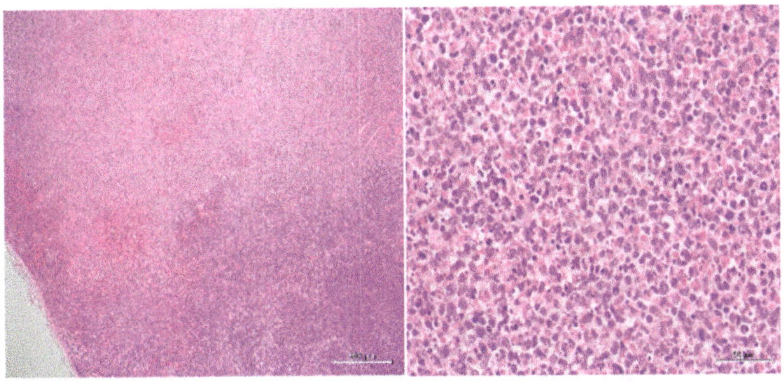

Fig. 3 Left cervical lymph node biopsy shows conspicuous apoptotic necrosis in paracortical and cortical areas with an abundance of macrophages and large lymphoid cells, which have irregular nuclei [hematoxylin-eosin staining × 4 (*left*), ×40 (*right*)]

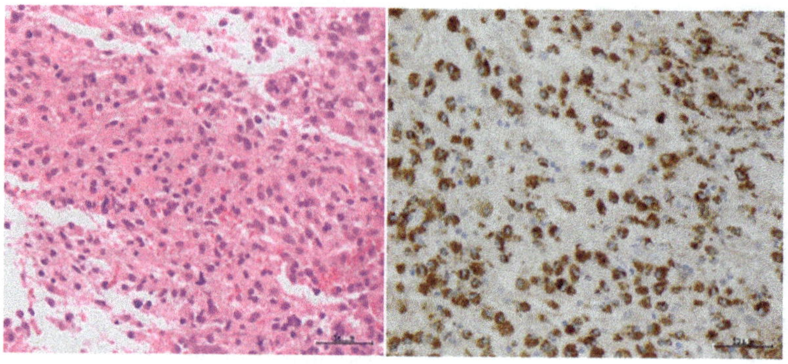

Fig. 4 Brain biopsy shows an abundance of CD68+ macrophages and histiocytes, as in the cervical lymph node. [hematoxylin-eosin × 40 (*left*), anti-CD68 (*right*)]

[8]. According to a review [3] that summarized 244 KFD cases, the mean age was 25 (1–64) years, and 70% were younger than 30 years; 33% were men, and 77% were women. Most of the cases were reported from East Asia and the Far East (50%), and the others were from Europe (27%) and America (7%). As in the present case, the most common symptoms were fever (35%), fatigue (7%), and cervical lymphadenomegaly (100%) [3]. Our case did not show any evidence of SLE, lymphoma, tuberculosis, arthritis, or viral disease based on laboratory findings and cervical lymph node biopsy.

Testitis has not been reported as a co-morbid disease in KFD. After diagnosing KFD based on results of the cervical lymph node biopsy, we could not explain the central nervous system (CNS) involvement in this case. Neurological involvement, including aseptic meningitis and encephalitis, is rare, and abnormal MRI findings in KFD usually show symmetrical, hyperintense T2 and FLAIR signals in the temporal lobes, pons, and periaqueductal gray matter [4–7]. Therefore, we considered the possibility of co-morbid ADEM. Avkan-Oguz et al. [6] reported the co-existence of KFD and ADEM based on brain MRI findings without a brain biopsy. Our case did not show symmetrical lesions, which were reported in the previous KFD reports with CNS involvement; hence, we evaluated brain pathology, and the results were consistent with those for KFD and showed a benign course. Although the etiology of the disease remains unknown, infectious or autoimmune pathogenesis is thought to be responsible. The factors that likely result in the infection include herpes simplex virus, EBV, CMV, human herpes virus 6, varicella zoster virus, HIV, rubella, measles, coronavirus, coxsackie virus, hepatitis A and B, *Yersinia enterocolitica*, toxoplasma, influenza viruses, mumps, streptococci, leptospira, and chlamydia. It has also been reported that the disease may occur after rabies, diphtheria-tetanus, poliomyelitis, hepatitis B, and influenza vaccines are injected [9]. KFD may initially be mistaken for various benign and malignant diseases, such as tuberculosis, lymphoma, SLE, limbic encephalitis, and sarcoidosis. On the other hand, with regards to clinical and laboratory presentations, KFD frequently mimics SLE, arthritis, mixed connective tissue disease, aseptic meningitis, encephalitis, tuberculous lymphadenitis, malignant lymphoma, and some other benign and/or malignant diseases [3, 10, 11]. In addition to painful cervical lymphadenopathies and aseptic meningitis, our case showed testitis and encephalitis, which are not typical MRI findings compared with those reported in a previous case report. Previous papers reported that most cases of KFD had a benign course; therefore, it was difficult to evaluate the effect of our therapies, such as prednisolone and intravenous immunoglobulin treatment. The definitive method for confirming the diagnosis of KFD is with a lymph node biopsy, and therefore, physicians should not hesitate to perform one in order to diagnose the condition. In addition, if progressive CNS involvement is observed, either steroid therapy or brain biopsy should be considered. Thus, KFD may exist on a wide spectrum of diseases, and we suggest that KFD should be included in the differential diagnosis of lymphadenopathy, encephalitis, testis, and fevers of unknown origin.

In conclusion, this is the first report of KFD involving testitis and pathologically proven asymmetrical brain regions.

Abbreviations

ADEM: Acute disseminated encephalomyelitis; CMV: Cytomegalovirus; CNS: Central nervous system; CSF: Cerebrospinal fluid; EBV: Epstein-Barr virus; FLAIR: Fluid-attenuated inversion recovery; HIV: Human immunodeficiency virus; KFD: Kikuchi-Fujimoto disease; MRI: Magnetic resonance imaging; PCR: Polymerase chain reaction; SLE: Systemic lupus erythematosus

Acknowledgments

None.

Funding

None.

Authors' contributions

Study concept and design: HK, OK. Acquisition of data: HK, OK, AH. HK, OK, AH, HM, YF, MN, CA, T. Takeda, FY, T. Tai, MK, K. Suzuki, NS, SS, MW, K. Shibuya, YI and YU examined and evaluated the patient. YT contributed to the CSF analysis. All authors read and approved the final manuscript.

Competing interests

The authors declare that they have no competing interests.

Author details

[1]Department of General Medicine and Emergency Care, Toho University School of Medicine, 6-11-1 Omorinishi Ota-ku, Tokyo 143-8541, Japan. [2]Division of Neurology, Department of Internal Medicine, Toho University School of Medicine, Tokyo, Japan. [3]Department of Neurosurgery Radiology, Toho University School of Medicine, Tokyo, Japan. [4]Department of Otorhinolaryngology, Toho University School of Medicine, Tokyo, Japan. [5]Department of Urology, Toho University School of Medicine, Tokyo, Japan. [6]Department of Radiology, Toho University School of Medicine, Tokyo, Japan. [7]Department of Pathology, Toho University School of Medicine, Tokyo, Japan. [8]Epilepsy Center, Shizuoka Institute of Epilepsy and Neurological, Tokyo, Japan.

References

1. Kikuchi M. Lymphadenitis showing focal reticulum cells hyperplasia with nuclear debris and phagocytosis: a clinicopathological study. Nippon Ketsueki Gakkai Zasshi. 1972;35:379–80.
2. Fujimoto Y, Kozima Y, Yamaguchi K. Cervical sub-acute necrotising lymphadenitis. A new clinicopathological entity. Naika. 1972;20:920–7.
3. Kucukardali Y, Solmazgul E, Kunter E, Oncul O, Yildirim S, Kaplan M. Kikuchi-Fujimoto disease: analysis of 244 cases. Clin Rheumatol. 2007;26:50–4.
4. Gonçalves LF, Debelenko LV, Bhambhani KJ, Scheid A, Altinok D. Histiocytic necrotizing lymphadenitis (Kikuchi-Fujimoto disease) with CNS involvement in a child. Pediatr Radiol. 2014;44:234–8.
5. Shafqat S, Memon SB, Hyder S, Hasan SH, Smego Jr RA. Brainstem encephalitis with Kikuchi-Fujimoto disease. J Coll Physicians Surg Pak. 2003; 13:663–4.
6. Avkan-Oguz V, Yapar N, Ozakbas S, Demir-Onder K, Aktas E, Alp-Cavus S, et al. A case of fever of unknown origin: co-existence of Kikuchi-Fujimoto disease and acute disseminated encephalomyelitis (ADEM). Intern Med. 2010;49:1823–6.
7. Guéguen A, Sené T, Maillart E, Gout O. Encephalitis and CSF increased level of interferon-alpha in Kikuchi-Fujimoto disease. BMJ Case Rep. 2012. 2012.
8. Pileri S, Kikuchi M, Helbron D, Lennert K. Histiocytic necrotizing lymphadenitis without granulocytic infiltration. Virchows Archiv A Pathol Anat Histol. 1982;395:257–71.
9. Sonneville R, Klein I, de Broucker T, Wolff M. Post-infectious encephalitis in adults: diagnosis and management. J Infect. 2009;58:321–8.
10. Sato Y, Kuno H, Oizumi K. Histiocytic necrotizing lymphadenitis (Kikuchi's disease) with aseptic meningitis. J Neurol Sci. 1999;163:187–91.
11. Lay-Son L, Espinoza-Martínez L. Encephalitis associated to Kikuchi-Fujimoto's disease in a young woman: a case report. Neurol Asia. 2011;16:81–3.

27

Long noncoding RNA papillary thyroid carcinoma susceptibility candidate 3 (PTCSC3) inhibits proliferation and invasion of glioma cells by suppressing the Wnt/β-catenin signaling pathway

Shujun Xia, Ri Ji and Weiwei Zhan*

Abstract

Background: The dysregulation of long noncoding RNAs (lncRNAs) has been identified in a variety of cancers. An increasing number of studies have found the critical role of lncRNAs in the regulation of cellular processes, such as proliferation, invasion and differentiation. Long noncoding RNA papillary thyroid carcinoma susceptibility candidate 3 (PTCSC3) is a novel lncRNA that was primarily detected in papillary thyroid carcinoma. However, the biological function and molecular mechanism of lncRNA PTCSC3 in glioma are still unknown.

Methods: The expression level of lncRNA PTCSC3 in human microglia and glioma cell lines was examined using quantitative real-time polymerase chain reaction (qRT-PCR). The influence of lncRNA PTCSC3 on cell proliferation were studied using the cell counting kit-8, and cell cycle and apoptosis were analyzed by flow cytometry assays. The migration and invasion abilities were investigated by transwell and wound healing assays. The target genes of lncRNA PTCSC3 were explored by qRT-PCR, immunofluorescence and western blot.

Results: LncRNA PTCSC3 was significantly downregulated in glioma cell lines. The overexpression of lncRNA PTCSC3 suppressed proliferation and induced apoptosis in U87 and U251 cells. Additionally, the overexpression of lncRNA PTCSC3 inhibited the migration and invasion of U87 and U251 cells. Moreover, lncRNA PTCSC3 inhibited the epithelial-mesenchymal transition of U87 cells. The study also demonstrated that LRP6, as a receptor of the Wnt/β-catenin pathway, was a target of lncRNA PTCSC3. By evaluating the expression levels of Axin1, active β-catenin, c-myc, and cyclin D1, the study indicated that lncRNA PTCSC3 inhibited the activation of the Wnt/β-cateninpathway through targeting LRP6.

Conclusions: LncRNA PTCSC3 inhibits the proliferation and migration of glioma cells and suppresses Wnt/β-catenin signaling pathway by targeting LRP6. LncRNA PTCSC3 is a potential therapeutic target for treatment of glioma.

Keywords: LncRNA PTCSC3, Glioma, Proliferation, Invasion, EMT, Wnt signal

* Correspondence: shanghairuijinus@163.com
Ultrasound Department, Rui Jin Hospital Shanghai Jiao Tong University School of Medicine, 197 Rui Jin Er Road, Huang Pu District, Shanghai Zip code: 200025, People's Republic of China

Background

Glioma appears to be one of the most common types of primary brain tumors in adults [1, 2]. Characterized by rapid progression, patients with glioma are most likely diagnosed at advanced stages, and the prognosis remains poor [3], posing a large threat to human health. Although some advances in comprehensive treatment as well as early diagnosis have been made, only a few patients have experienced the expected effects when translated to the clinic [4, 5]. Thus, it is imperative to explore the mechanisms concerning glioma formation and progression and to establish diagnostic and therapeutic targets for optimized management of glioma.

Long noncoding RNAs (lncRNAs) are defined as non-protein coding transcripts longer than 200 nucleotides. Recently, lncRNAs have gained much attention in the field of molecular biology. Increasing evidence indicates that lncRNAs are involved in diverse biological processes, including cell proliferation, differentiation, apoptosis, development and immune responses [6, 7]. Papillary thyroid carcinoma susceptibility candidate 3 (PTCSC3) is an intergenic long noncoding RNA gene (lincRNA) located at 14q.13.3, which was newly identified as thyroid specific [8]. Subsequently, lncRNA PTCSC3 was reported to be a tumor suppressor in thyroid cancer [9], and the mechanism study demonstrated that lncRNA PTCSC3 reduced cell motility and invasiveness by downregulating the S100A4 pathway [10]. However, little is known about the role of lncRNA PTCSC3 in other malignancies.

Our study was performed to assess the expression of lncRNA PTCSC3 in glioma cells and to evaluate its role and mechanism in tumor cell proliferation, invasion and migration. This is the first time that lncRNA PTCSC3 has been assessed in glioma. We assessed the expression level of lncRNA PTCSC3 in human microglia and glioma cell lines. Additionally, we demonstrated that lncRNA PTCSC3 overexpression suppressed proliferation, migration and invasion and inhibited the epithelial-mesenchymal transition (EMT) by suppressing the Wnt/β-catenin signaling pathway in glioma.

Methods

Cell culture

Several glioma cell lines (U87, U251, SHG44 & SHG139) were purchased from the Cell Bank Type Culture Collection of the Chinese Academy of Sciences (Shanghai, China). Human microglia was purchased from the Scinencell Research Laboratories (Carlsbad, CA, USA). Human astrocyte was purchased from Lonza (Basel, Switzerland) and cultured in AGM™ Astrocyte Growth Medium. Other cells were cultured in DMEM (Gibco, Carlsbad, CA, USA) supplemented with 10% of fetal bovine serum (Gibco) and 1% of penicillin-streptomycin at 37 °C, 5% CO_2 humidified atmosphere.

RNA extraction and quantitative reverse transcriptase-polymerase chain reaction (qRT-PCR)

Total RNA was extracted from cell lines with TRIzol reagent (Invitrogen, Carlsbad, CA, USA) and the concentration was measured by nanodrop spectrophotometer. One microgram of total RNA was reversely transcribed into first-strand cDNA using a Reverse Transcription Kit (Takara, Dalian, China). PCR was performed in VIIA7 system (Applied Biosystems, California, USA) with SYBR® Premix Ex Taq™ II Kit (Takara, Dalian, China). GAPDH was used as an internal control. Gene primers are listed in Table 1. Comparison Ct (2-△△Ct) method was used to analyze the data.

Table 1 Sequence of primers used for qRT-PCR

Gene		Sequence (5′–3′)
lncRNA PTCSC3	Forward Primer	GGCTTGAACAATCTTCCCACCTT
	Reverse Primer	TTTGGCAACACCCTCACAGACAC
MMP1	Forward Primer	AAAATTACACGCCAGATTTGCC
	Reverse Primer	GGTGTGACATTACTCCAGAGTTG
MMP2	Forward Primer	CCCACTGCGGTTTTCTCGAAT
	Reverse Primer	CAAAGGGGTATCCATCGCCAT
MMP9	Forward Primer	AGACCTGGGCAGATTCCAAAC
	Reverse Primer	CGGCAAGTCTTCCGAGTAGT
MMP13	Forward Primer	ACTGAGAGGCTCCGAGAAATG
	Reverse Primer	GAACCCCGCATCTTGGCTT
E-cadherin	Forward Primer	CGAGAGCTACACGTTCACGG
	Reverse Primer	GGGTGTCGAGGGAAAAATAGG
Fibronectin	Forward Primer	CGGTGGCTGTCAGTCAAAG
	Reverse Primer	AAACCTCGGCTTCCTCCATAA
Snail	Forward Primer	TCGGAAGCCTAACTACAGCGA
	Reverse Primer	AGATGAGCATTGGCAGCGAG
ZEB1	Forward Primer	GATGATGAATGCGAGTCAGATGC
	Reverse Primer	ACAGCAGTGTCTTGTTGTTGT
FZD8	Forward Primer	ATCGGCTACAACTACACCTACA
	Reverse Primer	GTACATGCTGCACAGGAAGAA
LRP6	Forward Primer	TTTATGCAAACAGACGGGACTT
	Reverse Primer	GCCTCCAACTACAATCGTAGC
Axin1	Forward Primer	GACCTGGGGTATGAGCCTGA
	Reverse Primer	GGCTTATCCCATCTTGGTCATC
C-myc	Forward Primer	GGCTCCTGGCAAAAGGTCA
	Reverse Primer	CTGCGTAGTTGTGCTGATGT
Cyclin D1	Forward Primer	TGGAGCCCGTGAAAAAGAGC
	Reverse Primer	TCTCCTTCATCTTAGAGGCCAC
GAPDH	Forward Primer	AAGGTGAAGGTCGGAGTCAAC
	Reverse Primer	GGGGTCATTGATGGCAACAATA

Lentivirus transfection

The lncRNA PTCSC3 was ligated into pLVX-IRES-puro to construct the lncRNA PTCSC3 overexpression plasmid. The pRUF-IRES-puro-PTCSC3 and pLVX-IRES-puro constructs were transfected into the HEK293T viral packaging cell line together with psPAX2 and pMD2.G plasmids. Forty-eight hours after transfection, the supernatant was collected and used to infect the cells.

CCK-8 assay

U87 and U251 were selected as the appropriate cell lines for gain-of-function experiments. The two cell lines were seeded into 96-well plates at a density of 1×10^4 cells/well 48 h after transfection and cultured at 37 °C, 5% CO_2 incubator. The viabilities of cells were assessed with the cell counting kit-8 (CCK-8; Dojindo Molecular Technologies, Japan) at four time points (12, 24, 48 & 72 h). The absorbance was detected by a TECAN infinite M200 plate reader at 450 nm.

Colony formation assay

For colony formation assay, 500 cells were seeded in each well of a six-well plate 48 h after transfection and cultured at 37 °C, 5% CO2 incubator with the medium being changed every 2 days. On the 7th day, the cultural media was removed, and cells were washed twice with PBS. After that, colonies were fixed in methanol for 20 min and stained with 1% crystal violet (Sigma) for 30 min, and then washed. Colonies were counted and photographed.

Flow cytometry assay

Fourty-eight hours after transfection, U87 and U251 cells were collected for cell cycle and apoptosis analysis. The cell cycle analysis was performed using the Cell Cycle Analysis Kit (Beyotime biotechnology, Jiangsu, China) according to the manufacturer's instructions. The apoptosis assay was performed using the Alexa Fluor® 488 Annexin V/Dead Cell Apoptosis Kit (Thermo Fisher Scientific, Waltham, MA, USA). The cells were detached by trypsinase, centrifuged at 1000 g for 5 min and then resuspended in 100 μL of binding buffer with 5 μL of Annexin v. After that, 1 μL of propidium iodide was added and mixed, followed by 15 min' incubation in dark. Subsequently, 400 μL of binding buffer was added to resuspend the cells, which were analyzed by Gallios Flow Cytometry (Beckman Coulter, USA). The experiments were repeated triple times.

Transwell assay

Cell invasion abilities were performed with transwell assay using transwell chambers with 8-μm pores (Costar, Corning, NY, USA). In invasion assay, the upper side of the insert membrane was coated with matrigel (BD Biosciences, New Jersey, USA). A number of 1×10^4 cells in 200 μl of serum-free medium were added into the upper chamber and 600 μl of medium with 5% FBS as chemoattractant was added into the lower chamber. After 24 h' incubation, the cells on the upper surface of the insert membrane were removed using cotton swab. The cells on the lower surface of the insert membrane were fixed in methanol for 20 min and then stained with 1% crystal violet for 30 min. The number of cells on the lower surface of the membrane was calculated with a microscope and then photographed. All experiments were performed in triplicate.

Scratch assay

Cells were seeded in each well of 6-well plates and cultured until 100% confluence. A scratch was performed using pipette tips and then serum-free medium was replaced. The scratch closing procedure was observed in 24 h and images were taken after 24 h' incubation.

Western blot analysis

Total protein was extracted from collected cells with RIPA buffer containing phenylmethanesulfonylfl uoride (PMSF). After a 30-min reaction on ice, the protein lysate was centrifuged at 13000 rpm for 15 min and the supernatant was collected. The protein concentration was measured by the BCA Protein Assay Kit (Pierce, Illinois, USA). Ten microgram of each protein was subjected to 8% SDS-PAGE and transferred to PVDF membranes, which was then blocked with 5% BSA in TBST (TBS containing 0.1% Tween-20) at room temperature for 1 h and incubated with the corresponding primary antibodies diluted in blocking buffer at 4 °C overnight. After washing with PBST (PBS containing 0.1% Tween), secondary antibodies was added for incubation at room temperature for 1 h. The western blot images were captured using the LI-COR Odyssey Scanner. Primary antibodies recognizing human E-cadherin, Fibronectin, LRP6, Axin1, active catenin, C-myc, Cyclin D1 (mouse mAb, 1:1000, Abcam, Cambridge, MA, USA) and GAPDH (rabbit mAb, 1:2000, Cell Signaling Technology, Danvers, MA, USA) were used.

Immunofluorescence assay

U87 cells were seeded in 35-mm cell culture dishes (NEST Biotech, Wuxi, China). The cells were fixed with 4% PFA in PBS for 20 min and permeabilized with 0.5% Triton X-100 for 5 min at room temperature. After washing in PBS, cells were blocked with 5% BSA for 1 h and incubated with primary antibodies against E-Cadherin and Fibronectin (1:200, Abcam, Cambridge, MA, USA) overnight at 4 °C, and then detected using Alexa fluor 546-conjugated anti-mouse IgG secondary antibodies, followed by a 2-mg/mL solution of 4′, 6-diamidino-2-

phenylindole (DAPI; Sigma–Aldrich, St. Louis, MO, USA) in PBS for nuclear staining. Cells were visualized under a confocal microscope (Leica, Solms, Germany).

RNAi

For RNAi-mediated knockdown experiment, lncRNA PTCSC3-specific siRNA and scramble negative control siRNA (ScrsiRNA) were purchased from GenePharma Co., Ltd (Shanghai, China). The sequences were as follow: lncRNA PTCSC3-siRNA, sense, 5′-AUCUUUUGCAUUA AUCUCCCU-3′, antisense, 5′-GGAGAUUAAUGCAAA AGAUGG-3′; ScrsiRNA, sense, 5′-UUCUCCGAACGUG UCACGUTT-3′, antisense, and 5′-ACGUGACACGUU CGGAGAATT-3′. U87 cells were transfected with 100 nM lncRNA PTCSC3 specific siRNA or scrsiRNA using Lipofectamine^{TM}2000 (Thermo Fisher Scientific, Waltham, MA, USA) according to the manufacturer's protocol. The transfection efficiency was confirmed by qRT-PCR (See Additional file 1: Figure S1).

Statistical analysis and quantification

All statistical analyses were performed using Statistical Program for Social Sciences 19.0 software (SPSS, Chicago, IL, USA) and GraphPad Prism 5.0 (GraphPad Software, LaJolla, CA, USA). Data were presented as the means ± SD. The significance of differences between groups was estimated by Student's *t*-test (two-sided, unpaired). $P < 0.05$ was considered to indicate a statistically significant difference. All experiments were repeated at least three times.

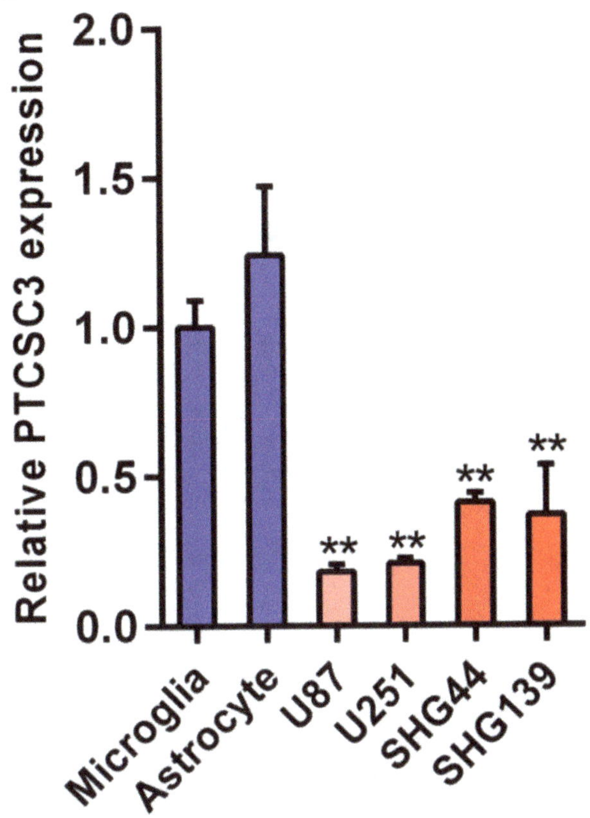

Fig. 1 Expression of lncRNA PTCSC3 in human microglia and glioma cell lines. qRT-PCR analysis of the expression levels of lncRNA PTCSC3 in human microglia, astrocyte and glioma cell lines (U87, U251, SHG44 & SHG139). The values were normalized to GAPDH mRNA expression. Data are expressed as the means ± S.D of three independent experiments. "**" indicates $P < 0.01$

Results

LncRNA PTCSC3 overexpression inhibits the proliferation and induces apoptosis in glioma cells

The expression level of lncRNA PTCSC3 in glioma was detected in human microglia cells, astrocyte and four glioma cell lines (U87, U251, SHG44 & SHG139) by qRT-PCR. LncRNA PTCSC3 was downregulated in glioma cell lines compared with human microglia cells and astrocyte (Fig. 1). Among the four glioma cell lines, U87 had the lowest expression level of lncRNA PTCSC3 compared with U251, SHG44 and SHG139 (Fig. 1). U87 and U251 were selected to investigate the biological function of lncRNA PTCSC3 in glioma cells. As lncRNA PTCSC3 was downregulated in glioma cell lines, the gain-of-function experiment was performed using lentivirus vector in the U87 and U251 glioma cell lines. The transfection efficiency was determined by qRT-PCR after 72 h of transfection. As shown in Fig. 2a, the expression levels of lncRNA PTCSC3 in U87 and U251 cells transfected with the lncRNA PTCSC3 overexpression vector were increased by 189.34-fold and 152.01-fold respectively, compared with control cells. In CCK8 assay, the cell viabilities of U87 and U251 cells were determined at five time points (0, 12, 24, 48, and 72 h) after being transfected with the lncRNA PTCSC3 overexpression vector. The viability of the U87 and U251 cells decreased significantly at 48, 72 h with overexpression of lncRNA PTCSC3 compared with the control (Fig. 2b, c). In cell cycle analysis, the proportions of cells in the G1 phase was significantly increased in U87 and U251 cells with lncRNA PTCSC3 overexpression compared with the control. Additionally, the proportion of cells in S and G2/M phases were reduced in the lncRNA PTCSC3 overexpression group (Fig. 3d-f). In colony formation assay, there were fewer colonies in the lncRNA PTCSC3 overexpression group compared with the control (Fig. 3g, i). Moreover, the apoptosis assay showed that lncRNA PTCSC3 overexpression promoted apoptosis in U87 and U251 cells (Fig. 4a–c). Our result indicated that lncRNA PTCS3 overexpression inhibited proliferation by inducing cell cycle arrest and apoptosis in glioma cells as well as suppressing cell viability.

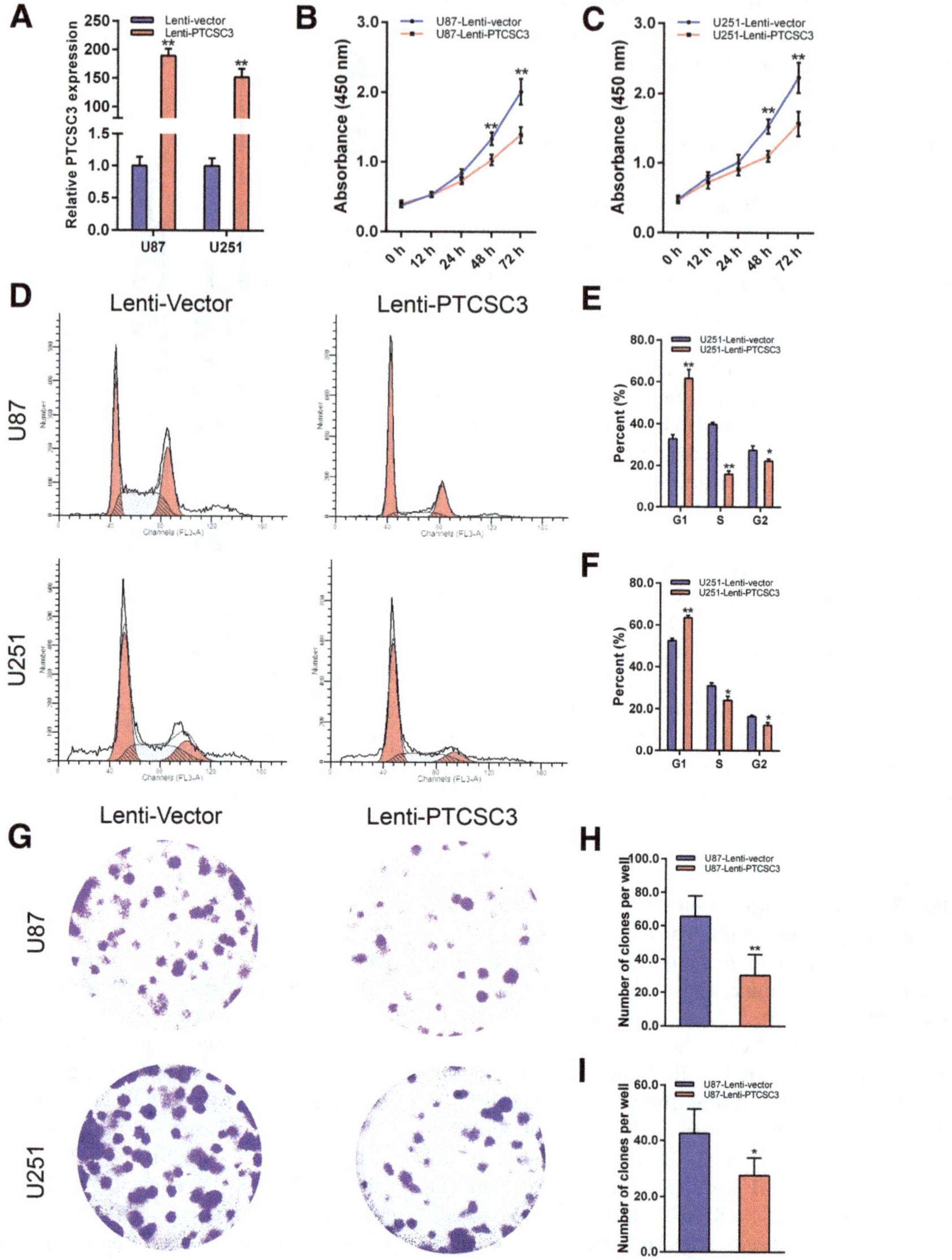

Fig. 2 LncRNA PTCSC3 overexpression inhibits the proliferation of U87 and U251. **a** qRT-PCR analysis of lncRNA PTCSC3 expression levels in U87 and U251 infected with Lenti-Vector or Lenti-PTCSC3. CCK-8 assays were performed to determine U87 (**b**) and U251 (**c**) cell proliferation after 12 h, 24 h, 48 h and 72 h infected with Lenti-Vector or Lenti-PTCSC3. **d** Representative flow cytometry images of the cell cycle in U87 and U251 cells infected with Lenti-Vector or Lenti-PTCSC3. The cell cycle results quantified in of U87 (**e**) and U251 (**f**) cells are presented as the percentage of total cells. **g** Colony formation assay was performed to determine the proliferation of U87 and U251 cells infected with Lenti-Vector or Lenti-PTCSC3. The colonies were captured and counted. Colony formation assay results of U87 (**h**) and U251 (**i**) cells are presented as histograms. Data are expressed as the means ± S.D of three independent experiments. "*" indicates $P < 0.05$, "**" indicates $P < 0.01$

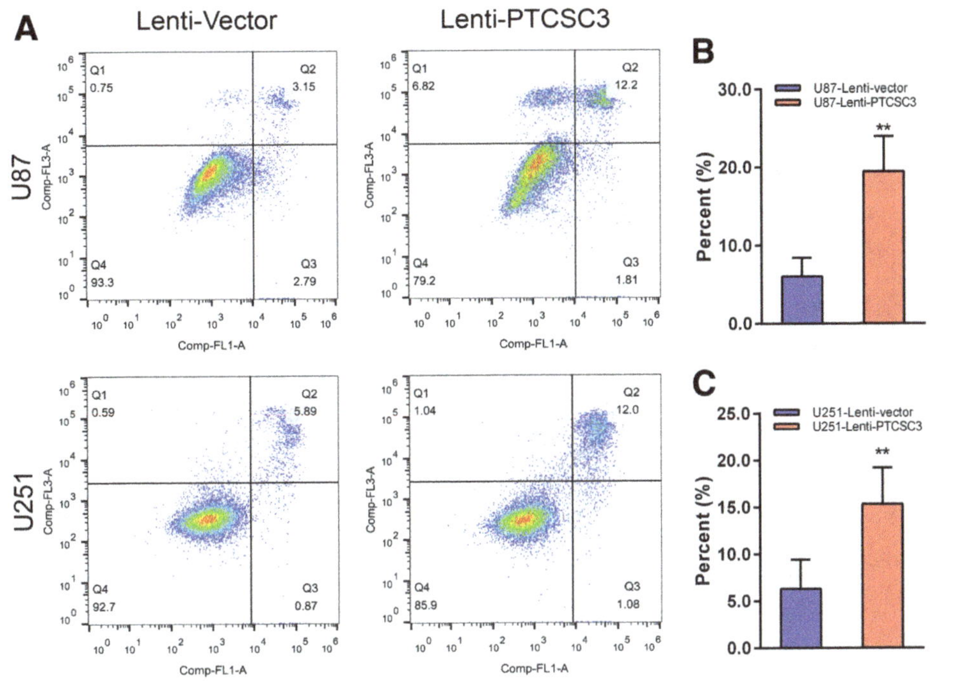

Fig. 3 LncRNA PTCSC3 overexpression induces apoptosis in U87 and U251. **a** Representative flow cytometry images of apoptosis of U87 and U251 cells infected with Lenti-Vector or Lenti-PTCSC3. The percentage of apoptotic U87 (**b**) and U251 (**c**) cells is presented as histograms. Data are expressed as the means ± S.D of three independent experiments. "*" indicates $P < 0.05$, "**" indicates $P < 0.01$

LncRNA PTCSC3 overexpression inhibits migration and invasion in glioma cells

Scratch test and transwell assay were used to evaluate the affect of lncRNA PTCSC3 on glioma cell migration and invasion respectively. The scratch test showed that lncRNA PTCSC3 overexpression remarkably inhibits U87 cell migration (Fig. 4a), which was quantified by the percentage of the wound area (Fig. 4c). The transwell invasion assay showed that overexpression of lncRNA PTCSC3 reduced the invasive capacity of U87 (Fig. 4b, d) and U251 cells (Fig. 4b, e). Further, the expression of matrix metalloproteinases (MMPs) in lncRNA PTCSC3 elevated cells were detected to investigate a potential mechanism for lncRNA PTCSC3 in the inhibition of migration and invasion, indicating that MMP2 and MMP9 expression were downregulated in lncRNA PTCSC3 overexpressed cells, while MMP1 and MMP13 remained unaffected (Fig. 4f–i). These data showed that lncRNA PTCS3 overexpression inhibited glioma cell migration and invasion via downregulating MMP2 and MMP9 expression.

LncRNA PTCSC3 overexpression inhibits the epithelial-mesenchymal transition of U87 cells

To investigate the affect of lncRNA PTCSC3 on the epithelial-mesenchymal transition of glioma cells, the study examined the mesenchymal markers and epithelial markers in U87 cells with or without lncRNA PTCSC3 overexpression. It showed that E-cadherin (epithelial marker) was upregulated (Fig. 5a) while Fibronectin, Snail and ZEB1 (mesenchymal markers) were downregulated in lncRNA PTCSC3 overexpressed cells (Fig. 5b-d). The function of lncRNA PTCSC3 increased the expression of E-cadherin and reduced the expression of Fibronectin was further confirmed by western blot (Fig. 5e and Additional file 2: Figure S2) and immunofluorenscence (Fig. 5f).

LncRNA PTCSC3 overexpression inhibits the Wnt/β-catenin signaling pathway by suppressing LRP6

The affect of lncRNA PTCSC3 on the Wnt/β-catenin signaling pathway was investigated in U87 cell line. Data indicated that the expression of LRP6, C-myc and Cyclin D1 were downregulated and the expression of Axin1 was upregulated when lncRNA PTCSC3 was overexpressed, wherease the expression of FZD8 remained unchanged (Fig. 6a–e). Conversely, the expression of LRP6, C-myc and Cyclin D1 were induced while that of Axin1 was reduced when lncRNA PTCSC3 was knocked down, wherease FZD8 expression remained unchanged (Fig. 6a–e). In western blot analysis, lncRNA PTCSC3 overexpression downregulated LRP6 expression, subsequently suppressing the expression of active β-catenin, C-myc and cyclin D1, while increasing Axin1 expression, and vice versa (Fig. 6f and Additional file 3: Figure S3).

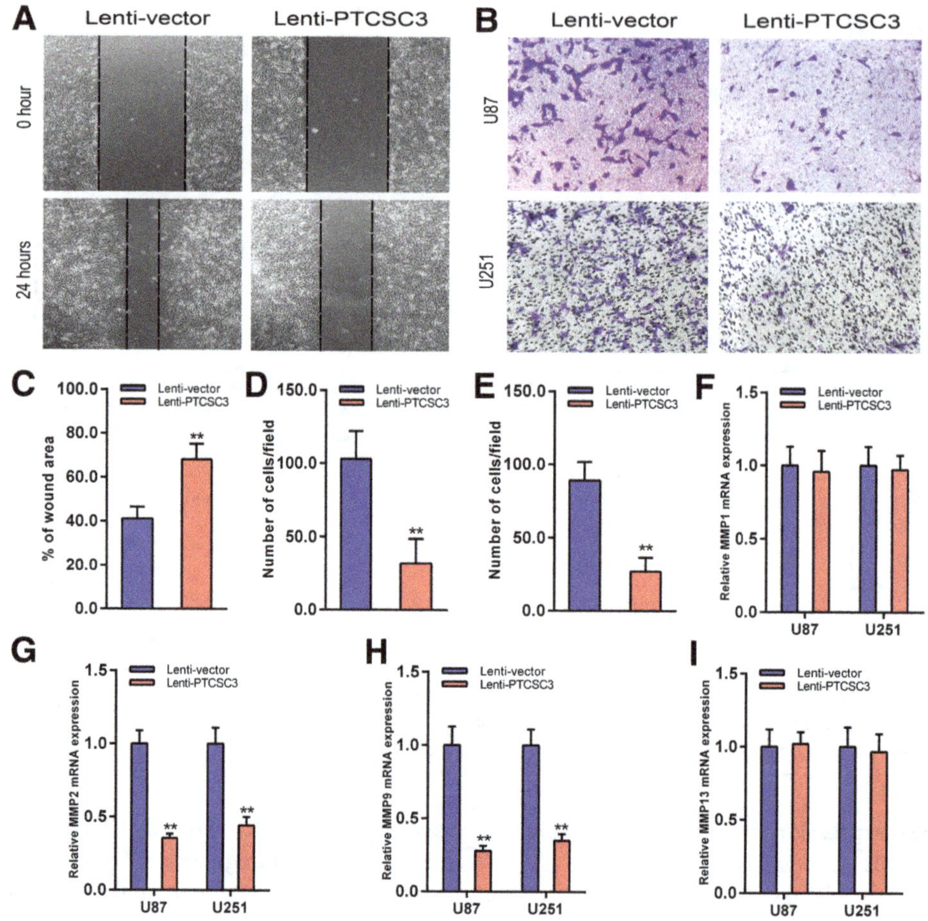

Fig. 4 LncRNA PTCSC3 overexpression inhibits the migration and invasion of U87 cells. **a** Wound healing assay was used to determine the migration ability of U87 cells with or without lncRNA PTCSC3 overexpression. Representative images of 0 h and 24 h of three repeated experiments are presented. **b** Transwell assay was performed to determine the invasion ability of U87 and U251 cells with or without lncRNA PTCSC3 overexpression. The representative images of invasive cells in the lower chamber stained with crystal violet. **c** The quantification of migration ability of U87 cells were presented as percentage of the wound area. The quantification of U87 (**d**) and U251 (**e**) cell invasion is presented as invasive cell numbers per field. qRT-PCR analysis of the mRNA expression levels of MMP1 (**f**), MMP2 (**g**), MMP9 (**h**) and MMP13 (**i**) in U87 and U251 cells with or without lncRNA PTCSC3 overexpression. Data are expressed as the means ± S.D of three independent experiments. "**" indicates $P < 0.01$

Discussion

It is well-known that lncRNAs are dysregulated in a variety of tumors and play important roles in carcinogenesis as well as cancer progression [11]. In the present study, we detected the expression level of lncRNA PTCSC3 in glioma. We demonstrated that lncRNA PTCSC3 was downregulated in glioma cells compared with normal brain cells. To investigate the biological function of lncRNA PTCSC3, we performed gain-of-function experiments in glioma cell lines. These experiments indicate that overexpression of lncRNA PTCSC3 inhibited proliferation, migration and invasion in glioma cells. For the mechanism study, we explored the influences of dysregulated lncRNA PTCSC3 in the EMT and Wnt/β-catenin signaling pathways, revealing a negatively regulatory mechanism between these pathways.

Evidences are accumulating that lncRNAs play pivotal roles in various maligancies. LncRNA H19 was reported to be overexpressed in pancreatic ductal adenocarcinoma and plays oncogenic role through promoting cancer cell proliferation [12]. It was also recognized as a novel biomarker for diagnosis of gastric cancer in plasma [13]. Urothelial Carcinoma Associated 1 (UCA1), which acts as oncogenic lncRNA and promotes bladder cancer progression [14], has been studied in a meta-analysis that up-regulated UCA1 was significantly corrected with LNM and poor OS in patients with various cancers [15]. In glioma, the exploration of lncRNAs is still superficial. LncRNA-ATB was abnormally upregulated in glioma and played an oncogenic role in glioma cells by inhibiting miR-200a and facilitating TGF-β2 [16]. LncRNA HULC, which was highly upregulated in liver cancer,

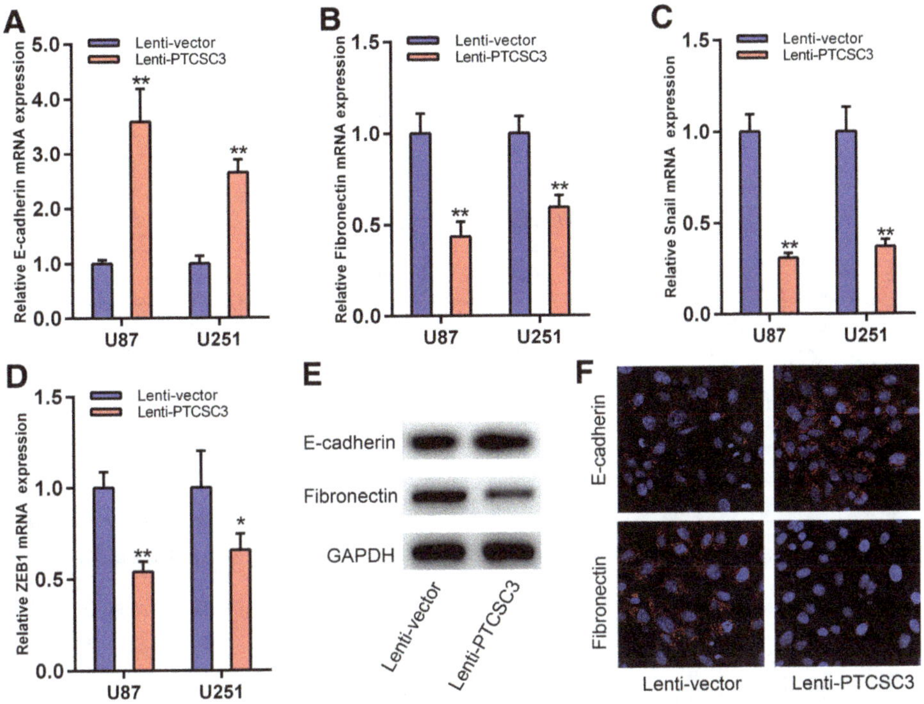

Fig. 5 LncRNA PTCSC3 overexpression inhibits the epithelial-mesenchymal transition of U87 cells. qRT-PCR analysis of the mRNA expression levels of E-cadherin (**a**), Fibronectin (**b**), Snail (**c**) and ZEB1 (**d**) in U87 and U251 cells with or without lncRNA PTCSC3 overexpression. **e** Western blot analysis of E-cadherin and Fibronectin in U87 cells. GAPDH was used as a loading control. Representative images of three repeated experiments are presented. **f** Representative images of immunofluorenscence analysis of E-cadherin and Fibronectin in U87 cells. Original magnification 400 ×. Data are expressed as the means ± S.D of three independent experiments. "*" indicates $P < 0.05$, "**" indicates $P < 0.01$

was discovered as an oncogene in glioma [17]. Another lncRNA MALAT1 (metastasis-associated lung adenocarcinoma transcript 1), which was initially found to be highly expressed in lung cancer and was a favorable prognostic factor for the survival of patients with stage I non-small-cell lung cancer (NSCLC), was demonstrated to have a tumor suppressive role in glioma by attenuating ERK/MAPK-mediated growth and MMP2-mediated invasiveness [18]. This is the first time that lncRNA PTCSC3 was reported in glioma. LncRNA PTCSC3 initially demonstrated that it was a susceptible gene in papillary thyroid carcinoma and that is also maintains the role of inhibition in thyroid cancer invasion [9, 10]. Our results showed that lncRNA PTCSC3 was downregulated in glioma cells. The analysis of tumor cell proliferation and invasion abilities in lncRNA PTCSC3-elevated cells showed the inhibitory role of lncRNA PTCSC3 in glioma, which is similar to its role in thyroid cancer.

To elucidate the possible mechanism by which lncRNA PTCSC3 regulates the proliferation and invasion of glioma cell, qRT-PCR and western blot analysis of the key molecular factors of EMT-associated biomarkers, including E-cadherin, fibronectin, Snail and ZEB1, were assessed in our study. EMT is a process involved in embryonic development, during which cells lose their epithelial features and adopt characteristics of mesenchymal cells. The EMT also plays a role in cancer invasion and metastasis in a sequence of discrete steps [19, 20]. Decreased expression of the epithelial marker E-cadherin and increased expression of mesenchymal markers, such as N-cadherin and fibronectin, are the most important features of EMT [21]. Transcriptional repressors Snail and ZEB have critical roles in regulating the EMT [22–24]. The activation of these transcriptional factors results in induction of the EMT phenotype [25]. Among the EMT markers we evaluated, the overexpression of lncRNA PTCSC3 led to the downregulation of E-cadherin and upregulation of Fibronectin, Snail and ZEB1, indicating that overexpression of lncRNA PTCSC3 represses the EMT.

EMT activation is induced by a variety of signaling pathways [26–28]. Here, we investigated the Wnt/β-catenin signaling pathway in glioma cell lines. Wnt signals are transduced across the membrane by low-density lipoprotein receptor–related protein (LRP) receptors [29]. According to our result, LRP6 was inactivated when lncRNA PTCSC3 was overexpressed. The APC/Axin/GSK/β-catenin-complex has been called a "destruction complex" in Wnt signaling [30]. In normal conditions, the complex remains stable. When Axin dissociates, β-catenin translocates to the nucleus and activates the

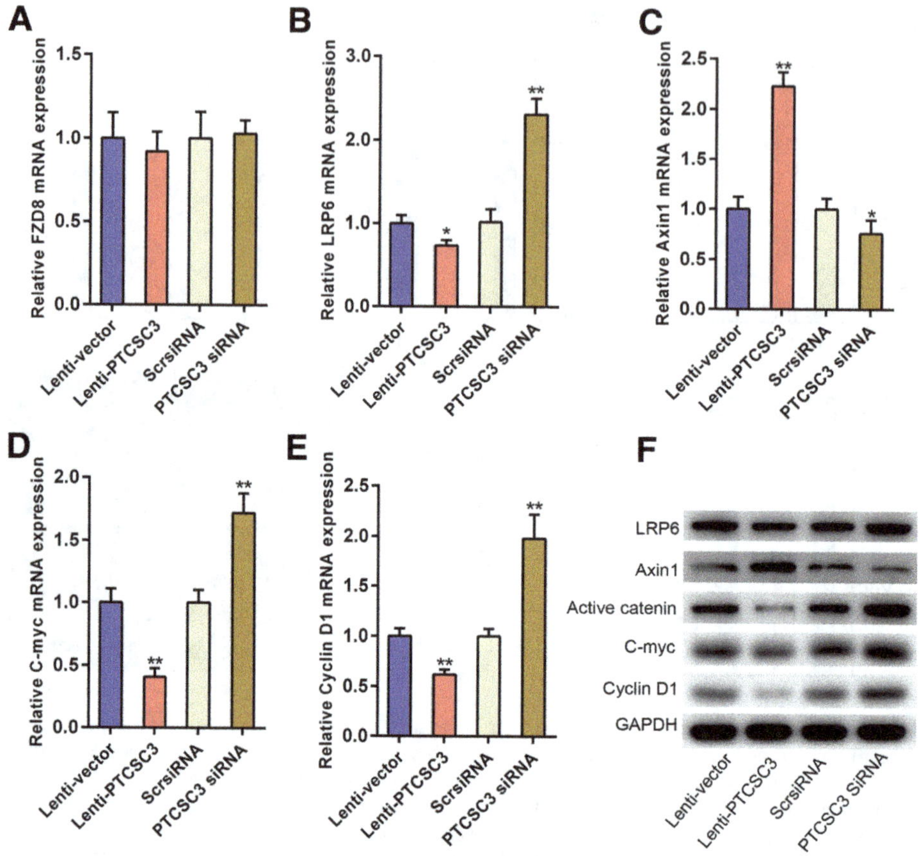

Fig. 6 LncRNA PTCSC3 overexpression inhibits the Wnt/β-catenin signaling pathway by suppressing LRP6. qRT-PCR analysis of the mRNA expression levels of FZD8 (**a**), LRP6 (**b**), Axin1 (**c**), C-myc (**d**) and Cyclin D1 (**e**) in cells with overexpression or knockdown of lncRNA PTCSC3. **f** Western blot analysis of LRP6, Axin1, Active catenin, C-myc and Cyclin D1 in U87 cells. GAPDH was used as loading control. Representative images of three repeated experiments are presented. Data are expressed as the means ± S.D of three independent experiments. "*" indicates $P < 0.05$, "**" indicates $P < 0.01$

transcription of specific target genes, such as c-Myc and cyclin D1 [31]. Previous reports indicate that the separation of the "destruction complex" leads to an increase in Axin1 protein expression and a concomitant decrease in β-catenin the cellular environment [32]. Our data revealed results similar to previous studies indicating that dissociation of the complex resulted in an increase in Axin1 and a reduction in active β-catenin as well as the subsequent inactivation of c-Myc and cyclin D1. The dissociation of the "destruction complex" was initiated by the inactivation of LRP6, which was primarily controlled by the overexpression of lncRNA PTCSC3.

Matrix metalloproteinases (MMPs) digest extracellular substrates and promote invasion of blood vessels and lymphatics in the spread of cancers [33]. MMP2 and MMP9 are induced by the EMT pathway and promote post-EMT invasion of underlying tissues [21]. Another study also generalized that MMP-2 and MMP-9 are activated by Snail [34]. Moreover, MMPs degrade E-cadherin, disrupting adhesive junctions, to facilitate the EMT [35]. Unsurprisingly, this study showed that MMP2 and MMP9 expression was downregulated in lncRNA PTCSC3-overexpressing cells, concomitant with the elevated expression of E-cadherin.

Our study illuminated a complicated mechanism network of how lncRNA PTCSC3 regulated glioma progression. As it was indicated, Wnt/β-catenin signaling pathway was initiated by LRP6, which was the target of lncRNA PTCSC3; the "destruction complex" was separated, resulting in a series of downstream alterations (Axin1, C-myc, Cyclin D1, etc.). The activation of Wnt/β-catenin signaling pathway induced EMT activation, which could also be regulated by Snail and ZEB1. The expression of MMP2 and MMP9 were downregulated, which was induced by the activation of EMT. In return, the decreased expression of MMP2 and MMP9 could also lead to an accumulation of E-cadherin.

Conclusion

In conclusion, lncRNA PTCSC3 is downregulated in glioma cells. The overexpression of lncRNA PTCSC3 inhibits proliferation, migration and invasion of glioma cells and suppresses the Wnt/β-catenin signaling pathway through targeting LRP6. LncRNA PTCSC3 is a potential novel therapeutic target for intervention of glioma.

Additional files

Additional file 1: Figure S1. qRT-PCR analysis of lncRNA PTCSC3 expression levels in U87 transfected with ScrsiRNA or PTCSC3 siRNA. Data are expressed as the means ± S.D of three independent experiments. "**" indicates $P < 0.01$.

Additional file 2: Figure S2. The protein expression level of E-cadherin and Fibronectin in U87 cells with or without lncRNA PTCSC3 overexpression was quantified. Data are expressed as the means ± S.D of three independent experiments. "**" indicates $P < 0.01$.

Additional file 3: Figure S3. The protein expression levels of LRP6 (A), Axin1 (B), Active catenin (C), C-myc (D) and Cyclin D1 in cells with overexpression or knockdown of lncRNA PTCSC3. Data are expressed as the means ± S.D of three independent experiments. "**" indicates $P < 0.01$.

Abbreviations

CCK-8: Cell counting kit-8; DMEM: Dulbecco's Modified Eagle Medium; EMT: Epithelial-mesenchymal transition; FBS: Fetal bovine serum; FZDI: Frizzled class receptor 8; GAPDH: Glyceraldehyde-3-phosphate dehydrogenase; LncRNA PTCSC3: Long noncoding RNA papillary thyroid carcinoma susceptibility candidate 3; LRP6: Low-density lipoprotein receptor–related protein 6; MMP: Matrix metalloproteinase; qRT-PCR: Quantitative reverse transcriptase-polymerase chain reaction; ZEB1: Zinc finger E-box binding homeobox 1

Acknowledgements

Not applicable.

Funding

National Natural Science Foundation of China (81471668 & 81671688). The funder had no role in study design, data analysis, decision to publish, and preparation of the manuscript.

Authors' contributions

SX and RJ performed the experiments. SX created the table and figures. SX wrote the primary manuscript. SX and WZ designed the experiments and modified the paper. WZ supervised the project. WZ provided funding for the entire project. All authors read and approved the final manuscript.

Competing interests

The authors declare that they have no competing interests.

References

1. Caruso G, Caffo M. Antisense oligonucleotides in the treatment of cerebral gliomas. Review of concerning patents. Recent Pat CNS Drug Discov. 2014; 9(1):2–12.
2. Taylor LP. Diagnosis, treatment, and prognosis of glioma: five new things. Neurology. 2010;75(18 Suppl 1):S28–32.
3. Omuro A, DeAngelis LM. Glioblastoma and other malignant gliomas: a clinical review. JAMA. 2013;310(17):1842–50.
4. Van Meir EG, Hadjipanayis CG, Norden AD, et al. Exciting new advances in neuro-oncology: the avenue to a cure for malignant glioma. CA Cancer J Clin. 2010;60(3):166–93.
5. Wen PY, Kesari S. Malignant gliomas in adults. N Engl J Med. 2008;359(5): 492–507.
6. Struhl K. Transcriptional noise and the fidelity of initiation by RNA polymerase II. Nat Struct Mol Biol. 2007;14(2):103–5.
7. Gupta RA, Shah N, Wang KC, et al. Long non-coding RNA HOTAIR reprograms chromatin state to promote cancer metastasis. Nature. 2010; 464(7291):1071–6.
8. Jendrzejewski J, He H, Radomska HS, et al. The polymorphism rs944289 predisposes to papillary thyroid carcinoma through a large intergenic noncoding RNA gene of tumor suppressor type. Proc Natl Acad Sci U S A. 2012;109(22):8646–51.
9. Fan M, Li X, Jiang W, et al. A long non-coding RNA, PTCSC3, as a tumor suppressor and a target of miRNAs in thyroid cancer cells. Exp Ther Med. 2013;5(4):1143–6.
10. Jendrzejewski J, Thomas A, Liyanarachchi S, et al. PTCSC3 Is Involved in Papillary Thyroid Carcinoma Development by Modulating S100A4 Gene Expression. J Clin Endocrinol Metab. 2015;100(10):E1370–7.
11. Huarte M. The emerging role of lncRNAs in cancer. Nat Med. 2015;21(11): 1253–61.
12. Ma L, Tian X, Wang F, et al. The long noncoding RNA H19 promotes cell proliferation via E2F-1 in pancreatic ductal adenocarcinoma. Cancer Biol Ther. 2016;17(10):1051–61.
13. Zhou X, Yin C, Dang Y, et al. Identification of the long non-coding RNA H19 in plasma as a novel biomarker for diagnosis of gastric cancer. Sci Rep. 2015;5:11516.
14. Xue M, Chen W, Li X. Urothelial cancer associated 1: a long noncoding RNA with a crucial role in cancer. J Cancer Res Clin Oncol. 2016;142(7):1407–19.
15. He A, Hu R, Chen Z, et al. Role of long noncoding RNA UCA1 as a common molecular marker for lymph node metastasis and prognosis in various cancers: a meta-analysis. Oncotarget. 2016.
16. Ma CC, Xiong Z, Zhu GN, et al. Long non-coding RNA ATB promotes glioma malignancy by negatively regulating miR-200a. J Exp Clin Cancer Res. 2016;35(1):90.
17. Zhu Y, Zhang X, Qi L, et al. HULC long noncoding RNA silencing suppresses angiogenesis by regulating ESM-1 via the PI3K/Akt/mTOR signaling pathway in human gliomas. Oncotarget. 2016;7(12):14429–40.
18. Han Y, Wu Z, Wu T, et al. Tumor-suppressive function of long noncoding RNA MALAT1 in glioma cells by downregulation of MMP2 and inactivation of ERK/MAPK signaling. Cell Death Dis. 2016;7, e2123.
19. Hanahan D, Weinberg RA. Hallmarks of cancer: the next generation. Cell. 2011;144(5):646–74.
20. Thiery JP. Epithelial-mesenchymal transitions in tumour progression. Nat Rev Cancer. 2002;2(6):442–54.
21. Kalluri R, Weinberg RA. The basics of epithelial-mesenchymal transition. J Clin Invest. 2009;119(6):1420–8.
22. Cano A, Perez-Moreno MA, Rodrigo I, et al. The transcription factor snail controls epithelial-mesenchymal transitions by repressing E-cadherin expression. Nat Cell Biol. 2000;2(2):76–83.
23. Vandewalle C, Comijn J, De Craene B, et al. SIP1/ZEB2 induces EMT by repressing genes of different epithelial cell-cell junctions. Nucleic Acids Res. 2005;33(20):6566–78.
24. Bracken CP, Gregory PA, Kolesnikoff N, et al. A double-negative feedback loop between ZEB1-SIP1 and the microRNA-200 family regulates epithelial-mesenchymal transition. Cancer Res. 2008;68(19):7846–54.
25. Davalos V, Moutinho C, Villanueva A, et al. Dynamic epigenetic regulation of the microRNA-200 family mediates epithelial and mesenchymal transitions in human tumorigenesis. Oncogene. 2012;31(16):2062–74.
26. Taipale J, Beachy PA. The Hedgehog and Wnt signalling pathways in cancer. Nature. 2001;411(6835):349–54.
27. Espinoza I, Miele L. Deadly crosstalk: Notch signaling at the intersection of EMT and cancer stem cells. Cancer Lett. 2013;341(1):41–5.
28. Katoh Y, Katoh M. FGFR2-related pathogenesis and FGFR2-targeted therapeutics (Review). Int J Mol Med. 2009;23(3):307–11.
29. MacDonald BT, Tamai K, He X. Wnt/beta-catenin signaling: components, mechanisms, and diseases. Dev Cell. 2009;17(1):9–26.
30. Behrens J, Jerchow BA, Wurtele M, et al. Functional interaction of an axin homolog, conductin, with beta-catenin, APC, and GSK3beta. Science. 1998; 280(5363):596–9.

31. Gehrke I, Gandhirajan RK, Kreuzer KA. Targeting the WNT/beta-catenin/TCF/LEF1 axis in solid and haematological cancers: Multiplicity of therapeutic options. Eur J Cancer. 2009;45(16):2759–67.
32. Schmitz Y, Rateitschak K, Wolkenhauer O. Analysing the impact of nucleo-cytoplasmic shuttling of beta-catenin and its antagonists APC, Axin and GSK3 on Wnt/beta-catenin signalling. Cell Signal. 2013;25(11):2210–21.
33. Willis AL, Sabeh F, Li XY, et al. Extracellular matrix determinants and the regulation of cancer cell invasion stratagems. J Microsc. 2013;251(3):250–60.
34. Qiao B, Johnson NW, Gao J. Epithelial-mesenchymal transition in oral squamous cell carcinoma triggered by transforming growth factor-beta1 is Snail family-dependent and correlates with matrix metalloproteinase-2 and –9 expressions. Int J Oncol. 2010;37(3):663–8.
35. Nistico P, Bissell MJ, Radisky DC. Epithelial-mesenchymal transition: general principles and pathological relevance with special emphasis on the role of matrix metalloproteinases. Cold Spring Harb Perspect Biol. 2012;4:2.

28

Subacute tetraplegia in an immunocompromised patient

Daniel Zeller[1*], Anke Heidemeier[2], Götz Ulrich Grigoleit[3] and Wolfgang Müllges[1]

Abstract

Background: Clinical reasoning in Neurology is based on general associations which help to deduce the site of the lesion. However, even "golden principles" may occasionally be deceptive. Here, we describe the case of subacute flaccid tetraparesis due to motor cortical lesions. To our knowledge, this is the first report to include an impressive illustration of nearly symmetric motor cortical involvement of encephalitis on brain MRI.

Case presentation: A 51 year old immunocompromized man developed a high-grade pure motor flaccid tetraparesis over few days. Based on clinical presentation, critical illness polyneuromyopathy was suspected. However, brain MRI revealed symmetrical hyperintensities strictly limited to the subcortical precentral gyrus. An encephalitis, possibly due to CMV infection, turned out to be the most likely cause.

Conclusion: While recognition of basic clinical patterns is indispensable in neurological reasoning, awareness of central conditions mimicking peripheral nervous disease may be crucial to detect unsuspected, potentially treatable conditions.

Keywords: Tetraparesis, Motor cortex, CMV encephalitis, Case report

Background

Connecting clinical findings to neuroanatomy is a basic principle of neurologists' thinking. One of the "golden principles" is the simple association flaccid paresis plus muscle atrophy pointing to peripheral nerve disease. However, even basic principles must be questioned occasionally. A rather common example is that of patients waking up with a drop hand – although clinically suggestive of a peripheral origin (i.e. radial nerve palsy), the alternative cause may be an acute central nervous system lesion (i.e. "hand knob" infarction) [1, 2]. The other way around, fulminant courses of inflammatory demyelinating polyneuropathy (Guillain-Barré syndrome, GBS) may mimic brain death [3]. Here, we describe the instructive case of a patient who subacutely developed flaccid tetraparesis due to bilateral motor cortical lesions, illustrated by striking findings on brain magnetic resonance imaging (MRI).

* Correspondence: zeller_d@ukw.de
[1]Department of Neurology, University of Würzburg, Josef-Schneider-Str. 11, 97080 Würzburg, Germany
Full list of author information is available at the end of the article

Case presentation

Six weeks after stem cell transplant for myelodysplastic syndrome, a 51 year old caucasian patient developed a high-grade pure motor flaccid tetraparesis within a few days. While cognitive and brainstem functions – including the function of facial muscles – were preserved, the patient was tetraplegic except for minimal finger movements of the left hand. The deep tendon reflexes were absent, and Babinski testing revealed mute soles on both sides. There was considerable generalized muscle atrophy which had already been noticed at first neurological assessment five days before transplant. At that occasion, however, the patient had presented without any paresis.

Development of tetraparesis within several days along with absent deep tendon reflexes might be indicative of GBS. However, the simultaneous and generalized rather than ascending development of tetraparesis is uncommon in GBS. In addition, ongoing strong immunosuppression by cyclosporine A and mycophenolate mofetil made the new occurrence of an autoimmune disorder unlikely. Therefore, taking into account that the patient had been treated in ICU for pneumonia with respiratory failure before, critical illness polyneuromyopathy was suspected.

A few days later, however, an acute confusional state prompted brain MRI. Fluid-attenuated inversion recovery (FLAIR) imaging revealed symmetrical hyperintensities strictly limited to the subcortical precentral gyrus (Fig. 1a). Correspondingly, diffusion-weighted imaging (DWI) showed signal hyperintensity (Fig. 1b), along with normal ADC and without any contrast enhancement. Six days before transplant, the patient had received cranial MRI without any pathological finding. Thus, tetraplegia was attributable to new symmetrical CNS lesions.

Stroke, for example due to cardiac embolism, was not supported by normal ADC. "Stroke mimics" with positive DWI, but without lesion hypointensity on the ADC map, include active MS plaques, cerebral abscess, and viral encephalitis [4]. The spatial pattern of the MRI lesions appeared virtually incompatible with MS, and the absence of a mass effect or rim enhancement rendered bacterial cerebritis or cerebral abscesses very unlikely [5]. Taken together, subacute development of tetraparesis along with new subcortical lesions in an immunocompromised patient were highly suggestive of infection by or reactivation of neurotropic viruses. Sole motor affection may make poliovirus highly suspicious [6], particularly in the light of recent reports of polio cases in Germany [7]. However, given the patient's vaccination against polio virus, this differential diagnosis was considered rather unlikely.

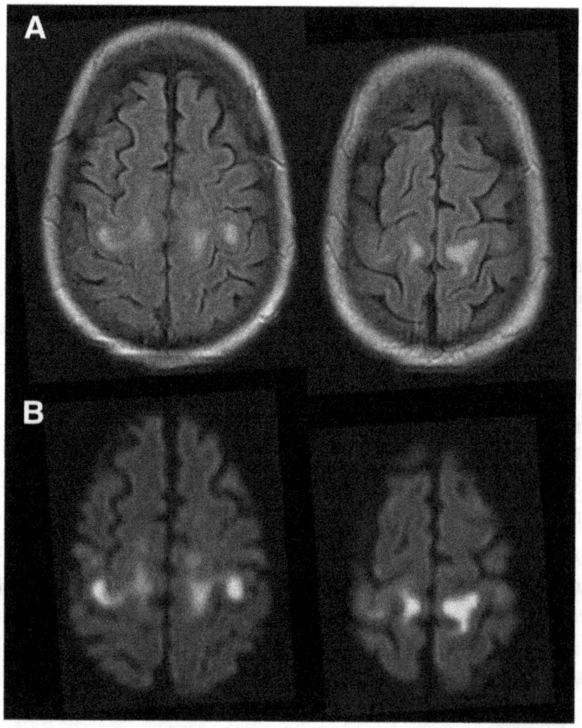

Fig. 1 Magnetic resonance imaging in a patient with subacute flaccid tetraplegia. FLAIR images show a hyperintense signal confined to subcortical precentral gyrus on both hemispheres **a.** This hyperintensity is associated with high signal on diffusion-weighted imaging **b**, without ADC correlate (not shown)

Spinal tap revealed a normal cell count (1 leucocyte/mm^3, normal range 0–4) along with slightly elevated protein (56.2 mg/dl, normal ≤50) and albumine (50.9 mg/dl, normal ≤35). CSF PCR was negative for herpes simplex virus type 1/2, varizella zoster virus, Epstein-Barr virus, cytomegalovirus, human herpes virus six, JC virus, adenovirus, enterovirus, poliovirus, and bacterial DNA (universal primer). However, repeat serum PCR for CMV showed a progressively increasing number of up to 8,600 copies/ml, starting shortly prior to the development of tetraparesis.

Sensitivity of CSF PCR for CMV encephalitis is generally believed to be high, yet unequal to 100% as far as known from comparison with viral isolation from autopsy samples [8]. Moreover, CSF virus PCR might initially be false-negative, with increasing probability of a positive PCR when there is a time frame of 3 – 14 days between symptom onset and lumbar puncture [9]. Therefore, while the laboratory findings were unable to prove CMV encephalitis, they were compatible with this suspected diagnosis. Accordingly, intravenous ganciclovir treatment (5 mg per kg per day over two weeks) was initiated. Over the following three weeks, serum PCR for CMV turned negative. Tetraparesis slowly improved, with still moderate pareses of the upper (between MRC 3 and 4), but severe pareses of the lower (between MRC 1 and 2) extremities at neurological reassessment four weeks after symptom onset. Unfortunately, in the further course the patient developed a septic syndrome, most likely owing to a pulmonary focus, and exspired due to septic multiple organ failure. Autopsy was prohibited.

Discussion and Conclusions

Though primarily suggestive for peripheral nervous disease, subacute flaccid tetraplegia may reflect pure motor cortical paresis [10, 11]. In our case, MRI pointed to an encephalitis limited to the bilateral subcortical precentral gyri. Thus, while recognition of basic patterns of clinical findings is indispensable in clinical reasoning, awareness of mimics may help to detect unsuspected treatable conditions.

Abbreviations

ADC: Apparent diffusion coefficient; CMV: Cytomegalovirus; CNS: Central nervous system; CSF: Cerebrospinal fluid; DNA: Deoxyribonucleic acid; DWI: Diffusion-weighted imaging; FLAIR: Fluid-attenuated inversion recovery; GBS: Guillain-Barré syndrome; MRI: Magnetic resonance imaging; MS: Multiple sclerosis; PCR: Polymerase chain reaction

Acknowledgements

Open access publication was funded by the German Research Foundation (DFG) and the University of Wuerzburg in the funding programme Open Access Publishing.

Funding

No funding was obtained.

Authors' contributions

DZ: conception of idea, manuscript writing and editing. AH: MR imaging, manuscript writing and editing. GUG: manuscript writing and editing. WM: manuscript writing and editing. All authors read and approved the final manuscript.

Competing interests

The authors declare that they have no competing interests.

Author details

[1]Department of Neurology, University of Würzburg, Josef-Schneider-Str. 11, 97080 Würzburg, Germany. [2]Department of Radiology, University of Würzburg, Josef-Schneider-Str. 11, 97080 Würzburg, Germany. [3]Department of Internal Medicine II, University of Würzburg, 97080 Würzburg, Germany.

References

1. Lee PH, Han SW, Heo JH. Isolated weakness of the fingers in cortical infarction. Neurology. 1998;50:823–4.
2. Jusufovic M, Lygren A, Aamodt AH, Nedregaard B, Kerty E. Pseudoperipheral palsy: a case of subcortical infarction imitating peripheral neuropathy. BMC Neurol. 2015;15:151.
3. Vargas F, Hilbert G, Gruson D, Valentino R, Gbikpi-Benissan G, Cardinaud JP. Fulminant guillain-barré syndrome mimicking cerebral death: case report and literature review. Intensive Care Med. 2000;26:623–7.
4. Roberts TP, Rowley HA. Diffusion weighted magnetic resonance imaging in stroke. Eur J Radiol. 2003;45:185–94.
5. Rath TJ, Hughes M, Arabi M, Shah GV. Imaging of cerebritis, encephalitis, and brain abscess. Neuroimaging Clin N Am. 2012;22:585–607.
6. Nagata N, Iwasaki T, Ami Y, Tano Y, Harashima A, Suzaki Y, Sato Y, Hasegawa H, Sata T, Miyamura T, Shimizu H. Differential localization of neurons susceptible to enterovirus 71 and poliovirus type 1 in the central nervous system of cynomolgus monkeys after intravenous inoculation. J Gen Virol. 2004;85:2981–9.
7. Böttcher S, Neubauer K, Baillot A, Rieder G, Adam M, Diedrich S. Stool screening of Syrian refugees and asylum seekers in Germany, 2013/2014: identification of sabin like polioviruses. Int J Med Microbiol. 2015;305:601–6.
8. Arribas JR, Clifford DB, Fichtenbaum CJ, Commins DL, Powderly WG, Storch GA. Level of cytomegalovirus (CMV) DNA in cerebrospinal fluid of subjects with AIDS and CMV infection of the central nervous system. J Infect Dis. 1995;172:527–31.
9. Davies NW, Brown LJ, Gonde J, Irish D, Robinson RO, Swan AV, Banatvala J, Howard RS, Sharief MK, Muir P. Factors influencing PCR detection of viruses in cerebrospinal fluid of patients with suspected CNS infections. J Neurol Neurosurg Psychiatry. 2005;76:82–7.
10. Darling WG, Pizzimenti MA, Morecraft RJ. Functional recovery following motor cortex lesions in non-human primates: experimental implications for human stroke patients. J Integr Neurosci. 2011;10:353–84.
11. Bertrand C, Martinez SN, Robert F, Bouvier G, Mathieu JP. Origin of the corticospinal motor fibers: a case of flaccid quadriplegia following bilateral cortical lesions. Rev Can Biol. 1972;31(Suppl):263–71.

29

Functional outcome and complications after the microsurgical removal of giant vestibular schwannomas via the retrosigmoid approach

Xiang Huang†, Jian Xu†, Ming Xu, Mingyu Chen, Kaiyuan Ji, Junwei Ren and Ping Zhong*

Abstract

Background: Intracranial vestibular schwannoma still remain to be difficulty for its unique microsurgical technique and preservation of neuro-function, as well as reducing common complications that may arise in surgery.

Methods: We consecutively enrolled 657 unilateral giant (>4 cm diameter) vestibular schwannoma patients treated in Huashan Hospital via the suboccipital retrosigmoid approach in the past 16 years. The extension of tumor removal, surgical mortality, facial nerve function, hearing, and the other main short and long-term complications were the studied parameters.

Results: Gross total resection was performed in 556 patients (84.6%); near-total resection was achieved in 99 patients (15.1%). The mortality rate is 0.6%. The main short-term complications included 'new' deafness (47.6%), intracranial infection (7.6%), lower cranial nerve defects (7.5%) and pneumonia (6.2%). The facial nerve was preserved anatomically in 589 cases (89.7%). Good facial nerve functional outcome (House-Brackmann Grades I and II) postoperatively was achieved in 216 patients (32.9%). Other 308 cases (46.9%) were House-Brackmann grade III, and 133 patients (20.2%) were House-Brackmann grade IV–VI. Follow-up data were available for 566 of the 657 patients (86.1%). The common long-term complications were hearing loss (85.2%), facial paralysis (HB grade IV–VI, 24.4%) and facial numbness (15.7%).

Conclusions: Trends in the data lead the authors to suggest that the microsurgical technique, intraoperative nerve monitoring, and multidisciplinary cooperation, were the keys to improving prognostic outcomes in giant intracranial vestibular schwannoma patients.

Keywords: Vestibular schwannoma, Neurosurgical procedures, Postoperative complications, Facial nerve injuries

* Correspondence: zhp228899@163.com
†Equal contributors
Department of Neurosurgery, Huashan Hospital, Fudan University, Shanghai 200040, People's Republic of China

Background

The giant vestibular schwannoma still remains to be the difficulty for the surgical treatment of intracranial vestibular schwannoma now. The giant tumor would oppress and shift most cranial nerves in posterior cranial fossa, including oculomotor nerve, trochlear nerve, trigeminal nerve, abducens and lower cranial nerves, causing severe clinical symptoms [1]. It is difficult to identify the meager facial nerve and cochlear nerve clearly and preserve their function during operation because of giant tumor compression and its abundant blood supply. Moreover, surgical operation would affect the function of cerebellum and brainstem during treatment because of giant tumor, which lead to many complications after surgery. Thus, it is still a great challenge for the neurosurgeons to remove tumors totally, preserve neural function, reduce the complications of patients and improve long-term survival quality of life. Compared to others approaches, it is more beneficial to choose suboccipital retrosigmoid approach for the full exposure of vestibular schwannoma and preservation of facial and hearing functions [2]. Therefore, suboccipital retrosigmoid approach has been widely applied in our department. From 1999 to 2014, 657 cases of giant tumors, which were all resected trans suboccipital retrosigmoid approach, were obtained in our department. After the collection of clinical data, we conducted a retrospective review on clinical symptoms, surgical outcomes, distribution of complications, and their possible causes and preventive measures for the expectation of providing the reference for future clinical treatment.

Methods

Patient population

There were 657 consecutive giant unilateral VSs (excluding neurofibromatosis type II cases) surgically treated via suboccipital retrosigmoid approach between January 1999 and December 2014 at Our Hospital. Clinical status and complications were assessed postoperatively with 14 days and at the time of follow-up. The patients' ages ranged from 12 to 80 years (mean age, 46.8 years). There were 289 male (44.0%) and 368 female (56.0%) patients. The peak incidence was between the ages of 40–60 years of age (366 cases, 55.7%) (Table 1). Patient charts were reviewed retrospectively for clinical status, operative findings, radiological results, and clinical outcomes. The data were analyzed with respect to tumor size, extent of resection, surgical results, and short- and long-term complications.

Tumor classification

Tumor size was categorized according to the international criteria using the largest extrameatal tumor diameter on the post-contrast axial magnetic resonance image (MRI). Giant tumors means >40 mm in the cerebellopontine angle (CPA) [3].

Table 1 Characteristics in 657 patients with intracranial giant vestibular schwannomas ($n = 657$)

Characteristics	
Age, year	
Range	12–80
Average	46.8
Sex, *N* (%)	
Female	289 (44.0%)
Male	368 (56.0%)
Extent of resection, *N* (%)	
Partial resection	2 (0.3%)
Near-total resection	99 (15.1%)
Gross total resection	556 (84.6%)
Managements during surgery	
Electrophysiological monitoring, *N* (%)	538 (81.9%)
External ventricular drainage, *N* (%)	15 (2.3%)
1/3 lateral cerebellum resection, *N* (%)	17 (2.6%)
Follow-up range, month	6–191
Average, month	59.6
Availability, *N* (%)	566 (86.1%)

Evaluation of facial nerve (FN)

FN function was evaluated according to the House-Brackmann (H-B) FN function grading scale immediately after surgery and at the time of last follow-up [4]. We classified FN function into 3 categories: good (H-B I + II), fair (H-B III), and poor (H-B IV + V + VI).

Evaluation of hearing nerve

The hearing function was evaluated by audiology examinations including pure tone audiometry (PTA) and speech discrimination score (SDS). The criteria used for the preoperative and postoperative hearing evaluations were provided by the classification method of the American Institute of Otolaryngology-Head and Neck Surgery (AAO-HNS), 1995 [5].

Surgical technique

The sub-occipital retrosigmoid approach was used in every case. Patients were settled in lateral position and a straight-incision behind ear was chosen. A surgical bone window was made to expose the connection of the transverse sinus and sigmoid sinus. The size of the craniotomy is independent of the tumor size because it is adjusted to the necessary cerebellar retraction. After dissecting the dural using a curved incision, the cerebrospinal fluid (CSF) was aspirated slowly from cerebellomedullary cistern to expose the tumor. Intraoperative electromyogram (EMG) monitoring was used in 538 cases (81.9%). EMG recordings of the orbicularis oris and oculi muscles were used to monitor FN function. A bipolar stimulus with an intensity of 1 mA to 0.05 mA and a duration of 0.1 ms was used to assess FN response.

Multidisciplinary cooperation

In recent 3 years, multidisciplinary cooperation strategy was used to treat giant vestibular schwannoma, which included diffusion tensor imaging (DTI) FN fiber tracking technology preoperatively, perioperative comprehensive assessment of facial and hearing function, perioperative psychological assessment, standard retrosigmoid approach technology, intraoperative EMG monitoring, facial function rehabilitation training and/or plastic surgery (Fig. 1).

Follow-up investigation

All patients were evaluated with contrast-enhanced MRI follow-up from 3 months to 1 year after operation. If the tumor was totally removed or the residual tumor was proved to be stable, patients were re-investigated yearly for at least 5 years clinically and radiologically using MRI. For evaluation we checked for facial symmetry at rest and in motion, separate movements of all three segments (forehead, eyes and mouth), and incidence of conjunctivitis and synkinesis, then graded the results by the H-B scale. If the patient could not come to the hospital a questionnaire was mailed to him/her 1 year postoperatively, questioning his/her perception of the functional recovery, as compared with the clinician's observation.

Analysis of postoperative complications

Postoperative complications were evaluated immediately perioperatively (within 2 weeks to detect short-term complications) and at the time of the last follow-up (to detect long-term complications). The results of FN outcome, hearing outcome, disequilibrium and tinnitus were reported, which were the important result intrinsic to the nature of the disease. Patients who complained of imbalance or unsteadiness after surgery were determined to have disequilibrium. Tinnitus is regarded as subjective and is therefore reported by patients. Facial numbness, taste disturbance, and lower cranial nerve deficits were categorized as cranial nerve complications. Other non-neurological complications included acute hydrocephalus postoperatively, hematoma in the brain, CSF leak and meningitis. Keratitis, labial herpes, occipital scalp hydrops and pneumonia were categorized as systemic complications. Categorical data were compared by the $\chi 2$ test with continuity correction if appropriate. Continuous variables were expressed as the mean ± SD, and were compared using Student's *t*-test. Two-tailed *P*-values <0.05 were considered to indicate a statistically significant difference. Statistical analysis was performed with the Stata software package (version 10.0).

Results

Clinical manifestation

All of those 657 patients were noticed some degree of hearing deficit and 248 patients (37.7%) experienced deafness. The other most frequent clinical symptoms were facial paresthesia (453 cases, 68.9%), tinnitus (296

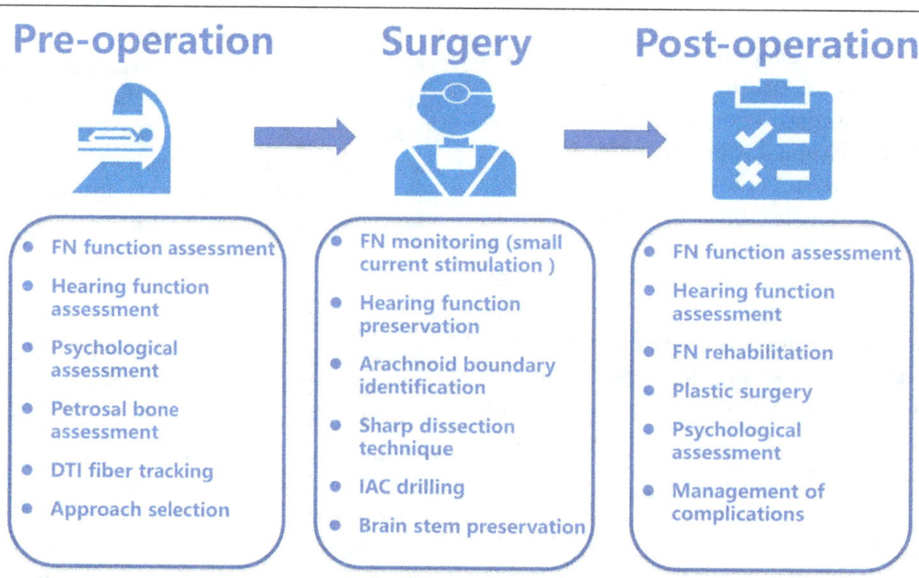

Fig. 1 Multi-disciplinary cooperation treatment and surgical technique for giant vestibular schwannomas. FN: facial nerve, DTI: Diffusion tensor imaging, IAC: internal auditory canal

cases, 45.1%), disequilibrium (293 cases, 44.6%), facial paralysis (HB III + IV 204 cases, 31.1%).

Surgical results

Of 657 cases of giant tumor, the external ventricular drainage from the occipital area was used in 15 cases (2.3%) before tumor resection because of hydrocephalus and 1/3 lateral cerebellum resection was used in 17 cases (2.6%). EMG monitoring was used in 538 cases (81.9%) during surgery. Gross total resection (GTR) was achieved in 556 cases (84.6%), near-total resection (NTR) was in 99 cases (15.1%) and only 2 cases (0.3%) had partial resection (Table 1). The FN anatomical preservation rate was 89.6%.

Mortality

Four patients died after the operation totally. The mortality rate is 0.6%. Two patients died because of the brain hemorrhage and acute hydrocephalus. One patient died of brain edema. One patient died of severe pneumonia due to low cranial nerve disturbance after the operation.

Follow-up outcome

Of 657 cases, 566 patients (86.1%) were successful followed up. Ninety-one patients (13.9%) were lost followed up. The follow-up range was 6 to 191 months (average 59.6 months).

Surgical complications

Of 657 cases within 2 weeks after surgery, disequilibrium was found in 186 cases (28.3%), new tinnitus in 61 cases (9.3%) and new hearing loss (AAO-HNS grade D) in 313 cases (47.6%). In follow-up data available for 566 patients (long-term results), disequilibrium was improved and only found in 38 cases (6.71%). Tinnitus was also improved and found in 14 cases (2.47%). However, loss of hearing (AAO-HNS grade D) seem to be not improved in long-term results and was found in 482 cases (85.2%). Other 67 patients (11.8%) were in grade C, 17 patients (3.00%) in grade B. Permanent facial paralysis (House-Brackmann III + IV + V) was in 250 cases (44.2%).

Other main short-term postoperative non-neurological complications included hematoma in 8 cases (1.2%), meningitis in 50 cases (7.6%), CSF leak in 18 cases (2.7%). The cranial nerve complication included lower cranial nerve deficit in 49 cases (7.5%). The systemic complications included keratitis in 8 cases (1.2%), labial herpes in 42 cases (6.4%), occipital scalp hydrops in 3 cases (0.5%) and pneumonia in 41 cases (6.2%).

However, for the main long-term complications, the condition was completely different. The incidence rate of long-term complications ranked from great to small as follows: facial numbness in 89 cases (15.7%), chronic headache in 18 cases (3.18%) and taste disturbance in 11 cases (1.94%), scar pain in 10 cases (1.77%), decreased vision in 7 cases (1.23%), delayed hydrocephalus in 6 cases (1.06%).

FN function

Short-term FN outcome

Of 657 patients, the facial nerve was preserved anatomically in 589 cases (89.7%). Immediately after surgery (within 2 weeks), good (H-B grade I or II) FN function was seen in 216 cases (32.9%), fair (H-B grade III) FN function was seen in 308 patients (46.9%), and poor FN function (H-B grade IV-VI) was seen in 133 patients (20.2%).

In 556 cases of GTR group, good (H-B grade I or II) FN function was seen in 170 cases (30.6%), fair (H-B grade III) FN function was seen in 271 patients (48.7%), and poor FN function (H-B grade IV–VI) was seen in 115 patients (20.7%).

In 99 cases of NTR group, 45 cases (45.5%) had good (H-B grade I or II) FN function, 36 cases (36.4%) had fair (H-B grade III) FN outcome, 18 cases (18.2%) had poor (H-B grade IV–VI) FN function outcome after surgery. Two patients received partial resection because their tumors were too large and had fair FN outcome (H-B grade III).

Long-term FN outcome

Of 566 patients who were successfully followed up after surgery, 316 cases (55.8%) had good (H-B grade I or II) FN function, 112 cases (19.8%) had fair (H-B grade III) FN outcome, 138 cases (24.4%) had poor (H-B grade IV–VI) FN function outcome in follow-up period.

The effect of multidisciplinary cooperation strategy

From 2012 to 2014, there were 154 patients received multidisciplinary cooperation strategy to treat giant vestibular schwannoma. The anatomical FN preservation rate is 98.1%. Immediately after surgery (within 2 weeks), good (H-B grade I or II) FN function was seen in 84 cases (54.5%), fair (H-B grade III) FN function was seen in 37 patients 24.0%), and poor FN function (H-B grade IV–VI) was seen in 33 patients (21.4%) (Table 2).

Hearing function

Before the operation, 248 patients (37.7%) suffered from grade D hearing loss, 101 patients (15.4%) suffered from grade C hearing loss, and 308 patients (46.9%) suffered from grade C hearing loss, according to the classification of AAO-HNS. After the surgical treatment, 561 patients (85.4%) lost hearing completely (AAO-HNS grade D), among them, 313 of whom were "new hearing loss" and were classified into grade B or C before operation. The other 74 patients (11.2%) were in grade C, 22 patients (3.35%) in grade B. The hearing preservation rate in

Table 2 The effect comparison of tradition and multidisciplinary cooperation group ($n = 657$)

Group	NO.	GTR (%)	FN preservation (%)	FN function 2 weeks after surgery (%)		
				H-B I or II	H-B II	H-B IV–VI
Tradition	503	402 (79.9)	438 (87.1)	132 (26.2)	271 (53.9)	100 (19.9)
MDC	154	154 (100.0)	151 (98.1)	84 (54.5)	37 (24.0)	33 (21.4)
Total	657	556 (84.6)	589 (89.6)	216 (32.9)	308 (46.9)	133 (20.2)

Abbreviations: *MDC* multidisciplinary cooperation group, *FN* facial nerve, *GTR* gross total resection

terms of the results of patients who had serviceable hearing pre-operatively was 7.14%.

Discussion

According to the literature review, although giant vestibular schwannoma accounts for only 2% of vestibular schwannoma, [6] the percentage of giant vestibular schwannoma is much higher in large neurosurgery center, such as German Hanover neuroscience center (12.5%) [7]. From 1999 to 2014, 1263 cases of vestibular schwannomas were treated in our department and giant tumor accounts for 52%(657 cases). One reason was that patients were comparatively centralized because Huashan hospital was a large neurosurgery center in China and the other was that it is not easy to diagnose vestibular schwannoma at its onset especially in developing country. Large or giant vestibular schwannoma was dominant in regions lacking checking means. So, More attention should be paid to the treatment of giant vestibular schwannoma.

The surgical strategy for giant vestibular schwannoma

We have reported that clinical manifestations of giant vestibular schwannoma were not only induced by the oppression of facial and auditory nerves from the tumor but also were caused by the oppressive effects of cranial nerves, cerebellum and brainstem from the tumor based on the conclusion of 1009 cases of large vestibular schwannoma [8]. Microsurgery was still an optimum choice for the treatment of giant vestibular schwannoma. The objective of the operation was not only to maximum extent more than tumor removal but also to protect the function of facial and auditory nerves and other cranial nerves and reduce complications. The mortality of operation obviously decreased with the rapid development of minimal invasive neurosurgery technology and electrophysiological monitor. For giant vestibular schwannoma, operative difficulty increased as the tumor size increased and there existed some problems including low rate of GTR and poor nervous function preservation [7, 9–12]. So, some researchers proposed different strategies such as multi-step operations and part removal of the tumor supplemented by stereotactic radiotherapy [13–15]. We thought both multi-step operations and different treatments in stages were supplementary approaches for unsatisfactory effects of single operation. If doctors could improve surgical outcome, single operation still was an optimum choice. In this study, 657 cases all adopted single operation of microsurgery. The anatomy preservation rate of facial nerves was 89.7%. The rate of GTR was 84.6%. The mortality was only 0.6%. In recent 3 years, we conducted multidisciplinary cooperation and improved microsurgical technology. We implemented the intraoperative monitoring of multiple groups of the cranial nerves and strengthened postoperative facial nerve function rehabilitation. There were 154 cases Involved, the rate of GTR: 100%. The mortality: 0%. The anatomy preservation rate of facial nerves increased to 98.1%. The facial nerve function preservation rate 2 weeks after operation: 78.5% (H-B I–III stage). All indicated that single operation could reach satisfactory effects.

The choice of surgical approach

So far, there were several surgical approaches for giant vestibular schwannoma including suboccipital retrosigmoid approach, middle cranial fossa approach and extended trans-labyrinthine approach. Middle cranial fossa approach seems more suitable for small and medium vestibular schwannoma. Extended trans-labyrinthine approach damaged the audition and its anatomy preservation rate of facial nerves was 74.6–87.8% [2, 16]. Suboccipital retrosigmoid approach was convenient and safe for neurosurgeons. It could provide spacious view of cerebellopontine angle and expose brainstem and cerebellopontine angle structure quickly, safely with multi-aspects. The operator could look directly at anterior inferior cerebellar artery (AICA) and facial and auditory nerves. Hence, it was an optimum approach for protecting intracranial segments of facial nerve. It has been reported that using suboccipital retrosigmoid approach, the anatomy preservation rate of FN was 86–92%. The function retention rate: 72–75% [1, 7]. In this study, 657 cases all adopted suboccipital retrosigmoid approach. The anatomy preservation rate of FN: 89.7%. The rate of GTR: 84.6%. In recent 3 years, the anatomy preservation rate of FN increased to 98.1%. The rate of GTR: 100%. The facial nerve function retention rate 2 weeks after operation: 78.5% (House-Brackmann I–III stage). We thought suboccipital retrosigmoid approach was appropriate for total removal of giant vestibular schwannoma.

Key operation points of suboccipital retrosigmoid approach

Exposure, decompression within the tumor and isolating tumor: During operation, the cerebrospinal fluid should be released slowly after open the dura. After retracting the cerebellum the tumor was exposed and its arachnoid boundary should be conducted sharp dissection. Resected tumor piece-by-piece and conducted sufficient intra-tumor decompression. Meanwhile, closely guarded subarachnoid space. Then separated tumor from its upper to lower pole and then the section of brainstem carefully and separated and protected petrosal vein appropriately. Key operation points should be noted during operation because of giant tumor: ① The decompression speed cannot be too fast during operation (either when released cerebrospinal fluid of cisterna magna or when resected tumor) to avoid bleeding of bridging veins. ② Intraoperative hemostasis should be immediate and effective and keep clear operation field to separate the tumor arachnoid boundary. Paid more attention to the areas close to brainstem segments of auditory nerve and trigeminal nerve, contiguous areas of tumor and the choroid plexus of the fourth ventricle and the brainstem ventral veins. Arachnoid boundary was not clear and needed to repeat confirmation before separation. ③ Intra-tumor decompression should be sufficient during operation. Then removed the tumor wall gradually. After sufficient decompression, thinner tumor wall (2–3 mm) was easier to be separated from arachnoid interval, which was more beneficial to identify and protect facial and auditory nerves. ④ Close protected petrosal vein during operation because the injury of petrosal vein could lead to bleeding directly and the obstacles of cerebellum backflow, further contributing to tissue edema and/or the hemorrhage induced by venous congestion. ⑤ Conducted thorough hemostasis for the broken blood vessels during operation and avoided hemorrhage after operation. Paid more attention to AICA. Sughrue et al. summarized and analyzed 32,870 cases of vestibular schwannomas from 100 articles. The statistical results showed that the most common cause to death of vestibular schwannoma was AICA hemorrhage [11]. Separated and retained all blood vessels as much as possible when we removing the tumor. The arteries or veins on the surface of the tumor should be retained if they did not supply tumor, which could avoid affecting blood supply of peripheral nerve tissues and venous reflux.

The search and preservation of FN: Auditory nerve would be firstly observed generally at the lower pole of tumor and should be assessed the reservation possibility. Tried to preserve the nerves if possible. The brainstem segment of FN could be found under the auditory nerve. Separated according to the distribution of nerves. Conducted sharp separation on the adhesion and tried to fully expose FN.

The management of internal auditory canal (IAC): Drilled and opened the IAC and exposed the tumor inside. Resected the tumor while separated and preserved FN. Finally, closed IAC appropriately. It might be not necessary or unable to open IAC in the following situations: ① There was no tumor in IAC. ② The opening of IAC was enlarged by the tumor and it was not necessary to be drilled. ③ There were nerves and vessels on the surface of the tumor at the opening of IAC and it was difficult to separate. ④ There was high jugular bulb or Overdeveloped mastoid air cells.

The hemostasis and close: Conducted precise hemostasis and close sutured dura and each layer of tissue.

FN preservation

The favorable postoperative function of FN was achieved in 47.6 to 92.8% of vestibular schwannoma patients trans-suboccipital retrosigmoid approach, even lower in giant tumors [8, 17–24]. In this study, 589 cases (89.7%) showed preserved FN. There were 216 cases (36.2%) showed good FN outcome 2 weeks after surgery, 308 cases (45.8%) showed fair prognosis. In 566 cases who were available for follow-up, most patients showed recovered function of FN. The favorable function of FN (H-B I–III stage) was achieved in 86.0% of patients. The difficulty for FN preservation includes: the distinguishing of FN during operation; the preservation of FN during resection of tumor and the rehabilitation of FN function after surgery. Hence, we recommended that the preservation of FN should be improved by multidisciplinary cooperation. The specific highlights include: 1. The location relationship between tumor and FN should be assessed by imaging before surgery. 2. The microsurgical technology should be improved and monitoring of electrophysiology should be enhanced during surgery. 3. The plastic surgeon collaborates to do rehabilitation of FN function and repairing of FN.

The location relationship between tumor and facial nerve should be assessed by imaging before surgery

DTI helps us to determine the diffusion tension of water molecules in white matter. DTI-based fiber tracking technology (DTT) helps us to visualize the direction where fiber bundle of the white matter in brain travels [25]. Many reports of vestibular schwannoma revealed that FN could be imaged and fiber tracking technology for FN has been considered as a novel, non-invasive accurate method to predict the location and direction of FN in large vestibular schwannoma. The success rate of DTT was reported to be 62.5–100% [26–28].

The microsurgical technology should be improved and monitoring of electrophysiology should be enhanced during surgery

We believe that 2 key factors should be managed to preserve the FN during removal of tumor: 1. The blunt dissection should be combined with sharp dissection during dissection of FN. The FN themselves and blood supply should be preserved. 2. Accurate judgment of FN function during surgery: The EMG monitoring should be continuously given to determine the location and function of FN during surgery.

Some proposed to alternate the total resection with near-total or partial resection in order to preserve FN. However, Nonaka et al. [24] analyzed 410 cases of vestibular schwannoma and found that there was no significant difference in the anatomical and functional preservation of facial nerves in the GTR group and NTR group. In this study, 79.3% of 556 cases who underwent GTR showed good or fair prognosis of FN. 81.8% of 99 cases who underwent NTR showed good or fair prognosis of FN. Subsequent chi-squared analysis showed that good and fair FN outcomes did not correlate with the extent of resection ($P = 0.569$). We hence strengthened that preserving the FN at the condition of maximal resection of tumor. The continuous monitoring of electrophysiology should be performed to confirm the location of FN. Meanwhile, the decision on GTR or not should be made when the monitoring data of electrophysiology significantly change.

Early rehabilitation of FN function and repairing of FN after surgery

Although we take many measures to preserve the FN, the preservation rate of FN is less than 100%. In this study, the anatomical preservation of FN was achieved in 589 cases (89.7%). What should be done to repair the ruptured FN? Sammi et al. [19, 29] suggested that the ruptured nerve should be immediately repaired if it was ruptured during the surgery. The methods to reconstruct the nerve included end-to-end anastomosis, intracranial-temporal bone nerve graft reconstruction and intracranial-extracranial graft reconstruction (intracranial-stylomastoid foramen). If the proximal and residual end of FN with impairment or complete degeneration is located in the brainstem, the hypoglossal nerve or contralateral FN can be used as donors to resuscitate the FN. The resuscitation should be done as early as possible. Early rehabilitation should be carried out after surgery.

Based on our experience, the ruptured nerve should be immediately repaired if it was ruptured during the surgery. The end-to-end anastomosis or nerve transplantation is the most common method. For patients with poor prognosis of FN function, if it was not possible to perform anatomical preservation during surgery, FN plastic surgery is recommend to repair the nerve (masseter nerve-facial nerve anastomosis). If the anatomical preservation was done during surgery, the strict rehabilitation should be strengthened and the recovery of FN function should be persistently observed. If the prognosis is poor, early intervention such as FN plastic surgery should be applied. For the time window of intervention, 1 year after surgery is the best period to predict whether the FN plastic surgery function is recovered or not (sensitivity 97%, specificity 97%) [30]. Therefore, we recommend early FN plastic surgery in the period of 1 year after tumor removal surgery for those who had poor prognosis despite anatomical preservation of facial nerves.

Among 566 cases who were successfully follow-up, 37 patients whose post-operative immediate FN function showed poor prognosis received only rehabilitation and recovered to HB I or II stage 1 year after surgery, 36 cases received masseter nerve-facial nerve anastomosis in plastic surgery and showed satisfactory outcome [31].

Hearing preservation

The most relevant factor for preservation of hearing is the tumor size. The smaller tumor has the higher preservation possibility of hearing function after surgery. On the contrary, the larger tumor has the lower preservation possibility of hearing function after surgery [32]. Glasscock et al. [33] showed that patients with tumor bigger than 2 cm had highly low possibility of hearing preservation and early detection was critical for hearing preservation. We demonstrated that about 10% of patients with large vestibular schwannoma had hearing function [8]. For those patients, the acoustic nerve should be anatomically preserved with maximum effort. The preservation of hearing is still the goal of the surgery, which is dependent on normal internal auditory artery, structure of cochlea and cochlear nerve. Two problems should be solved to preserve the hearing: First, ensure the continuity of cochlear nerve and internal auditory artery. This requires the surgeon should have the ability to determine which one is cochlear nerve under the pathological state. Secondly, the effective monitoring of electrophysiology during the surgery is critical to complete preservation of cochlear nerve. The use of assistant-endoscopic surgery is helpful for preservation of hearing during resection of vestibular schwannoma. In this study, the hearing preservation rate was low because all the neuromas were giant. The preservation of hearing after surgery remains a highlighted issue for giant vestibular schwannomas.

Other complications

Other complications included CSF leak, ataxia, tinnitus, facial numbness, taste disturbance, low cranial nerve deficit, post-operative hemorrhage, brain edema, meningitis etc. In this study, the incidence of CSF leakage is lower than literature report. Only 18 cases (2.7%) developed CSF leakage. However, CSF leakage is a common complication with incidence of 6.2–20% due to resection of large vestibular schwannomas, which is characterized by otorrhea, rhinorrhea and incision leakage of cerebrospinal fluid [34–39]. Sughrue et al. believed the most common factor for CSF leakage was associated with approach. It is not true that bigger tumors are more prone to leak of CSF. Instead, the trans-labyrinthine approach is more likely to cause CSF leakage than trans-retrosigmoid approach [11]. We concluded the following experience to avoid this complication: 1. It is best not to open the mastoid cells during operation. When it has to be open, bone wax and biogel should be used to rigorously seal it. 2. The opening of IAC shall not be excessively big. It should be big enough as long as the tumor in the canal is well exposed. During resection of tumor, the dura in the canal should be completely preserved. After resection of tumor, the canal should be carefully closed. 3. Strict suturing of dura is essential. The muscle and skin shall be rigorously sutured in organized layers. 4. The treatment of reducing intracranial pressure should be applied after surgery. The leakage of CSF should be immediately treated if it is happen. The mild incision leakage of CSF and scalp hydrops can be treated with subcutaneous puncture and pressure dressing. If it is not improved or it is suspected to be caused by poor closing of air chamber in the back wall of IAC, the exploration of CSF leakage and repairing procedures should be performed as soon as possible. For CSF rhinorrhea and otorrhea, cisternography or head MRI T2-weight imaging should be performed to confirm the location of leakage. The repairing should be immediately performed to avoid life-threatening complications such as intracranial infection caused by prolonged leakage of CSF. Meanwhile, the potent, sufficient antibiotics easy to pass blood brain barrier should be used to prevent and control infection. All cases with leakage of CSF in this study improved after treatment and discharged from the hospital.

In this study, 50 cases (7.6%) developed meningitis and the incidence was higher than literature report, which should be pay abundant attention to. Meningitis has two types, including bacterial meningitis and aseptic meningitis. The bacterial meningitis was more likely due to contamination during surgery, probably because of insufficient conformance with aseptic procedure and long surgery. The reasons for aseptic meningitis remained unknown. We found that the bacteria were often not considered in cases with meningitis after surgery of vestibular schwannomas. CSF samples were cultured for all the 50 cases of meningitis in this study. However, only 3 of them were bacteria-positive meningitis. Among these 3 cases, only 1 case was correlated with CSF leakage. Lebowitz et al. [40] suggested that most cases of meningitis after surgery of vestibular schwannomas were considered as aseptic meningitis and associated with filling the mastoid cells with bone wax. Therefore, we recommended the following key steps to reduce aseptic meningitis: 1. Carefully protect subarachnoid space, especially avoid hemorrhage during operation which flows into the surrounding subarachnoid space. 2. Reduce implants (such as glue, artificial dura matter, bone wax and hemostatic material), on the premise that the surgical outcome can be ensured. When closing cranium, each layer should be repeatedly washed with sterile normal saline to remove scraped bone substances and bone wax particles.

Conclusions

To accumulate surgical experience and to master the clinical anatomy of the suboccipital retrosigmoid approach to vestibular schwannoma surgery, intraoperative nerve monitoring, preoperative study of the imaging and clinical data, and multidisciplinary cooperation, were the keys to improving prognostic outcomes in giant intracranial vestibular schwannoma patients.

Abbreviation

AICA: Anterior inferior cerebellar artery; CPA: Cerebellopontine angle; CSF: Cerebrospinal fluid; DTI: Diffusion tensor imaging; DTT: Diffusion tensor imaging-based fiber tracking technology; EMG: Electromyography; FN: Facial nerve; GTR: Gloss total resection; H-B: House-Brackmann scale; IAC: Internal auditory canal; NTR: Near-total resection; STR: Subtotal resection

Acknowledgements

Not applicable.

Funding

This study is part of the medical project supported by Shanghai Science and Technology Commission, China (Grant No. 134119a4700) and "Yang Fan" project (15YF1401500). The study is also part of "China Spark Program"supported by Ministry of Science and Technology, China (Grant No. S2013C000013).

Authors' contributions

XH and JX analyzed and interpreted the patient data, and were major contributors in writing the manuscript. MX, MYC, KYJ and JWR recorded and collected patients' information, and also participated in writing the manuscript. PZ performed surgeries for most of cases and designed this study. All authors read and approved the final manuscript.

Competing interests

The authors declare that they have no competing interests.

References

1. Silva J, Cerejo A, Duarte F, Silveira F, Vaz R. Surgical removal of giant acoustic neuromas. World Neurosurg. 2012;77(5–6):731–5.
2. Ansari SF, Terry C, Cohen-Gadol AA. Surgery for vestibular schwannomas: a systematic review of complications by approach. Neurosurg Focus. 2012;33(3):E14.
3. Kanzaki J, Tos M, Sanna M, Moffat DA, Monsell EM, Berliner KI. New and modified reporting systems from the consensus meeting on systems for reporting results in vestibular schwannoma. Otol Neurotol. 2003;24(4):642–8. discussion 648–649.
4. House JW, Brackmann DE. Facial nerve grading system. Otolaryngol Head Neck Surg. 1985;93(2):146–7.
5. Committee on Hearing and Equilibrium guidelines for the evaluation of hearing preservation in acoustic neuroma (vestibular schwannoma). American Academy of Otolaryngology-Head and Neck Surgery Foundation, INC. Otolaryngol Head Neck Surg. 1995;113(3):179–180.
6. Tos M, Stangerup SE, Caye-Thomasen P, Tos T, Thomsen J. What is the real incidence of vestibular schwannoma? Arch Otolaryngol Head Neck Surg. 2004;130(2):216–20.
7. Samii M, Gerganov VM, Samii A. Functional outcome after complete surgical removal of giant vestibular schwannomas. J Neurosurg. 2010;112(4):860–7.
8. Huang X, Xu J, Xu M, Zhou LF, Zhang R, Lang L, Xu Q, Zhong P, Chen M, Wang Y, et al. Clinical features of intracranial vestibular schwannomas. Oncol Lett. 2013;5(1):57–62.
9. Anderson DE, Leonetti J, Wind JJ, Cribari D, Fahey K. Resection of large vestibular schwannomas: facial nerve preservation in the context of surgical approach and patient-assessed outcome. J Neurosurg. 2005;102(4):643–9.
10. Angeli RD, Ben Ammar M, Sanna M. Perioperative complications after translabyrinthine removal of large or giant vestibular schwannoma: outcomes for 123 patients. Acta Otolaryngol. 2011;131(11):1237–8.
11. Sughrue ME, Yang I, Aranda D, Rutkowski MJ, Fang S, Cheung SW, Parsa AT. Beyond audiofacial morbidity after vestibular schwannoma surgery. J Neurosurg. 2011;114(2):367–74.
12. Wanibuchi M, Fukushima T, Mcelveen Jr JT, Friedman AH. Hearing preservation in surgery for large vestibular schwannomas. J Neurosurg. 2009;111(4):845–54.
13. Fuentes S, Arkha Y, Pech-Gourg G, Grisoli F, Dufour H, Regis J. Management of large vestibular schwannomas by combined surgical resection and gamma knife radiosurgery. Prog Neurol Surg. 2008;21:79–82.
14. Iwai Y, Yamanaka K, Ishiguro T. Surgery combined with radiosurgery of large acoustic neuromas. Surg Neurol. 2003;59(4):283–9. discussion 289–291.
15. Satyarthee GD, Kumar S. Is staged surgery for giant vestibular schwannomas always better in improving outcome: Needs socioeconomic consideration? J Neurosci Rural Pract. 2014;5(4):437–9.
16. Zhang Z, Wang Z, Huang Q, Yang J, Wu H. Removal of large or giant sporadic vestibular schwannomas via translabyrinthine approach: a report of 115 cases. ORL J Otorhinolaryngol Relat Spec. 2012;74(5):271–7.
17. Sterkers JM, Morrison GA, Sterkers O, El-Dine MM. Preservation of facial, cochlear, and other nerve functions in acoustic neuroma treatment. Otolaryngol Head Neck Surg. 1994;110(2):146–55.
18. Gormley WB, Sekhar LN, Wright DC, Kamerer D, Schessel D. Acoustic neuromas: results of current surgical management. Neurosurgery. 1997;41(1):50–8. discussion 58–60.
19. Samii M, Matthies C. Management of 1000 vestibular schwannomas (acoustic neuromas): the facial nerve—preservation and restitution of function. Neurosurgery. 1997;40(4):684–94. discussion 694–685.
20. Lanman TH, Brackmann DE, Hitselberger WE, Subin B. Report of 190 consecutive cases of large acoustic tumors (vestibular schwannoma) removed via the translabyrinthine approach. J Neurosurg. 1999;90(4):617–23.
21. Darrouzet V, Martel J, Enee V, Bebear JP, Guerin J. Vestibular schwannoma surgery outcomes: our multidisciplinary experience in 400 cases over 17 years. Laryngoscope. 2004;114(4):681–8.
22. Jain VK, Mehrotra N, Sahu RN, Behari S, Banerji D, Chhabra DK. Surgery of vestibular schwannomas: an institutional experience. Neurol India. 2005;53(1):41–5. discussion 45.
23. Samii M, Gerganov V, Samii A. Improved preservation of hearing and facial nerve function in vestibular schwannoma surgery via the retrosigmoid approach in a series of 200 patients. J Neurosurg. 2006;105(4):527–35.
24. Nonaka Y, Fukushima T, Watanabe K, Friedman AH, Sampson JH, Mcelveen Jr JT, Cunningham 3rd CD, Zomorodi AR. Contemporary surgical management of vestibular schwannomas: analysis of complications and lessons learned over the past decade. Neurosurgery. 2013;72(2 Suppl Operative):115. discussion ons115.
25. Hodaie M, Quan J, Chen DQ. In vivo visualization of cranial nerve pathways in humans using diffusion-based tractography. Neurosurgery. 2010;66(4):788–95. discussion 795–786.
26. Gerganov VM, Giordano M, Samii M, Samii A. Diffusion tensor imaging-based fiber tracking for prediction of the position of the facial nerve in relation to large vestibular schwannomas. J Neurosurg. 2011;115(6):1087–93.
27. Roundy N, Delashaw JB, Cetas JS. Preoperative identification of the facial nerve in patients with large cerebellopontine angle tumors using high-density diffusion tensor imaging. J Neurosurg. 2012;116(4):697–702.
28. Taoka T, Hirabayashi H, Nakagawa H, Sakamoto M, Myochin K, Hirohashi S, Iwasaki S, Sakaki T, Kichikawa K. Displacement of the facial nerve course by vestibular schwannoma: preoperative visualization using diffusion tensor tractography. J Magn Reson Imaging. 2006;24(5):1005–10.
29. Samii M, Matthies C. Management of 1000 vestibular schwannomas (acoustic neuromas): surgical management and results with an emphasis on complications and how to avoid them. Neurosurgery. 1997;40(1):11–21. discussion 21–13.
30. Rivas A, Boahene KD, Bravo HC, Tan M, Tamargo RJ, Francis HW. A model for early prediction of facial nerve recovery after vestibular schwannoma surgery. Otol Neurotol. 2011;32(5):826–33.
31. Wang W, Yang C, Li Q, Li W, Yang X, Zhang YX. Masseter-to-facial nerve transfer: a highly effective technique for facial reanimation after acoustic neuroma resection. Ann Plast Surg. 2014;73 Suppl 1:S63–9.
32. Samii M, Matthies C. Management of 1000 vestibular schwannomas (acoustic neuromas): hearing function in 1000 tumor resections. Neurosurgery. 1997;40(2):248–60. discussion 260–242.
33. Glasscock 3rd ME, Hays JW, Minor LB, Haynes DS, Carrasco VN. Preservation of hearing in surgery for acoustic neuromas. J Neurosurg. 1993;78(6):864–70.
34. Bani A, Gilsbach JM. Incidence of cerebrospinal fluid leak after microsurgical removal of vestibular schwannomas. Acta Neurochir (Wien). 2002;144(10):979–82. discussion 982.
35. Brennan JW, Rowed DW, Nedzelski JM, Chen JM. Cerebrospinal fluid leak after acoustic neuroma surgery: influence of tumor size and surgical approach on incidence and response to treatment. J Neurosurg. 2001;94(2):217–23.
36. Hoffman RA. Cerebrospinal fluid leak following acoustic neuroma removal. Laryngoscope. 1994;104(1 Pt 1):40–58.
37. Selesnick SH, Liu JC, Jen A, Newman J. The incidence of cerebrospinal fluid leak after vestibular schwannoma surgery. Otol Neurotol. 2004;25(3):387–93.
38. Sade B, Mohr G, Dufour JJ. Vascular complications of vestibular schwannoma surgery: a comparison of the suboccipital retrosigmoid and translabyrinthine approaches. J Neurosurg. 2006;105(2):200–4.
39. Stieglitz LH, Giordano M, Gerganov V, Raabe A, Samii A, Samii M, Ludemann WO. Petrous bone pneumatization is a risk factor for cerebrospinal fluid fistula following vestibular schwannoma surgery. Neurosurgery. 2010;67(2 Suppl Operative):509–15.
40. Lebowitz RA, Hoffman RA, Roland Jr JT, Cohen NL. Autologous fibrin glue in the prevention of cerebrospinal fluid leak following acoustic neuroma surgery. Am J Otol. 1995;16(2):172–4.

Permissions

All chapters in this book were first published in NEUROLOGY, by BioMed Central; hereby published with permission under the Creative Commons Attribution License or equivalent. Every chapter published in this book has been scrutinized by our experts. Their significance has been extensively debated. The topics covered herein carry significant findings which will fuel the growth of the discipline. They may even be implemented as practical applications or may be referred to as a beginning point for another development.

The contributors of this book come from diverse backgrounds, making this book a truly international effort. This book will bring forth new frontiers with its revolutionizing research information and detailed analysis of the nascent developments around the world.

We would like to thank all the contributing authors for lending their expertise to make the book truly unique. They have played a crucial role in the development of this book. Without their invaluable contributions this book wouldn't have been possible. They have made vital efforts to compile up to date information on the varied aspects of this subject to make this book a valuable addition to the collection of many professionals and students.

This book was conceptualized with the vision of imparting up-to-date information and advanced data in this field. To ensure the same, a matchless editorial board was set up. Every individual on the board went through rigorous rounds of assessment to prove their worth. After which they invested a large part of their time researching and compiling the most relevant data for our readers.

The editorial board has been involved in producing this book since its inception. They have spent rigorous hours researching and exploring the diverse topics which have resulted in the successful publishing of this book. They have passed on their knowledge of decades through this book. To expedite this challenging task, the publisher supported the team at every step. A small team of assistant editors was also appointed to further simplify the editing procedure and attain best results for the readers.

Apart from the editorial board, the designing team has also invested a significant amount of their time in understanding the subject and creating the most relevant covers. They scrutinized every image to scout for the most suitable representation of the subject and create an appropriate cover for the book.

The publishing team has been an ardent support to the editorial, designing and production team. Their endless efforts to recruit the best for this project, has resulted in the accomplishment of this book. They are a veteran in the field of academics and their pool of knowledge is as vast as their experience in printing. Their expertise and guidance has proved useful at every step. Their uncompromising quality standards have made this book an exceptional effort. Their encouragement from time to time has been an inspiration for everyone.

The publisher and the editorial board hope that this book will prove to be a valuable piece of knowledge for researchers, students, practitioners and scholars across the globe.

List of Contributors

Sung-Ju Hsueh, Han-I Lin and Chin-Hsien Lin
Department of Neurology, National Taiwan University Hospital, No. 7, Chung-Shan South Road, Taipei 100, Taiwan

Ni-Chung Lee
Department of Medical Genetics, National Taiwan University Hospital, Taipei 100, Taiwan

Shu-Hua Yang
Department of Orthopedics, National Taiwan University Hospital, No. 7, Chung-Shan South Road, Taipei 100, Taiwan

Shin Iida, Masataka Nakamura, Shinya Asayama, Takenobu Kunieda, Satoshi Kaneko and Hirofumi Kusaka
Department of Neurology, Kansai Medical University, 2-5-1, Shinmachi, Hirakata, Osaka 5731010, Japan

Hitoshi Osaka
Department of Pediatrics, Jichi Medical School, 3311-1, Yakushiji, Shimotsuke-shi, Tochigi 3290498, Japan

Luciano Vieira de Araujo and Fernando Henrique Inocêncio Borba Ferreira
School of Arts, Sciences and Humanities, University of São Paulo, Av. Arlindo Béttio, 1000, Ermelino Matarazzo, São Paulo 03828-000, Brazil

Luiz Carlos de Abreu and Claudio Leone
School of Public Health, University of São Paulo, São Paulo, Brazil

Carlos Bandeira de Mello Monteiro
School of Arts, Sciences and Humanities, University of São Paulo, Av. Arlindo Béttio, 1000, Ermelino Matarazzo, São Paulo 03828-000, Brazil
School of Public Health, University of São Paulo, São Paulo, Brazil

Talita Dias da Silva
School of Arts, Sciences and Humanities, University of São Paulo, Av. Arlindo Béttio, 1000, Ermelino Matarazzo, São Paulo 03828-000, Brazil
Harvard School of Public Health, Harvard University, Boston, MA, USA

Felipe Fregni
Center for Neurosciences (NEC), University of São Paulo, São Paulo, Brazil
Spaulding Rehabilitation Hospital and Massachusetts General Hospital, Harvard Medical School, Boston, MA, USA

Ravindra Kumar Garg, Imran Rizvi, Rajan Ingole, Hardeep Singh Malhotra, Neeraj Kumar and Dhruv Batra
Department of Neurology, King George's Medical University, UP, Lucknow 226003, India

Amita Jain
Department of Microbiology, King George's Medical University, UP, Lucknow 226003, India

Lili Wang, Yun Zhang and Maolin He
Department of Neurology, Beijing Shijitan Hospital, Capital Medical University, Beijing 100038, People's Republic of China

Vanesa Bochkezanian
Exercise Medicine Research Institute, Edith Cowan University, Perth, Australia
Centre for Sports and Exercise Science, School of Medical and Health Sciences, Edith Cowan University, Joondalup 270 Joondalup Drive, Joondalup, WA 6027, Australia

Timothy S. Pulverenti and Anthony J. Blazevich
Centre for Sports and Exercise Science, School of Medical and Health Sciences, Edith Cowan University, Joondalup 270 Joondalup Drive, Joondalup, WA 6027, Australia

Robert U. Newton
Exercise Medicine Research Institute, Edith Cowan University, Perth, Australia
Centre for Sports and Exercise Science, School of Medical and Health Sciences, Edith Cowan University, Joondalup 270 Joondalup Drive, Joondalup, WA 6027, Australia
UQ Centre for Clinical Research, University of Queensland, Brisbane, Australia

Gabriel S. Trajano
School of Exercise and Nutrition Sciences, Queensland University of Technology, Brisbane, Australia

Amilton Vieira
UDF-University Centre, Brasilia, Brazil

Bolin Hu, Pengcheng Wu, Yan Peng, Weijiang Ding, Ming Zhang and Xueliang Qi
Department of Neurology, The Second Affiliated Hospital of Nanchang University, No. 1, Minde Road, Nanchang, Jiangxi 330006, People's Republic of China

Yibiao Zhou
Department of Orthopedics, The First Affiliated Hospital of Nanchang University, Nanchang, Jiangxi 330006, People's Republic of China

Xiaoping Tang
Department of MRI, The Second Affiliated Hospital of Nanchang University, Nanchang, Jiangxi 330006, People's Republic of China

Ying Du, Chuan Li, Dai-di Zhao, Jia-rui Lu, Wei Zhang and Zhu-yi Li
Department of Neurology, Tangdu Hospital, Fourth Military Medical University, Xi'an City, Shaanxi Province 710038, China

Crystal Stinson, Larry L. Bellinger and Phillip R. Kramer
Department of Biomedical Sciences, Texas A&M University College of Dentistry, 3302 Gaston Avenue, Dallas, TX 75246, USA

Michael B Yee and Paul R. Kinchington
Dept Ophthalmology and of Molecular Microbiology and Genetics, 203 Lothrop St., Pittsburgh, PA 15213, USA

Mohong Deng
Department of Oral and Maxillofacial Surgery, The State Key Laboratory Breeding Base of Basic Science of Stomatology & Key Laboratory of Oral Biomedicine Ministry of Education, School & Hospital of Stomatology, Wuhan University, Wuhan, People's Republic of China

Hanna M. Volpert, Jan Pfeiffenberger, Wolfgang Stremmel, Daniel N. Gotthardt, Mark Schäfer and Karl Heinz Weiss
Department of Internal Medicine IV, Heidelberg University Hospital, Im Neuenheimer Feld 410, Heidelberg, Germany

Markus Weiler
Department of Neurology, Heidelberg University Hospital, Im Neuenheimer Feld 400, 69120 Heidelberg, Germany

Jan B. Gröner
Department of Internal Medicine I, Heidelberg University Hospital, Im Neuenheimer Feld 410, Heidelberg, Germany

Miao Liu, Jianhua Wang and Jing Zeng
Institute of Geriatrics, Chinese PLA General Hospital, 28 Fuxing Road, Beijing 100853, China
Beijing Key Laboratory of Aging and Geriatrics, Beijing, China

Yao He
Institute of Geriatrics, Chinese PLA General Hospital, 28 Fuxing Road, Beijing 100853, China
Beijing Key Laboratory of Aging and Geriatrics, Beijing, China
State Key Laboratory of Kidney Disease, Chinese PLA General Hospital, 28 Fuxing Road, Beijing 100853, China

Oliver Höffken, Özüm S. Özgül, Elena K. Enax-Krumova and Martin Tegenthoff
Department of Neurology, Berufsgenossenschaftliches Universitätsklinikum Bergmannsheil GmbH, Ruhr-University Bochum, Bürkle-de-la-Camp-Platz 1, 44789 Bochum, Germany

Christoph Maier
Department of Pain Medicine, Berufsgenossenschaftliches Universitätsklinikum Bergmannsheil GmbH, Ruhr-University Bochum, Bürkle-de-la-Camp-Platz 1, 44789 Bochum, Germany

Ying Wang, Pei Shang, Meiying Xin, Jing Bai and Chunkui Zhou
Neuroscience Centre, Department of Neurology, the First Hospital of Jilin University, Xinmin Street 71#, Changchun 130021, China

Hong-Liang Zhang
Neuroscience Centre, Department of Neurology, the First Hospital of Jilin University, Xinmin Street 71#, Changchun 130021, China Department of Life Sciences, the National Natural Science Foundation of China, Beijing, China

Yanguang Shen, Yan Zhong, Haiyi Wang, Lu Ma, Yingwei Wang and Huiyi Ye
Department of Radiology, Chinese PLA General Hospital, Fuxing Road 28, Beijing 100853, China

Kun Zhang
Department of Radiology, Chinese Navy General Hospital, Beijing, China

Zhonghua Sun
Department of Medical Radiation Sciences, Curtin University, Perth 6102, Australia

Geert Jan Biessels
Department of Neurology, G03.232 Brain Center Rudolf Magnus, University Medical Cente, 3508, GA, Utrecht, the Netherlands

Jolien Janssen
Department of Neurology, G03.232 Brain Center Rudolf Magnus, University Medical Cente, 3508, GA, Utrecht, the Netherlands
Julius Center for Health Sciences and Primary Care, University Medical Center Utrecht, Utrecht, the Netherlands

Esther van den Berg
Department of Neurology, G03.232 Brain Center Rudolf Magnus, University Medical Cente, 3508, GA, Utrecht, the Netherlands
Department of Neurology, Erasmus MC - University Medical Center, Rotterdam, the Netherlands

Bernard Zinman
Lunenfeld-Tanenbaum Research Institute, Mount Sinai Hospital, Toronto, Canada, Division of Endocrinology, University of Toronto, Toronto, Canada

Mark A. Espeland
Department of Biostatistical Sciences, Wake Forest School of Medicine, Winston-Salem, NC, USA

Michaela Mattheus
Global biometrics and datamanagement, Boehringer Ingelheim, Ingelheim, Germany

Odd Erik Johansen
Clinical development, Therapeutic Area Metabolism, Boehringer Ingelheim, Asker, Norway

Vera Spatenkova
Neurocenter, Neurointensive Care Unit, Regional Hospital, Husova 357/10, Regional Hospital, 46063 Liberec, Czech Republic

Ondrej Bradac
Department of Neurosurgery, Military University Hospital and First Medical School, Charles University, Prague, Czech Republic

Daniela Fackova and Zdenka Bohunova
Department of Clinical microbiology and immunology, Antibiotic Centre, Regional Hospital, Liberec, Czech Republic

Petr Suchomel
Neurocenter, Department of Neurosurgery, Regional Hospital, Liberec, Czech Republic

Sujata P. Thawani
Department of Neurology, New York University School of Medicine, New York, NY, USA

Thomas H. Brannagan
Peripheral Neuropathy Center, Neurological Institute, Columbia University, College of Physicians and Surgeons, New York, NY, USA

Peter H. R. Green
Celiac Disease Center, Department of Medicine, Columbia University College of Physicians and Surgeons, New York, NY, USA

Benjamin Lebwohl
Celiac Disease Center, Department of Medicine, Columbia University College of Physicians and Surgeons, New York, NY, USA
Department Medical Epidemiology and Biostatistics, Karolinska Institutet, 171 77 Stockholm, Sweden

Jonas F. Ludvigsson
Department Medical Epidemiology and Biostatistics, Karolinska Institutet, 171 77 Stockholm, Sweden
Department of Pediatrics, Örebro University Hospital, Örebro University, Örebro, Sweden
Division of Epidemiology and Public Health, School of Medicine, University of Nottingham, Nottingham, UK

Tomasz Litwin, Karolina Dzieżyc and Michal Karliński
2nd Department of Neurology, Institute of Psychiatry and Neurology, 02 957 Warsaw, Poland

Anna Członkowska
2nd Department of Neurology, Institute of Psychiatry and Neurology, 02 957 Warsaw, Poland
Department of Experimental and Clinical Pharmacology, Medical University of Warsaw, Warsaw, Poland

Johan Bring
Statisticon AB i Uppsala, Uppsala, Sweden

Carl Bjartmar
Wilson Therapeutics AB, Stockholm, Sweden

Preet Singh, Kavitha Kongara, Neil Ward, Venkata Sayoji Rao Dukkipati, Craig Johnson and Paul Chambers
Massey University, Institute of Veterinary, Animal and Biomedical Sciences, Palmerston North, New Zealand

David Harding
Massey University, Institute of Fundamental Sciences, Palmerston North, New Zealand

Panitha Jindahra, Charungthai Dejthevaporn and Pimjai Niparuck
Department of Medicine, Faculty of Medicine Ramathibodi Hospital, Mahidol University, 270 Rama VI Road, Bangkok 10400, Thailand

Jariya Waisayarat
Department of Pathology, Faculty of Medicine Ramathibodi Hospital, Mahidol University, 270 Rama VI Road, Bangkok 10400, Thailand

Piyaphon Cheecharoen
Department of Radiology, Faculty of Medicine Ramathibodi Hospital, Mahidol University, 270 Rama VI Road, Bangkok 10400, Thailand

Thanatporn Threetong, Purit Petpiroon, Tharikarn Sujirakul, Anuchit Poonyathalang and Kavin Vanikieti
Department of Ophthalmology, Faculty of Medicine Ramathibodi Hospital, Mahidol University, 270 Rama VI Road, Bangkok 10400, Thailand

Fumie Hayashi, Shintaro Hayashi, Dai Matsuse, Ryo Yamasaki and Jun-ichi Kira
Department of Neurology, Neurological Institute, Graduate School of Medical Sciences, Kyushu University, 3-1-1 Maidashi, Higashi-ku, Fukuoka 812-8582, Japan

Keiji Yonekura
Department of Pediatrics, Kure Medical center, Hiroshima, Japan

Yun Yuan
Department of Neurology, Peking University First Hospital, #8 Xishiku St, Xicheng District, Beijing 100034, China

Jing Miao, Fei-fei Su, Xue-mei Liu and Xiao-jing Wei
Department of Neurology and Neuroscience Center, First Affiliated Hospital of Jilin University, Changchun, 130021 Jilin, People's Republic of China

Xue-fan Yu
Department of Neurology and Neuroscience Center First Affiliated Hospital of Jilin University, Changchun, 130021 Jilin, People's Republic of China

Taku Hatano, Shin-Ichi Ueno, Arisa Hayashida, Kazuaki Kanai and Nobutaka Hattori
Department of Neurology, Juntendo University Graduate School of Medicine, 2-1-1 Hongo, Bunkyo-ku, Tokyo 113-8421, Japan

Masashi Takanashi
Department of Neurology, Juntendo University Graduate School of Medicine, 2-1-1 Hongo, Bunkyo-ku, Tokyo 113-8421, Japan
Department of Neurology, Juntendo Koshigaya Hospital, 560 Fukuroyama, Koshigayashi, Saitama 343-0032, Japan

Hitoshi Tsuchihashi
Department of Dermatology, Juntendo University Graduate School of Medicine, 2-1-1 Hongo, Bunkyo-ku, Tokyo 113-8421, Japan

Yutaka Tsukune
Department of Internal Medicine, Division of Hematology, Juntendo University Graduate School of Medicine, 2-1-1 Hongo, Bunkyo-ku, Tokyo 113-8421, Japan

Yasushi Shimo
Department of Neurology, Juntendo University Graduate School of Medicine, 2-1-1 Hongo, Bunkyo-ku, Tokyo 113-8421, Japan
Department of Research and Therapeutics for Movement Disorders, Juntendo University Graduate School of Medicine, 2-1-1 Hongo, Bunkyo-ku, Tokyo 113-8421, Japan

Jeanne Benoit
Peripheral Nervous System, Muscle & ALS Department, University of Nice and Côte d'Azur (UCA), Nice, France

Osamu Kano and Yasuo Iwasaki
Division of Neurology, Department of Internal Medicine, Toho University School of Medicine, Tokyo, Japan

Angela Puma
Peripheral Nervous System, Muscle & ALS Department, University of Nice and Côte d'Azur (UCA), Nice, France
UMR7370 CNRS, LP2M, Faculté de Médecine, University Côte d'Azur, Nice, France

Sabrina Sacconi
Peripheral Nervous System, Muscle & ALS Department, University of Nice and Côte d'Azur (UCA), Nice, France
Université Côte d'Azur, Centre National de la Recherche Scientifique, Institut de Pharmacologie Moléculaire et Cellulaire, Valbonne, France

Antonino Uncini
Department of Neuroscience, Imaging and Clinical Sciences, University "G. d'Annunzio", Chieti-Pescara, Italy

Mingqin Zhu, Xuefan Yu, Caiyun Liu, Chenchen Duan, Chunxiao Li and Ying Zhang
Department of Neurology and Neuroscience Center, First Hospital of Jilin University, Xinmin Street No 71, Changchun 130000, China

Jie Zhu
Division of Neurodegerneration, Department of Neurobiology, Care Sciences & Society, Karolinska Institutet, SE 14157, Huddinge, Stockholm, Sweden

Hidenori Kido, Asami Hamai and Yoshihisa Urita
Department of General Medicine and Emergency Care, Toho University School of Medicine, 6-11-1 Omorinishi Ota-ku, Tokyo 143-8541, Japan

Hiroyuki Masuda, Yutaka Fuchinoue and Masaaki Nemoto
Department of Neurosurgery Radiology, Toho University School of Medicine, Tokyo, Japan

Chiaki Arai and Teppei Takeda
Department of Otorhinolaryngology, Toho University School of Medicine, Tokyo, Japan

Fumihito Yamabe, Toshihiro Tai and Mizuki Kasahara
Department of Urology, Toho University School of Medicine, Tokyo, Japan

Kenichi Suzuki and Nobuyuki Shiraga
Department of Radiology, Toho University School of Medicine, Tokyo, Japan

Sota Sadamoto, Megumi Wakayama and Kazutoshi Shibuya
Department of Pathology, Toho University School of Medicine, Tokyo, Japan

Yukitoshi Takahashi
Epilepsy Center, Shizuoka Institute of Epilepsy and Neurological, Tokyo, Japan

Shujun Xia, Ri Ji and Weiwei Zhan
Ultrasound Department, Rui Jin Hospital Shanghai Jiao Tong University School of Medicine, 197 Rui Jin Er Road, Huang Pu District, Shanghai Zip code: 200025, People's Republic of China

Daniel Zeller and Wolfgang Müllges
Department of Neurology, University of Würzburg, Josef-Schneider-Str. 11, 97080 Würzburg, Germany

Anke Heidemeier
Department of Radiology, University of Würzburg, Josef-Schneider-Str. 11, 97080 Würzburg, Germany

Götz Ulrich Grigoleit
Department of Internal Medicine II, University of Würzburg, 97080 Würzburg, Germany

Xiang Huang, Jian Xu, Ming Xu, Mingyu Chen, Kaiyuan Ji, Junwei Ren and Ping Zhong
Department of Neurosurgery, Huashan Hospital, Fudan University, Shanghai 200040, People's Republic of China

Index